ultrasound in
gynecology
and obstetrics

Sam N. Hassani

ultrasound in gynecology and obstetrics

(in collaboration with R. L. Bard)

includes 337 illustrations

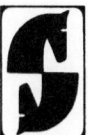

Springer-Verlag
New York Heidelberg Berlin

S. N. Hassani, M.D.
Assistant Professor of Radiology
State University of New York at Stony Brook and
Physician in Charge, Ultrasound Division, Department of Radiology
Queens Hospital Center
Jamaica, New York 11432

R. L. Bard, M.D.
New York City

Library of Congress Cataloging in Publication Data

Hassani, N., 1938–

    Ultrasound in gynecology and obstetrics.
    Includes bibliographies and index.
    1. Diagnosis, Ultrasonic. 2. Generative organs, Female—Diseases—
Diagnosis. 3. Ultrasonics in obstetrics. I. Bard, Robert Laurence. II. Title.
RG1075.U4H37   618.2′07′54   77-28316

9 8 7 6 5 4 3 2 1

ISBN-13: 978-1-4612-6256-5   e-ISBN-13: 978-1-4612-6254-1
DOI: 10.1007/978-1-4612-6254-1

To Our Families

foreword

by Dr. Donald L. King

The past decade has seen the ascent of ultrasonography to a preeminent position as a diagnostic imaging modality for obstetrics and gynecology. It can be stated without qualification that modern obstetrics and gynecology cannot be practiced without the use of diagnostic ultrasound, and in particular, the use of ultrasonography. Ultrasonography quickly and safely provides detailed, high-resolution images of the pelvic organs and gravid uterus. The quality and quantity of diagnostic information obtained by ultrasonography far exceeds anything previously available and has had a revolutionary impact on the management of patients. High-resolution static images permit the intrauterine diagnosis of fetal growth retardation and fetal abnormalities. In addition to traditional images, newer dynamic imaging techniques allow observation of fetal motion, cardiac pulsation, and respiratory efforts. The use of ultrasonography for guidance has greatly augmented the safety and utility of amniocentesis.

One of the great virtues of diagnostic ultrasound has been its apparent safety. At present energy levels, diagnostic ultrasound appears to be without any injurious effect. Although all the available evidence suggests that it is a very safe modality and that the benefit to risk ratio is very high, the actual safety margin for its use as yet remains unknown. As a consequence, practitioners are urged to limit its use only to those situations in which genuine clinical indications exist and real benefit to the patient is likely to result.

The future will bring with it greater understanding not only of the biologic effects of ultrasound but many new techniques for its application in diagnosis and therapy. One of these, the use of pulse-Doppler ultrasound, will almost certainly be valuable to assess and eventually measure blood flow in the uterine arteries, placenta, and within the fetus itself. The vast potential of diagnostic ultrasound as yet has hardly been exploited. The great growth of the past decade will eventually be overshadowed by even greater progress in the future.

Donald L. King, M.D.
Associate Professor of Radiology
Columbia University
New York, New York

foreword

by Dr. Jan J. Smulewicz

In his recent book, Dr. Hassani did a very thorough exploration and an excellent explanation of the wide variety of examinations in the field of obstetrics and gynecology with the ultrasonography method. I found the book very easy to read, the interpretation very clear, and the large volume of material excellently chosen. I am sure that the book will be of great interest to practitioners, especially obstetricians and gynecologists. This method being noninvasive and eliminating the danger of ionizing radiation, should find its way into every hospital or center where good medical care is provided.

Jan J. Smulewicz, M.D.
Professor of Radiology
Mount Sinai School of Medicine
Director of Radiology
Beth Israel Medical Center
New York, New York

preface

Ultrasound imaging has reached a stage of sophistication whereby diagnostic information can be gained without discomfort to the patient and with complete absence of morbidity and mortality. The procedure is quick, safe, noninvasive, and, in many instances, supercedes and obviates more time-consuming procedures requiring catheterization, injection of a contrast material, and radiographic imaging. In obstetric problems, the danger of ionizing radiation to the fetus is eliminated. In debilitated and very ill patients this simple and painless method becomes the procedure of choice.

Unique features of ultrasound equipment allow for pinpoint localization of lesions and direct visual guidance of percutaneous puncture techniques for aspiration and biopsy. The accuracy of ultrasound-guided cystic punctures and the absence of side effects make this modality far superior to percutaneous invasive techniques performed with other imaging systems. Renal cyst puncture and amniocentesis are but two of the procedures in which ultrasonic guidance is the method of choice. Since this modality is noninvasive, it may be performed serially and at any given time.

This sequential observation of pathophysiology in the fetus and the mother provides important data on the progression of acute and chronic diseases and their response to treatment. The unusual accuracy of ultrasound in differentiating cystic from solid masses and its ability to localize the lesion in a three-dimensional representation have rendered other diagnostic procedures unnecessary for the practicing obstetrician and gynecologist. The standard radiologic evaluation for abdominal masses has generally included the plain x-ray film of the abdomen, intravenous urography, barium enema, gastrointestinal series, cholecystography, and radioisotopic procedures. Invasive and time-consuming studies such as lymphangiography and arteriography have also been used, sometimes without adding further diagnostic information. Sonography is safe and relatively inexpensive and should be included in the workup of a mass lesion. Since ultrasound may give a specific diagnosis, its application should follow the plain x-ray film. This simple and rapid study may eliminate the need for a prolonged hospital stay and the discomfort of further examinations. Diagnostic ultrasound has greatly reduced the patient time spent in the x-ray department, giving the obstetrician and gynecologist faster and more reliable diagnostic information, and generally speeding up the patient turnover at the hospital. With the economic emphasis on the cost reduction of medical services and hospitalization expense, the ultrasound department serves a vital function in facilitating diagnostic services.

The purpose of this book is to introduce the physician to the essential principles of ultrasound physics and the practical aspects of scanning procedures. Important concepts are clearly and thoroughly presented. Mathematical formulas and advanced physics principles beyond the scope of the clinician have been omitted. The text is limited to the pelvis and medically related areas in order to concentrate on each area in sufficient depth so as to be valuable to the specialist who must be familiar with the diagnostic capabilities of atraumatic scanners in his field. The methods of examination and diagnostic findings are detailed to be useful to the obstetrician, gynecologist, radiologist, and general surgeon.

The comprehensive scope serves as a general reference for both the family practitioner and the student in training.

In the sections on physical and practical applications, precise directions for examination are given and scanning pitfalls with the production of artifacts have been underscored. The evolution of scanning systems has been traced so that the potential features and limitations of each imaging unit are recognized. Representations of each type of scanning device are illustrated and their inherent advantages discussed.

Examination of each area has been arranged so that the reader may review the pertinent regional anatomy before studying the ultrasonic presentation of normal structures. The pathology of each organ is presented as a disease spectrum and the evolution of the disorder is discussed. Correlation between sonographic findings and the histopathologic changes is emphasized. The combination of real-time and gray-scale scanning offers the reader a comprehensive understanding of ultrasonic pathology.

Where controversy exists, the opinions of various authorities are cited and compared with our experience. The diagnostic versatility of the various imaging systems are evaluated for each organ complex and the investigative method of choice is suggested for each disorder.

Considerable attention has been given to clinical and pathologic aspects. The practice of ultrasonic scanning requires a thorough knowledge of the diagnostic problems of obstetrics and gynecology and their related specialties. The text is designed as a bridge between sonographic imaging and general obstetric and gynecologic principles.

acknowledgments

I wish to express my deep appreciation to Drs. Hugh Barber, Fred Benjamine, George Blinick, Philip Bresnick, Alfred Brockunier, Bernard Diamond, Hilliard Dubrow, Fritz Fuchs, Martin Kurman, James Nelson, Seymour Sussman, Martin Stone, Michael Tafreshi, and Maurice Abitbol for their support of our academic efforts in the application of ultrasonography to the field of obstetrics and gynecology.

We are also very grateful to Akram Hassani, Nat Lewis, John H. Grant, Marie Snailer, Judy Sharpe, Lee Weingarten, R.D.M.S., and Sonia Suga for their technical assistance.

The investigative efforts of our many colleagues in the field of ultrasonography have greatly facilitated the evolution of this textbook. The support of the publishers and the collaboration of the Editorial Staff are warmly acknowledged.

contents

4 ultrasonography of gynecologically and obstetrically related medical and surgical disorders 33

introduction

Diagnoses are missed not because of lack of knowledge on the part of the examiner, but rather because of lack of examination.

Sir William Osler

The field of diagnostic ultrasound has expanded in application so rapidly over the past few years that it has become part of the routine diagnostic workup. The history of ultrasonography is vastly different from the evolution of X rays. After the discovery of the X ray in 1885, it was rapidly accepted by the medical community and many radiologic societies soon appeared. The imaging potential of X rays was so exciting that many patients and their physicians received massive exposure to this form of highly penetrating electromagnetic energy. The dreadful sequelae of radiation-induced injuries and malignancies subsequently appeared.

The development of ultrasonography is quite different. In spite of the absence of demonstrable side effects and the ease and accuracy of the study, its use did not become fashionable until very recently. The nature of the sound beam is that of mechanical energy and its possible long-term biologic effects still remain unclear. However, it is known that the ionizing effects of X rays make even small doses potentially harmful. Sonar mechanical vibrations are such that energy below the level that breaks tissue bonds will not produce any tissue damage. Our experience to date with low intensity ultrasound suggests that no hazardous effects will occur in the short or long term in patients.

The field of ultrasonography has assumed such importance primarily as a result of the harmless nature of the modality. Also, the tireless efforts of a large number of investigators from varied medical fields and allied services have developed sonography into one of the best diagnostic tools. The pioneers in ultrasound, using only A-mode to combat the skepticism of their colleagues, must have been exceptionally dedicated and patient. Scanning the abdomen and mentally integrating thousands of A-mode spikes to give an answer to the clinician in need of a firm diagnosis must have produced great frustration. This problem was alleviated by the introduction of B-mode scanning units. Soon this technique was followed by the time-motion– or M-mode.

My personal experience with ultrasonography began with the late Dr. Lajos von Micsky and his experiments conducted in a water tank. This type of study was mainly intended to produce higher quality pictures in order to improve diagnostic accuracy. The introduction of Doppler ultrasound proved to be an instant success with clinicians in the evaluation of the fetal heart. The idea of scanning the pelvis with a full bladder opened the ultrasonic door to the visualization of the deep pelvic organs and dramatically improved diagnostic accuracy in this region.

The true revolution in ultrasonography began with the development of the scan converter with its sophisticated logarithmic compression amplifiers. This presentation of a scan in various shades of gray related to echo amplitude opened new horizons in the study of tissue signatures. Soon we were imaging the medium-sized arteries and veins in the upper abdomen and, comparing these with our anteroposterior (AP) and cross-table lateral angiograms, we were able to sonographically map the organs in relation to the vascular anatomy.

The fundamentals of ultrasound, like those of any other branch of medicine, require the user to be familiar with the effects and limitations of the method. By this technique we are able to locate different organs and tissues and measure the interfaces between them, and to cut in cross sections through different structures. In contrast to other examinations which yield indirect information, ultrasound enables us to outline the lesion directly and to investigate its relationship with neighboring structures. There is no need for the administration of any radiologic contrast, possibly harmful to the function of the impaired organ. Ultrasound, both as a screening and diagnostic modality, is a noninvasive and atraumatic procedure and is complimentary to angiography in many cases. The unique feature of ultrasound is the ability to recognize and differentiate deep body organs and lesions having similar density on conventional X-ray studies.

The information gained through ultrasound, as in other imaging procedures, is optimized when coupled with the patient's clinical picture. At present, parenchymal lesions of the lung cannot be evaluated by ultrasound since the air-containing lung will not transmit sound waves.

The history of ultrasonography is a long one and the procedure has suffered from many setbacks in its attempt for acceptance by the medical profession. Its inherently harmless nature has accounted for a significant portion of its popularity in modern medical practice. Whether the sophisticated electronic technology that spawned high resolution ultrasound will cause the growing field of ultrasound to supersede other diagnostic modalities, or create nonultrasonic imaging systems that will phase out ultrasonography, remains to be determined.

The pioneers of ultrasonography had much difficulty in applying sonar to diagnosis since they were using first generation scanners based on ultrasonic technology used in industry and military pursuits. In later years newer ultrasonic units designed to meet specific clinical purposes have been constructed. Cooperation of physicists, engineers, and physicians dedicated to ultrasonic imaging has led to development of diagnostic systems of considerable practical value. Since the early days of the application of sonar principles in medicine, there have been continual new innovations in this field. The progress of acoustic waves in diagnostic imaging has been aided by the development of special ultrasonic transducers, sophisticated amplifiers, and sensitive electronic displays. The introduction of recently perfected scan converter systems adds a new dimension to the field of ultrasonography.

The word sonar is an acronym of sound navigation and ranging. Historically, ultrasound was developed during World War I. Langevin (1) used the principle of sonar to detect and locate submarines. Sounding of the ocean floor to provide depth measurements was employed in 1918 to aid in shipping and navigation (1). Further improvement in technology created more extensive usage of sonar in industry and military situations. Military sonar used by the navy could measure the depth of a reflecting surface and also track an object in motion. In 1930 ultrasound was used in industry to detect flaws in iron castings. Prior to World War II, Dussik (2) used ultrasound in the field of medicine. His attempt to visualize the ventricular system of the brain was unsuccessful. However, in 1937, he designed an ultrasonic device for application to the brain (3). The first ultrasonic instrument, called the supersonic reflectoscope, was introduced in 1940 (4). This practical instrument, based on the pulse-echo technique, measured distance on the principle of transmission of very short pulses of sonic energy. During World War II the application of radar principles in military imaging further helped to develop the sonar technique. The conjoint use of both imaging systems speeded progress in each field and led to the availability of the first medical sonar units in the late 1940s and early 1950s.

Continuing new developments in ultrasound were spurred on by dedicated researchers. The application of new electronic circuitry and rapid reporting data retrieval systems changed the use of ultrasound from that of a research tool to an essential diagnostic modality. The fields of echoencephalography and then of M-Mode echocardiography were developed. Next, unidimensional and two-dimensional ultrasonic scanning were combined.

As various medical teams cooperated in the development of ultrasonic scanners, smaller and more practical ultrasonographic units became available. Pioneer work in the use of ultrasonography in obstetrics and gynecology was done by Thompson (5) and Gottesfeld (6). W. L. Wright designed a hand-operated ultrasonic unit. Subsequently many compact commercial ultrasonographic units became available. J. J. Wild made great contributions to the field of ultrasonography. In particular, he devoted his work to the differentiation of benign and malignant tumors (7).

When the prototype of the contact ultrasonic scanner became more popular, since the transducer could now be placed on the patient's skin with direct contact, many further advances in equipment design became possible. Water bath scanning of the eye (8) was another technical development, and was soon followed by the application of time-motion displays (9). By using two-dimensional real-time scanning systems respiratory and vascular motion can be detected and pathological conditions evaluated, in addition to detection and evaluation of their three-dimensional images.

At present, use of ultrasonography is spreading into many branches of medicine. It has become an integral part of many subspecialties, such as obstetrics and gynecology and urology, since it is one of the most accurate diagnostic tools in many disorders involving soft tissue pathology.

Modern electronics has given the medical sonographer high-resolution equipment which is relatively simple to use. The application of ultrasonography has been so rapid that it is now the preferred diagnostic test in many clinical problems. In certain disorders, such as placenta previa, it is virtually the only diagnostic tool that is available.

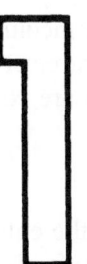

principles of ultrasonography

CHARACTERISTICS OF ULTRASOUND

NATURE OF ULTRASONIC WAVES

Sound is a mechanical vibration of particles in a medium around an equilibrium position. Sonic waves require a medium of a molecular nature in order to propagate. The highest frequency audible to the human ear is 20,000 cycles per second or 20 kiloHertz (KHz). Sound waves above this frequency are described as ultrasound. Unlike electromagnetic waves, sound cannot travel across a vacuum (10).

The wavelength of audible sound in air varies from a few inches to a few feet. Ultrasonic waves are usually produced by a continuous series of contractions and relaxations of substances that have piezoelectric properties. The waves generated are carried as condensations and rarefactions in the transmitting medium. The frequency range used in diagnostic medicine is approximately 1 million cycles per second, with a wavelength of about 1.5 millimeters (mm) in water.

PIEZOELECTRIC PRINCIPLE

The piezoelectric effect is fundamental to the development of ultrasound. "Piezo" is derived from the Greek word *piesis,* ie, to press. Piezoelectric actually means "pressure electric." Quartz has piezoelectric qualities, since its size and shape change under the influence of an electric field. When an electric current is passed through quartz, the crystal expands and contracts according to the polarity of the current. Sound waves are generated as a result of these compressions and rarefactions. On the other hand, mechanical energy, in the form of sound waves applied to the crystal, produces an electric current. This is known as the piezoelectric principle (Fig. 1.1a and b). Several other substances are known to have piezoelectric properties, such as barium titanate, lithium sulfate, and lead zirconate (11). The titanates are the more commonly used crystal (10) for sonography.

SOUND WAVES

Sonic waves travel through a medium as alternate condensations and rarefactions. The following practical definitions are commonly used (Fig. 1.1c).

1. Cycle. One cycle is the entire condensation and rarefaction phase.

2. Wavelength. The length of one cycle is a wavelength, or, a complete condensation and rarefaction zone is a wavelength.

3. Frequency. The number of cycles per unit time. The frequency of sound waves is described in terms of hertz (cycles per second).

4. Velocity. Velocity is the speed of sound in the medium through which sound is propagated.

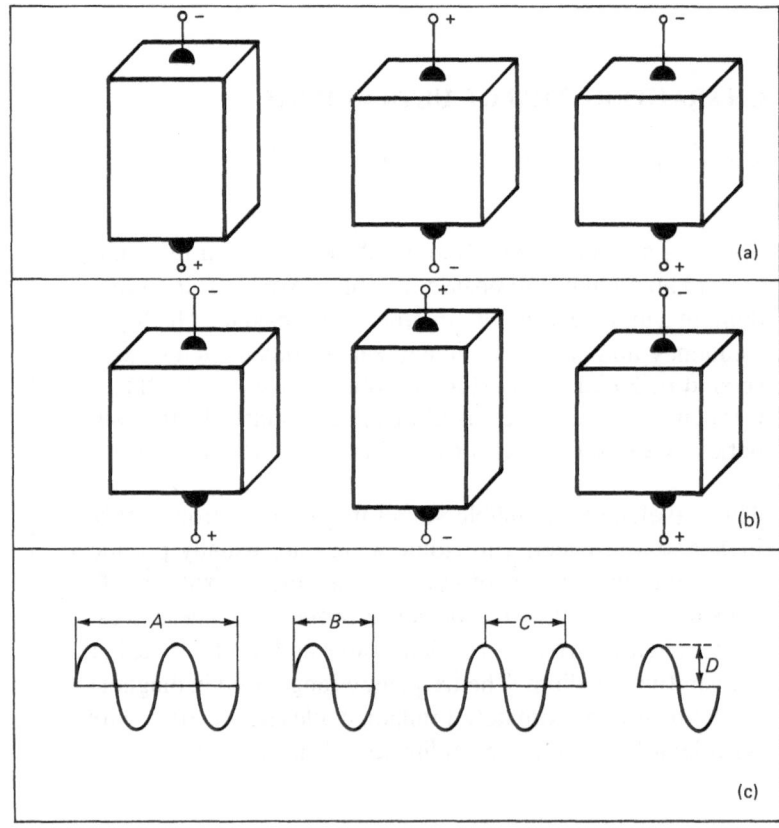

FIGURE 1.1
Piezoelectric effect. (a) Mechanical stress deforming crystal and producing current. (b) Expansion of crystal as current is applied and contraction of crystal as current polarity is reversed. (c) Wave pattern produced by alternate compressions and rarefactions. A, spatial pulse length; B, full cycle; C, wavelength; D, amplitude.

The relationship between velocity, wavelength, and frequency is as follows:

$$V = \lambda \times F$$
$$\text{Velocity} = \text{Wavelength} \times \text{Frequency}$$

EFFECT OF MEDIUM

In any given medium the velocity of sound remains constant, but its frequency varies inversely with wavelength. The higher the frequency, the smaller the wavelength. High-frequency sound waves are more directional than low-frequency sound. However, the attenuation of high-frequency waves is greater than that of low-frequency waves, since the absorption of sound is greater at high frequency (10). In medical work, frequencies above 1 MHz are employed. At a frequency of 2 MHz, the wavelength of sound in water is approximately 0.75 mm.

Velocity depends on the density and elasticity of the medium. The elasticity of the medium is significant, since the velocity of sound changes in media of different inherent elastic properties. In a homogeneous medium, ultrasound travels in a straight line at a velocity dependent on the properties of the medium but independent of wavelength.

INTENSITY

The intensity of the ultrasound beam is a measure of the strength of its energy and is defined as power per unit area. The intensities used in commercially available medical units usually are between 1 and 40 milliwatts per square centimeter (mW/cm^2). Tissue damage may occur at 4 W/cm^2 (11,18); thus, currently used intensity levels are roughly 100 to 1000 times lower in energy than the potentially damaging level. The safety margin is much greater, since the acoustic pulse is active less than 1 percent of the scanning time.

The decibel (db) is the practical unit for the measurement of sound intensity. The ratio of signal amplitudes must be expressed logarithmically due to the wide range of echo energies. The formula for the ratio of echo amplitude in terms of decibels is as follows:

$$db = 20 \log A_1/A_2$$

where A_1 is the echo amplitude and A_2 the incident sound amplitude.

BEAM WIDTH AND ECHO PATTERN

The beam width is related to the diameter of the crystal. Ultrasonic waves transmitted from the transducer have a diverging beam width. In this path, any echo received is registered as if it were in the central beam axis (12). A target on the edge of the beam is recorded in the same way as a target in the middle.

The appearance of the displayed point is important. The echo is registered as a dot or line. The dots lie in the center of the beam and the lines are perpendicular to the beam axis of the transducer. The length of each line is proportional to the width of the beam. The apparent beam width is wider if the target is located obliquely to the incident beam. The effective beam width changes with the sensitivity of the ultrasound machine. By increasing the sensitivity of the machine, low-amplitude echoes from the edge of the beam are registered. However, the target is displayed as lines instead of dots and resolution is decreased. Also, the geometry of the target is extremely important (Fig. 1.2a,b, and c). If the transmitted beam is stationary and at right angles to the target, the shape of the returned echo is specified by the electric characteristics of the transducer (12). If the transmitted beam is not stationary or strikes the target obliquely, the shape of the returned echo is elongated due to a greater effective beam width with respect to the target. Thus, the echoes appear as small lines instead of dots (Fig. 1.3a,b, and c).

ATTENUATION

When a sonic beam is passed through a medium, a decrease in the intensity of the sound, ie, *attenuation,* may be expressed as a half-value layer. The half-value layer is the distance the

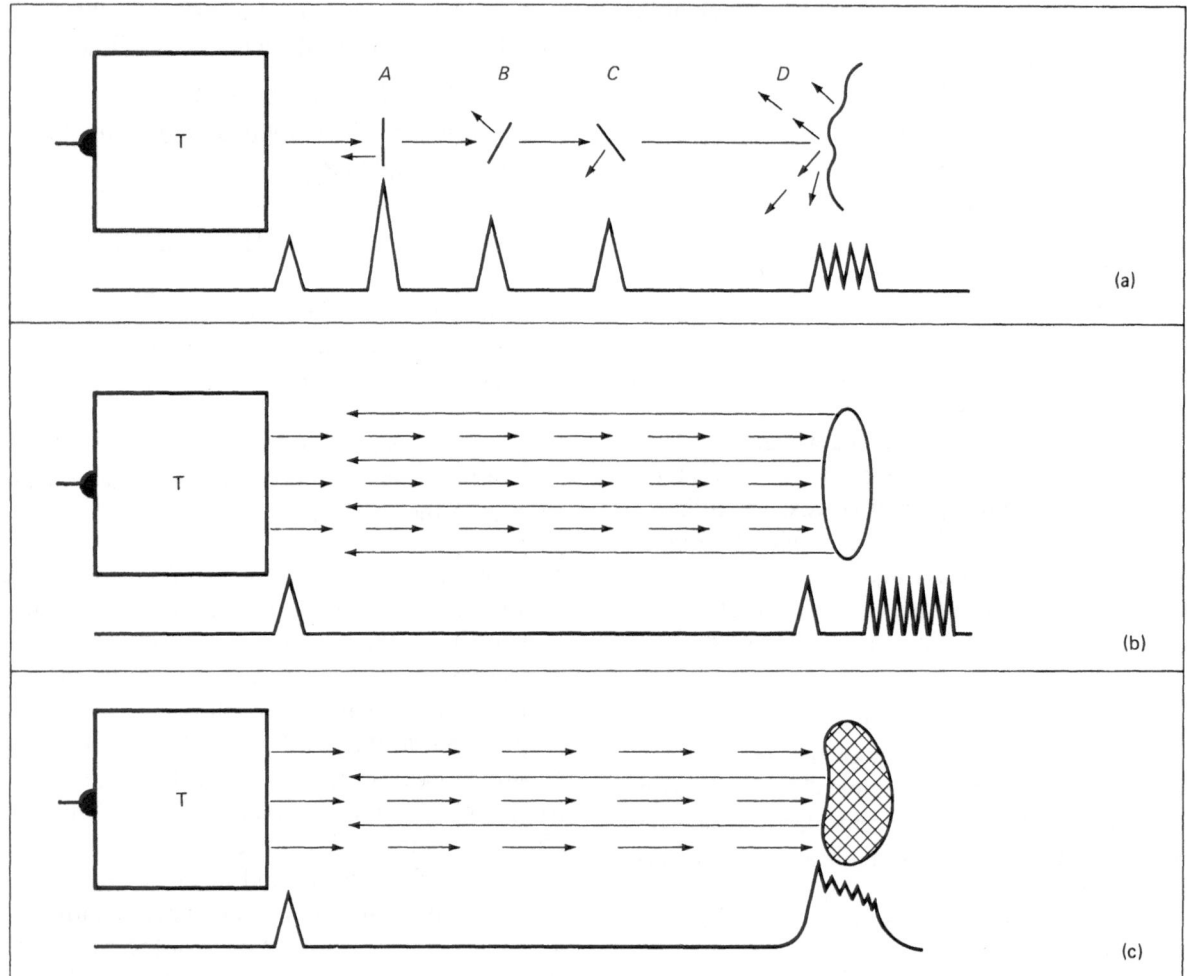

FIGURE 1.2
Reflection processes. (a) Strong echo generated by perpendicular interface (A). Weaker echoes due to sound reflected away from receiving transducer (B,C). Diffuse low-level echoes from irregular reflecting interface (D). (b) No echoes produced as sound beam passes through homogeneous medium of cystic structure. Note high through transmission represented as multiple echoes distal to the posterior wall. (c) Echo production by solid, nonhomogeneous medium. Note poor through transmission with no echoes distal to the posterior wall. T, transducer.

transmitted sound must travel before its initial intensity is reduced by one-half. For example, bone has a smaller half-value layer than does soft tissue (10). However, energy loss is also caused by beam divergence, scattering, and absorption of sound by tissue. The amount of sound absorbed is proportional to the depth of the tissue and the square of the frequency of sound. Attenuation of the sonic beam has many practical applications. For example, cystic and solid masses can be differentiated since cystic masses have a much greater half-value layer than do solid structures. In general, soft tissue attenuation is 1 db/MHz/cm. Attenuation of bony structures is about 20 times greater than that of soft tissue. For this reason, a low-frequency transducer must be used when scanning through bony structures such as the ribs.

ACOUSTIC IMPEDANCE

The transmissivity of the ultrasonic beam depends upon sound velocity (V) and the density (D) of the medium. The overall transmission is defined as acoustic impedance (*Z*). Consequently, acoustic impedance is directly related to the product of the speed of sound in a given medium and the tissue density (11). Thus,

$$Z = DV$$

where Z is the impedance, D the density, and V the sound velocity. If the interface between two media is a region of acoustic impedance mismatch, a reflection will take place proportional to the impedance differential. Each tissue has a characteristic acoustic impedance.

RESOLUTION

Resolution is the minimum distance between two point targets required to register each point as a distinct entity. The greater the resolving power,

the closer the two objects may be and still be individually recognized. The resolution of any wave form is directly related to the frequency of oscillation. Higher frequency sound usually has better resolution but its intensity falls off rapidly as it passes through a given medium (11). Lower frequency sound usually has excellent transmission but poor resolution characteristics. The frequency range between 2 and 3.5 MHz has the best balance between resolution and transmission for abdominal scanning. However, equipment available at present does not allow identifi-

FIGURE 1.3
Echo shape and beam path. (a) Narrow beam. Point target displayed as sharp dot. (b) Wide beam. Point target displayed as short line perpendicular to beam. (c) Narrow beam. Oblique linear target displayed as short line. T, transducer.

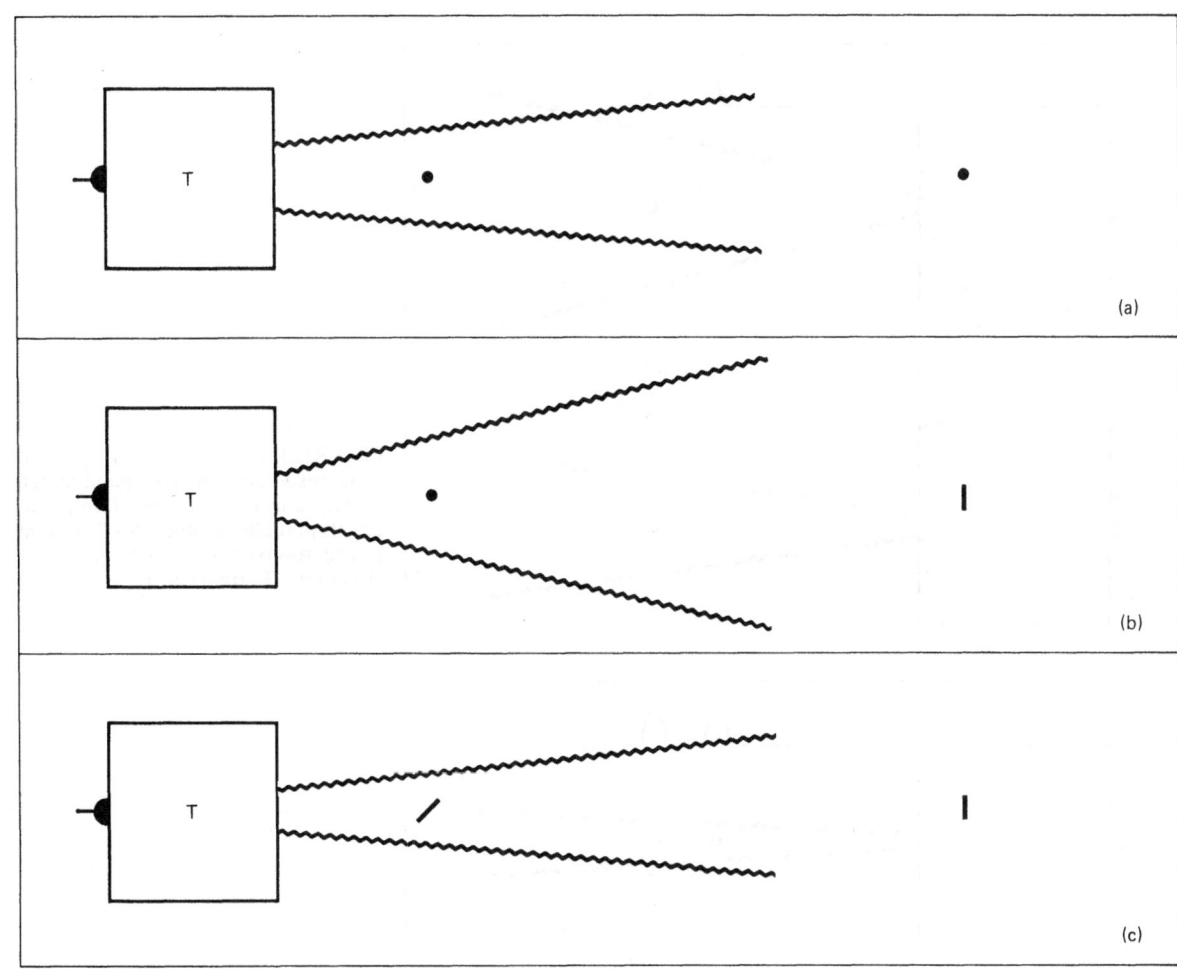

cation of very deep-seated abdominal structures below a certain size. Recognition of a smaller lesion depends on the overall resolution of the equipment.

In ultrasound we are concerned with axial and lateral resolution. Axial or depth resolution is the ability to distinguish two points along the beam axis (Fig. 1.4a,b, and c). The minimum resolvable distance is measured as the axial resolution and depends on wavelength, since objects separated by less than one wavelength cannot be resolved. Although the wavelengths of current transducers vary from 0.1 to 1.5 mm, the resolution of the oscilloscope, or scan converter tube, may not be sufficient to separate very closely spaced echoes. The display system must be sensitive enough to match the transducer frequency. Lateral or azimuthal resolution is the ability to distinguish two points located perpendicular to the beam axis (Fig. 1.5a,b, and c). The minimum resolvable side-by-side distance between two objects is measured as the lateral resolution. This distance is inversely proportional to the width of the beam and depends on the diameter of the crystal, the wavelength, and the degree of beam divergence with distance.

REPETITION RATE

The rate at which bursts of ultrasonic energy are emitted is called the repetition rate. Most commercially available instruments emit 200 to 2000 repetitions per second. This high repetition rate requires extremely sensitive receivers capable of detecting a signal that has less than 1 percent of the incident ultrasonic beam energy reflected back to the transducer.

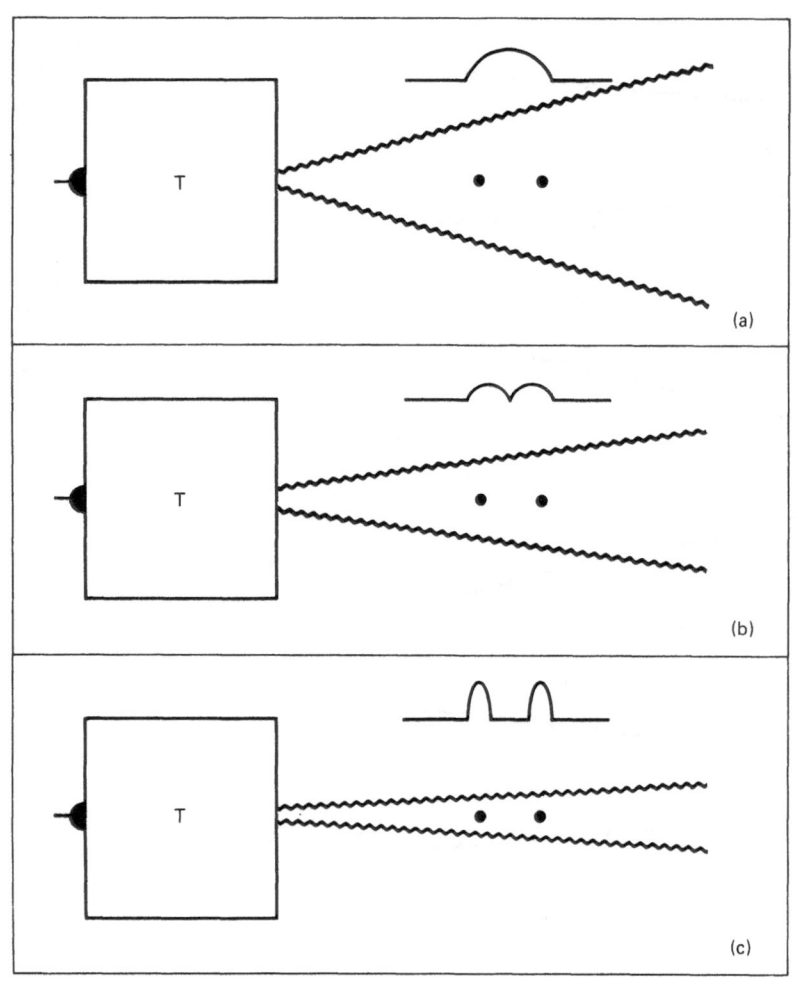

FIGURE 1.4
Axial resolution. (a) Two point targets displayed as one echo. (b) Two point targets partially resolved. (c) Two point targets resolved as two distinct structures. T, transducer.

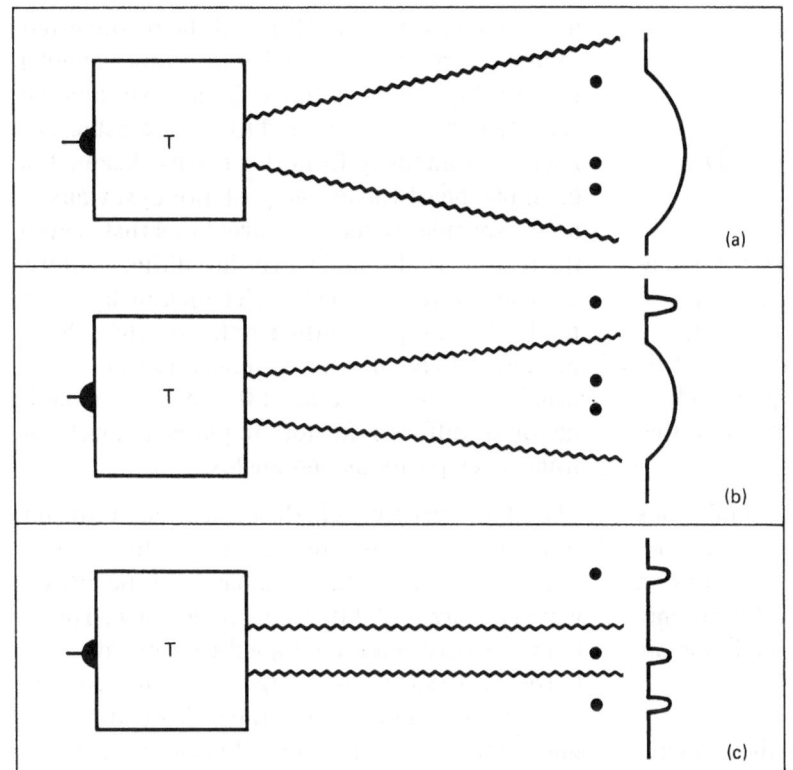

FIGURE 1.5
Lateral resolution. (a) Three point targets displayed as one point. (b) Two point targets shown as one point with better azimuthal resolution due to narrower beam width. (c) Optimal resolution distinguishing two closely spaced targets. T, transducer.

REVERBERATION

The face of the transducer may act as a reflecting surface to returning sound waves. Consequently, the sound beam may bounce back from the surface of the transducer, follow its original course, and, in return, hit the transducer a second time to be displayed on the oscilloscope at a distance twice as far from the transducer as the original echo. This pattern may be repeated with progressively weaker echoes. This phenomenon is called reverberation and may produce confusing and troublesome artifacts (Fig. 1.6).

DISTANCE MEASUREMENT OF REFLECTING INTERFACE

By knowing the velocity of sound in the medium being examined and the time it takes for the sonic pulse to strike an interface and return as a reconverted echo, it is possible to measure the distance between the reflecting interface and the transducer. After the sonograph is calibrated for

FIGURE 1.6
Reverberation phenomenon. The face of the transducer acts as a reflecting surface to the returning sound beam. The echo bounced back appears on the oscilloscope as a series of progressively weaker echoes. Note the reverberation artifact in abdominal scanning.

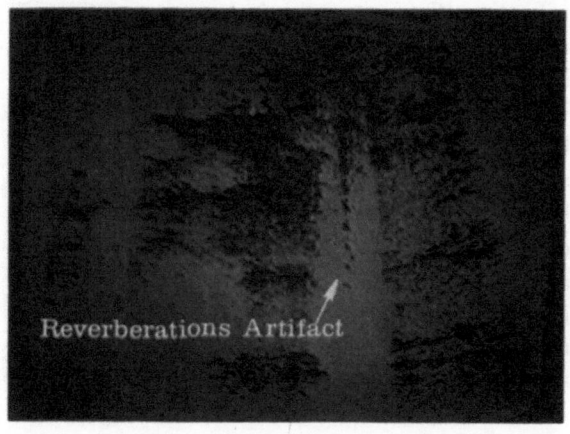

the velocity of sound in the medium examined, time is converted to distance automatically.

DIRECTIVITY, REFLECTIVITY, AND TRANSMISSIVITY

Ultrasonography is based on the pulse-echo relationship. Short electric pulses produced by a generator are converted by a transducer into bursts of acoustic energy. The sound beam emitted proceeds in a typical divergent path and produces different echoes, depending upon the interacting media.

High-frequency ultrasound has many similarities to light energy. In its course of travel, ultrasound will be reflected and refracted when it strikes an interface between two acoustically different media. If physiologic and geometric conditions are suitable, diffraction also occurs.

Reflection of ultrasound depends on the acoustic impedance mismatch of two media. The greater the difference in impedance, the greater the reflection. That portion of the sound wave not reflected is transmitted through the medium. If the incident beam is not perpendicular to the interface, sound will be reflected and refracted, depending on the angle of incidence (11). The incident beam should be normal to the interface studied to achieve maximum reflection back to the transducer. Snell's law of optical refraction applies to the refraction effect of the incident beam and Huygen's principle of optical diffraction applies to diffraction of the sonic beam.

The principal advantage of high-frequency sound is that it can be aimed toward specific organs. Study by ultrasound is optimal when the beam strikes at an angle perpendicular to the reflecting interface. If the beam is not quite perpendicular to the object of interest, a portion of reflected sound will not return to the crystal. Therefore, correlation between directivity and reflectivity is necessary for a good examination.

Certain structures have high reflecting qualities for ultrasound waves. Flat and concave surfaces are specular reflectors (12), and the reconverted waves return as a narrow beam. Proper angular relationships between transmitted waves and the reflected beam are required to receive echoes of maximum intensity from this narrow beam. For example, heart valves and posterior cyst walls act as specular reflectors. Structures that scatter the reconverted sound waves in a diffuse pattern are called diffuse reflectors. The parenchyma of the liver is a typical diffuse reflector; the echoes produced do not depend on angulation and are usually of low amplitude (13). Adequate examination of diffuse reflectors requires a variety of transducer positions and angles.

Fluid-filled structures in the body cavity transmit sound well and are detectable by the fact that reflection occurs at the boundaries of the cavity, which are areas of differential impedance. The interface between a fluid-filled cavity and bordering tissue yields a large impedance change and strong echoes are returned. Acoustic mismatch is much greater between tissue and bone. For example, at the interface between soft tissue and bone, more than 50 percent of the transmitted sound waves will be reflected. At an air–soft tissue interface, 100 percent reflection occurs.

Different organs in the body have different acoustic impedances. Therefore, the transmissivity of sound will change as it travels through various tissues. Every time the transmitted beam of ultrasound strikes an interface, an ultrasonic wave (echo) is reflected back and displayed on an oscilloscope. The greater the acoustic impedance mismatch at the interface between two media, the greater the reflection. Consequently, in heterogeneous media, many echoes are produced; in homogeneous media there are few or no echoes. Therefore, heterogeneous structures are said to be echogenic, whereas homogeneous regions are echo-free or anechoic. A fluid-filled cavity is homogeneous and thus echo-free. Fluid-filled cysts and solid masses are differentiated by the absence or presence of echo-producing interfaces within the lesions. This principle is used to diagnose pericardial effusions, ascites, and normal blood pools, such as the aorta.

The acoustic impedance of bone and high–atomic number elements is very great, while that of air is low. Therefore, the incident beam at a soft tissue–air interface is totally reflected. Since there is no penetration, lung scanning with ultrasound is impossible at present. At soft tissue–bone interfaces, significant quantities of ultrasound are absorbed. Thus, the ribs may produce some difficulty when the liver or spleen is scanned. The bony structures of children, however, cause fewer problems because these structures are smaller and contain less calcium.

DISPLAY MODES

The reflected echoes may be displayed by A-mode, B-mode, or M-mode presentations.

A-MODE (AMPLITUDE MODE)

The A-mode ultrasound system displays the electrically converted echo pattern as a vertical deflection (Fig. 1.7a). The amplitude of each deflection is proportional to the reflected energy received by the transducer. The deflections occur at different points on a calibrated tracing, corresponding to the distance of the reflecting surface from the face of the transducer. The

FIGURE 1.7
Display modes. (a) A-mode. Echo-producing interfaces produce vertical deflections proportional to echo amplitude. (b) B-mode. Vertical deflections converted into dots of brightness may be used for scanning. Brightness of dots is proportional to echo amplitude. (c) M-mode. Motion of objects recorded by moving the B-mode tracing along the time axis. T, transducer.

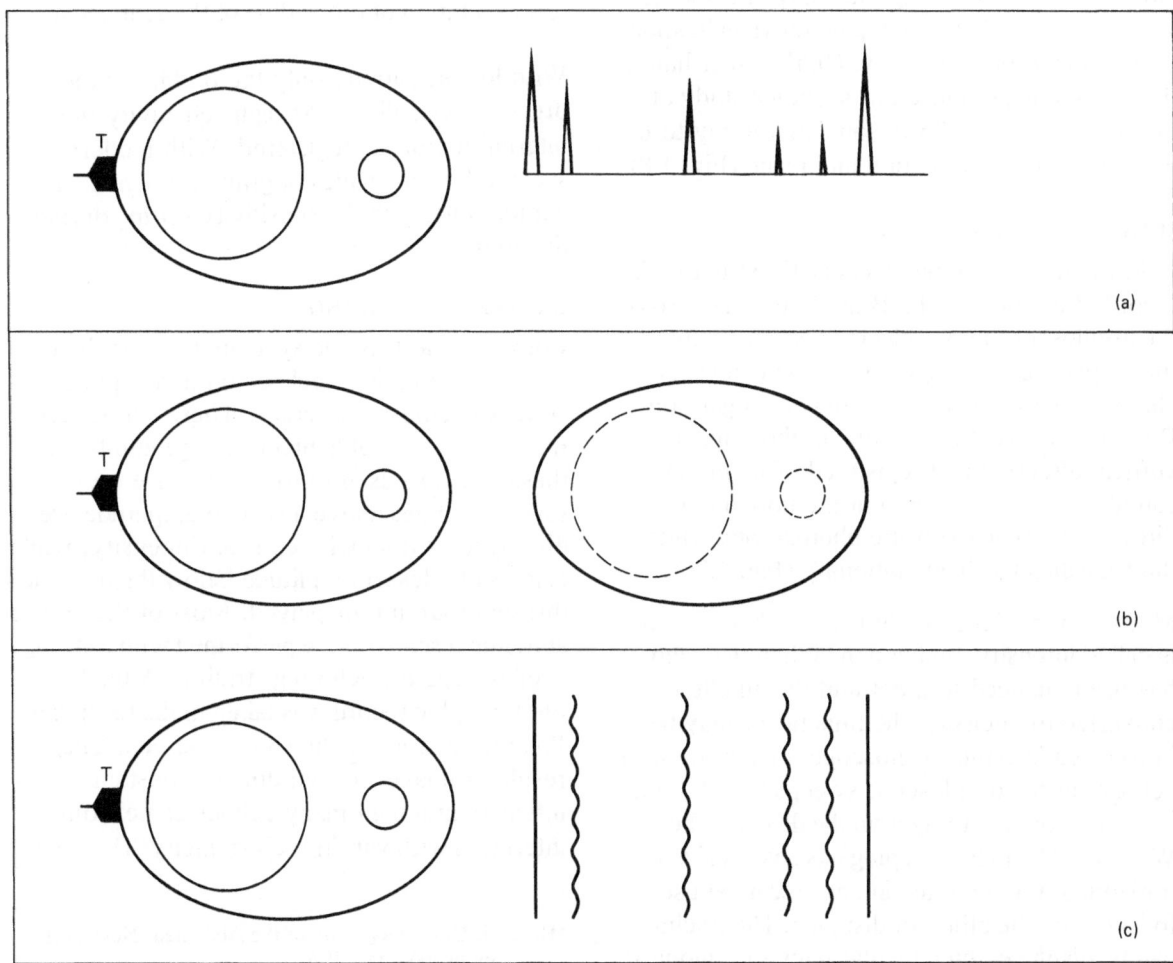

(a)

(b)

(c)

number, shape, location, and amplitude of the echo spikes furnish detailed information of the structure examined. The horizontal distance between registered echoes is proportional to the depth of the tissue which produced reflection.

B-MODE (BRIGHTNESS MODE)

With B-mode, echoes are displayed on the oscilloscope as a series of dots and lines, the brightness of which varies with the intensity of the reflected waves, since the echoes are projected as a linear series of bright dots (Fig. 1.7b). The second dimension of the oscilloscope can be used for acoustic section or sonolaparotomy of an organ by moving the transducer in the desired planes. This technique is called B-mode. Consequently, a single sonolaparotomy produces a two-dimensional representation. In B-mode, a great deal of information is lost during the study of a specific area as a result of attempting better visualization of the topographic anatomy. On the other hand, this technique permits cross-sectional study of the body and also allows sonolaparotomy to be performed in any direction and plane (Fig. 1.8).

M-MODE (MOTION MODE)

In M-mode, the motion of a pulsatile structure is recorded by moving the B-mode tracing across the oscilloscope at preselected speeds. Actually, the display of the amplitude of the echoes is changed to dots. The dots of moving organs on B-mode are swept across the oscilloscope in a vertical direction and registered. This motion can also be demonstrated in the horizontal direction by time exposure photography while the transducer is held stationary (Fig. 1.7c).

Modification of the amplitude of echoes to dots is called intensity modulation. When the echo has been changed to a dot and the amplitude converted to intensity, the time factor may be introduced into the oscilloscope tracing. In most echograms the oscilloscope sweeps from bottom to top or from left to right on the display tube. When the M-mode sweeping has a vertical and horizontal motion, one dimension can be used for time and the other for distance. The tracing can be displayed on a regular television monitor as a black-and-white or a gray scale by using a scan converter.

The M-mode presentation may be recorded on Polaroid film or on a cathode-ray tube. A strip chart recorder affords better detail.

MECHANISM OF CROSS-SECTIONAL IMAGE PRODUCTION

As the transducer moves over stationary structures a cross-sectional image will be built up from the organ of interest. The scanning is performed through a specially designed arm which holds the ultrasonic transducer. The arm motion is followed by a computer which spatially orients the transducer position and echo pattern on the monitor screen. As the transducer moves the returned echo signals will appear on the oscilloscope (Fig. 1.8). The final image is the representation of the outline of the scanned area.

With low sensitivity only the outline of the organs is visualized. At high sensitivity the internal texture is registered. With modern gray scale, different shades of gray are seen clearly without changing the sensitivity setting during the study.

GRAY-SCALE IMAGING

Conventional B-mode systems use threshold detection to register echoes on a phosphor storage oscilloscope screen. These echoes are recorded as dots of light and a large number of these dots are used to form an image on the screen. Echoes above a certain amplitude are displayed as dots with constant intensity, while echoes of a lesser amplitude below the detection threshold are not displayed. Most of the earlier abdominal scans* were performed with a storage oscilloscope for echo registration. A final photographic record was taken in the form of a Polaroid picture of the storage screen. The resultant image showed dots of constant intensity although many echoes came from interfaces with varying echogenicity. The final

*Hassani, Ultrasonography of the Abdomen. New York, Springer-Verlag, 1976.

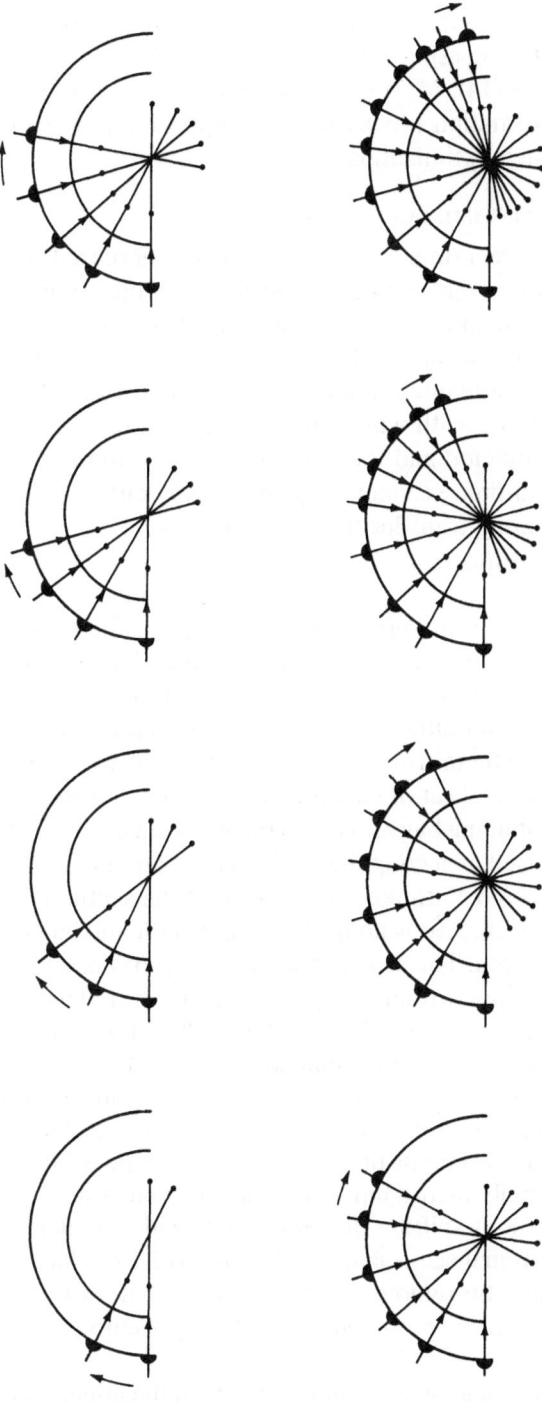

FIGURE 1.8
Spatial orientation of the scan. As the transducer traverses the body contour, the echoes returning from the region being scanned are aligned on the oscilloscope in exact depth with respect to the sound beam. The series of echoes returned are oriented in a two-dimensional arrangement over a 180° scan arc.

sonogram with the storage or bistable unit consisted of a black-and-white photograph without information regarding echo amplitude. There is good representation of the size, shape, and position of the lesion and also whether it is cystic or solid. However, the internal echo pattern may only be evaluated in a qualitative manner since it involves manipulation of the sensitivity settings.

Gray scale displays a dynamic range of echo amplitudes simultaneously as varying shades of gray. High-intensity echoes appear dark gray and low-intensity echoes light gray. Anechoic areas are colorless with current registration methods. Usually, the sensitivity setting need not be adjusted to evaluate tissue echo characteristics. For example, echoes from the renal collecting system appear dark gray while those from the surrounding parenchyma are light gray.

Early gray-scale techniques used photographic film to record scans. Film was exposed to a scan pattern composed of amplitude-modulated echoes presented to a short-persistence oscilloscope. Usually four shades of gray were obtained with this method. Disadvantages included a complicated area scanning technique to prevent overwriting echoes, and a longer scanning time inherent with this maneuver. In addition, the camera F-stop setting, oscilloscope intensity, and film speed influenced the gray-scale effect (14). After the scan was completed, the film had to be developed before the picture could be interpreted. Current commercial systems in which a scan converter is used offer eight to ten shades of gray displayed on a television tube (Fig. 1.9). The scan converter tube detects all echo intensities and is connected to a closed circuit television system providing an instant visual display of the area scanned. The technique is the same as for conventional B-scanning methods. Scanning time is reduced due to better resolution and simultaneous display of weak and strong echoes, eliminating the need to vary sensitivity settings during sectioning. The image developed on the monitor tube may then be recorded with Polaroid, 35 mm film, or multiformat imaging using a

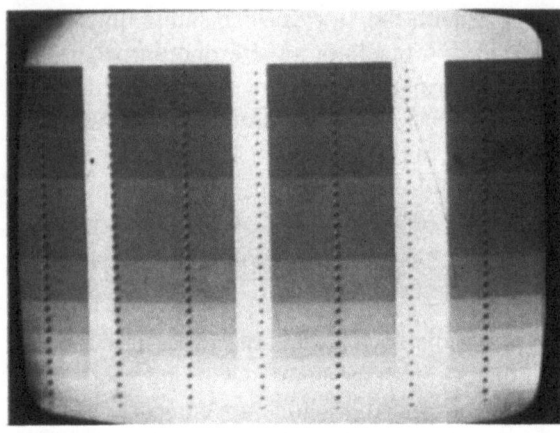

FIGURE 1.9
Demonstration of multiple shades of gray.

microprocessor. Moderate differentiation of signal processing enhances contrast at tissue interfaces (14). Most scan converter systems offer information processing techniques for postscan image optimization (Fig. 1.10).

REAL-TIME SCANNING

The real-time scanner has greatly increased the scope of information available from ultrasonic examination. This modality has been applied to numerous areas of the body (15–17). The two main advantages of real-time scanning are the rapidity with which the examination can be completed and the ability to observe motion. Real-time scanners usually employ either a rotating transducer or a linear array of transducers.

There are several commercially available real-time scanners. One of the earliest real time scanners (Fig. 1.11) uses two 2.5-MHz transducers that emit ultrasonic beams toward a parabolic acoustic mirror (Fig. 1.12a). The reflector sends a parallel set of sound waves through a water-containing bag applied to the body surface. A gel is used as a coupling agent. The scanning field is covered 15 times per second and the sectional view studied is about 14 cm in length and 20 cm in depth. This field is built up to approximately 120 lines within 70 milliseconds (msec). The width of the section is a few millimeters. The unit produces instantaneous sectional images and displays them simultaneously on an oscilloscope and television monitor. This immediate and continuous presentation makes it possible to visually record movement of a desired structure. Without shifting the applicator head, parallel sectional scans can be taken up to 3.5 cm laterally by remote control of the motion of the transducer mounted within the applicator head.

The linear array scanner, in which the applicator has a linear array of 64 transducers, firing four at a time, to produce approximately 60 lines of information (Fig. 1.12b), has been available commercially for a few years. Presently, many types of real-time units have been developed.

Most machines are equipped with depth compensation controls which amplify the near, far,

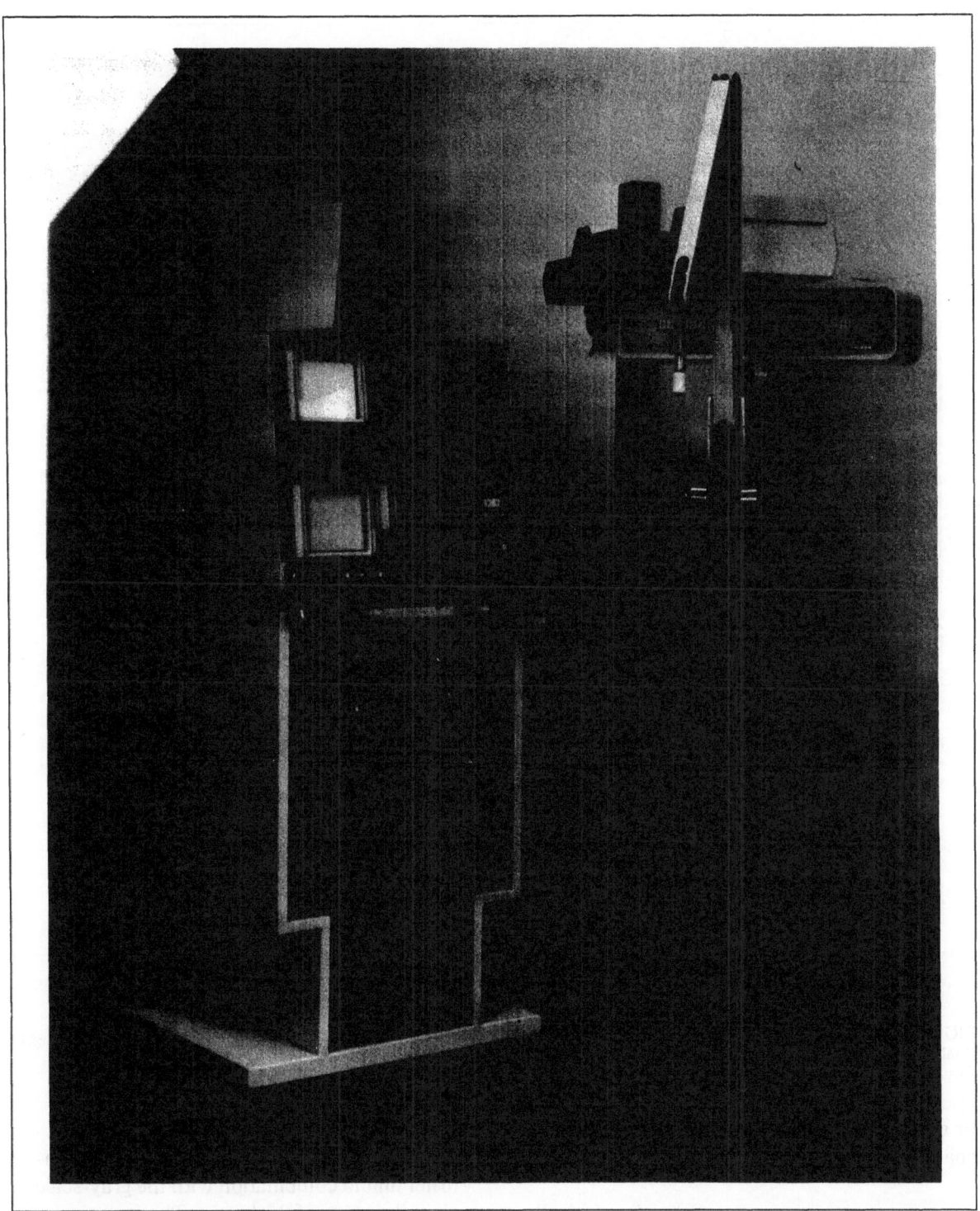

FIGURE 1.10
Contact diagnostic ultrasound scanner.
Courtesy of Picker Corporation.

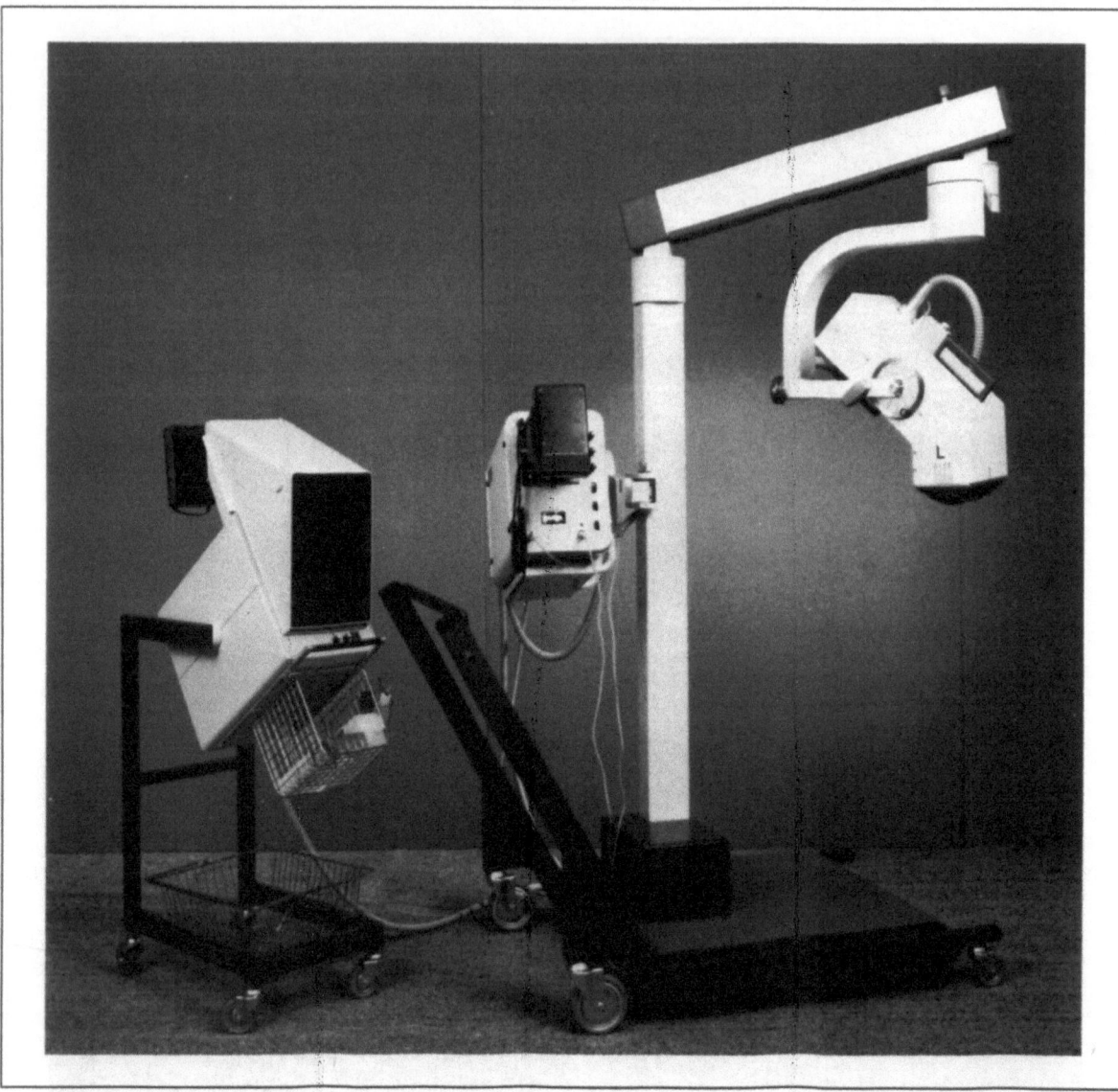

FIGURE 1.11
Real-time scanner.
Courtesy of Siemens Company.

or overall field. Another device adjusts the shades of gray on the monitor.

Linear transducer arrays may be electronically phased by pulsing each of the multiple transducer crystals as a separate unit. The wave front formed follows the pattern of transducer excitation. The wave pattern may be made to produce a sector scan with a variable scan angle

of up to 90°. The wave front may also be focused to different depths. Resolution with current systems varies (Fig. 1.12c).

We use the commercially available Bronson-Turner unit in combination with the gray-scale unit in the study of the breast. The scanning part of the Bronson-Turner consists of a handpiece and a small chamber which contains the transducer and acts as a water bag. The transducer has a 10 MHz frequency and is enclosed in a housing that is held against the area

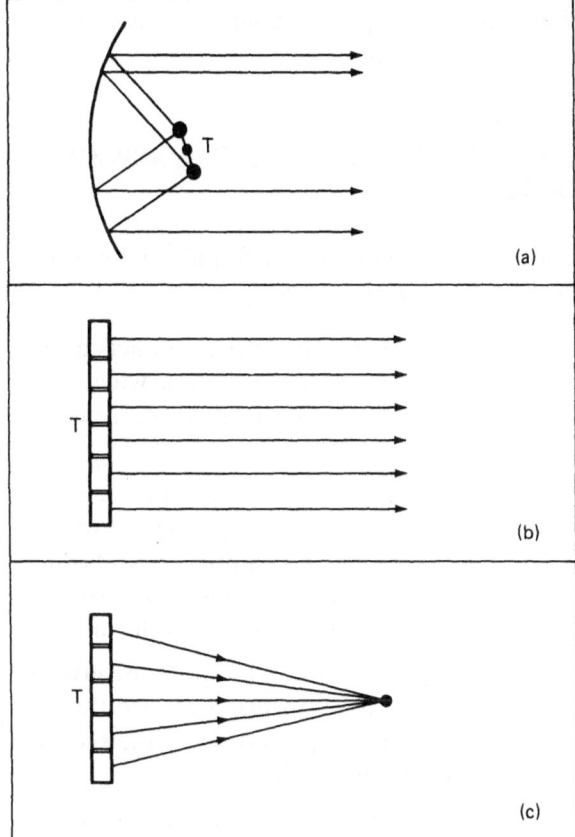

FIGURE 1.12
Real-time scanning systems. (a) Rotating transducer reflects sound waves from parabolic surface to generate parallel beam. (b) Linear transducer array. Multiple transducers being pulsed in sequence to produce parallel beam. (c) Phased linear array. Variable wavefront generated by coordinated pulsing of each transducer element. T, transducer.

of interest. The transducer of the Bronson-Turner unit is about 0.25 inch in diameter and 1.5 inches long. This unit has a rapid scanning rate of 11 sweeps per second. It produces a dynamic display of successive cross sections that appear on a television monitor. The transducer moves in a sector and the image appears linearly. The scanning part is coupled through a flexible cable to the cathode-ray tube.

The cathode-ray tube resembles a 12-inch television set. The section of the tissue being studied appears on the monitor and is represented in dark and light areas which directly correspond to the amount of reflected sound beam. There are two controls: One selects the depth of field and covers the ranges of 0 to 3 cm, 1.5 to 4.5 cm, and 3 to 6 cm. The second varies the sensitivity setting of the unit (gain setting) and can be manipulated from 40 to 80 db (standarized with reference to an echo returned from a plain glass plate); it is calibrated in 10-db steps.

DOPPLER EFFECT

The frequency change of mechanical waves due to the relative motion of either sound source or observer is called the Doppler effect. It is named after Christian Doppler who first described this phenomenon. The measurement of sound frequency is obtained by computing the pressure peaks that cross an observer in a unit of time or in 1 second. If the sound source moves toward the observer during measurement a greater number of peaks will be counted and the calculated frequency will be greater than the "true" frequency. On the other hand, if the sound source moves away from the observer the calculated frequency will be lower than the "true" frequency. This phenomenon also occurs if the observer moves toward or away from the source. The Doppler effect can be used in the detection of the moving organ by using two crystals, one crystal generating a continuous ultrasonic beam emitted toward the organ of interest and second receiving the reflected echo. The stationary organ does not change the frequency of the reflected sound, while the moving organ does change the frequency of the reflected ultrasonic beam.

DOPPLER TECHNIQUE

The operation of Doppler instruments is based on transmitting and receiving an ultrasonic beam that hits moving structures or fluids, such as blood in the cardiovascular system. The simplest Doppler has a transducer with two crystal elements. One crystal transmits a continuous sonic beam and the second receives the reflected waves. The transmitting crystal is excited through a low-power oscillator which operates in the range of 3 to 8 MHz. The sound intensities are usually under 50 mW/cm².

The transmitted and received signals occur at the surface of the transducer and the returned information appears in electronic form at the receiving amplifier. The end result is called amplitude-modulated or AM waves. These AM waves are similar to radiowaves in that the amplitude of the modulation is proportional to the amplitude of the returned signal. A radio frequency amplifier with a special detector may be used to clarify the returning Doppler signal.

With modern Doppler instruments we are able to listen to the Doppler signal range for almost all physiologic flow patterns. As we gain more experience, a great deal of information can be obtained regarding the blood flow. For example, areas of stenosis in a blood vessel produce a high-velocity–type jet flow which yields a high-frequency Doppler signal. These signals are clearly differentiated from those either distal to or proximal to the stenotic signal. As previously described, structures in motion can easily be detected. For example, fetal heart motion can be identified as early as 8 to 10 weeks after conception.

The most modern Doppler equipment incorporates features of continuous-wave Doppler combined with pulse-echo type ultrasound, and has the capability to determine the location or depth of an interface as well as the velocity of the flow.

EQUIPMENT AND PRACTICAL ASPECTS OF USE

The essential part of a sonographic unit consists of the following elements.

1. Transducer. The transducer acts as a sender and receiver of sonic waves. It functions as a receiver 99.9 percent of the time.
2. Transmitter. The transmitter regulates the sonic waves through the transducer. A timer in the transmitter controls the frequency and duration of ultrasonic pulses emitted by the transducer.
3. Receiver. Returning echoes reconverted through the transducer to electric impulses are picked up by the receiver and signal amplifier.
4. Signal amplifier. The signal amplifier, located between the receiver and cathode-ray tube, increases the voltage of the signal.
5. Cathode-ray tube. The cathode-ray tube receives the amplified impulses of the returning echo. The processed impulses are displayed on the cathode-ray tube or oscilloscope.

The transducer is the only element discussed in this section.

TRANSDUCER

COMPONENTS

The transducer has a lead zirconate crystal with piezoelectric properties, which can expand and contract in response to electric pulses (Fig. 1.1). The piezoelectric crystal has a small cylindrical shape and is generally 1 to 2 cm wide and 1 mm thick. The electrodes providing the electric potential are connected to both sides of the crystal. The vibrating crystal causes compressions and rarefactions in all directions. To provide a unidirectional ultrasonic beam, a backing material is used to absorb the waves in unwanted directions. The backing material acts as an acoustic as well as a mechanical damper for the crystal.

The frequency of oscillation controls the resolution capability of the system. After transmission, the acoustic energy of reflected sound is reconverted into electric impulses for data analysis, since the same crystal generates electric currents when exposed to returning high-frequency waves. The transducers usually used in clinical work have different frequency ranges, from 1 to 15 MHz. Approximately 99.9 percent of the time the transducer acts as a receiver.

To vary the frequency of the sound, the transducer must be changed. For example, a frequency of 2.25 MHz is used in abdominal studies. For echocardiography, a transducer frequency of 3.5 MHz is utilized (18). The characteristics of the system depend on the frequency of the transducer and the choice of frequency depends on the region to be studied (18). Transducers of low frequency have longer wavelengths, resulting in greater beam penetration and better depth of study. However, increasing the wavelength decreases the resolution of the system. High frequency offers high resolution. In ophthalmology, the transducer frequency varies from 7.5 to 20 MHz. As a result, the higher frequency provides optimal definition of small objects but the depth of penetration is limited.

MOUNTING

The disc of piezoelectric crystal in the transducer has a suitable mounting arrangement for optimal resolution (19–21). To produce continuous waves a thin layer of a matching wave is used to improve the sensitivity (18). In the back of the transducer is a loading or backing material, which absorbs sound energy directed or transmitted backward. Consequently, the quality and shape of forward energy, especially of short pulses, are improved.

NEAR FIELD AND FAR FIELD

Divergence of the beam from the transducer is of extreme importance. In a circular transducer, the beam emitted from the face is cylindrical. During the course of propagation, the sound waves run parallel for a certain distance and then gradually begin to diverge. That portion of the beam close to and parallel with the transducer is called the near field and that extending from the divergent point is called the far field (Fig. 1.13a,b, and c). At the end of the near field, the intensity of sound is maximal in the axis of the beam. Thus, maximum information is obtained when the object is located in the near field because the sound beam is parallel to the transducer and more perpendicular to the target. Consequently, the intensity of the reconverted echo is greater.

OPTIMAL CRYSTAL SIZE

To increase the resolution of the ultrasonic beam (12), its width should be as small as possible. To enlarge the near field and obtain better information, the size of the crystal is increased or wavelength decreased. Reducing the diameter of the crystal narrows the width of the beam but decreases the length of the near field and increases the divergent angle of the far field (12).

To obtain the optimum size of the transducer crystal, the beam width should be constructed in such a way that the near field is half the desired operating range of the transducer. To obtain higher resolution, frequency should be increased. In practice, the highest frequency consistent with maximum penetration for the required study is utilized (Fig. 1.14a,b, and c).

FOCUS

Resolution can also be improved by using focused or collimated transducer to reduce beam width within the focal zone. By applying a focusing lens with a concave surface, the focus of the ultrasonic beam will be narrowed to a predetermined distance from the face of the transducer (Fig. 1.13). The focused transducer has helped to improve resolution of deep abdominal structures.

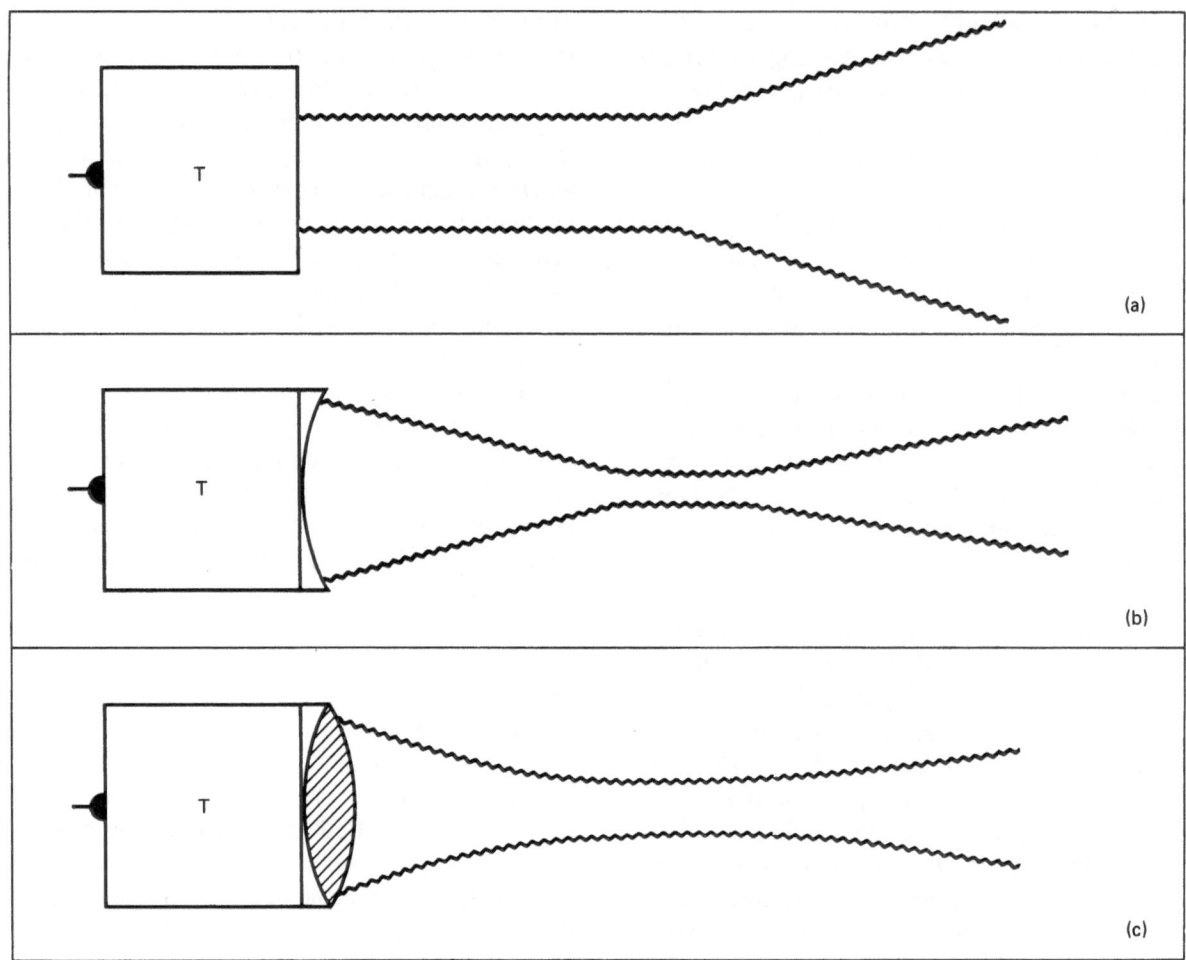

FIGURE 1.13
Transducer beam patterns. (a) Nonfocused transducer. Parallel wavefront forms the near field. Divergent beam in far field. (b) Focused transducer. Narrowest beam width at focal zone. (c) Collimated transducer. Elongated near field and less far field beam divergence. T, transducer.

FUNCTION

As previously described, piezoelectric crystals emit ultrasound pulses as short as 1 second in duration. After the sonic burst has been emitted, the transducer then acts as a receiver, picking up the reflected sonic waves. After this period of time, another burst of ultrasound is emitted and the cycle repeated. There are different types of transducers.

PULSE CHARACTERISTICS AND THE DAMPING SYSTEM

The optimal spatial pulse length is between 1 and 2.5 cycles. The excited crystal has a tendency to oscillate for a long time, producing a prolonged spatial pulse length too long to provide adequate axial resolution. The damping system controls crystal oscillation by mechanical and electronic means (Fig. 1.15a,b, and c). Damping may be adjusted manually or built into the electronic circuity. Overdamping produces a short spatial pulse length and the pulse may lack sufficient energy to be useful. Thus, a properly spaced pulse depends on a well-adjusted damping system.

SIGNAL PROCESSING

Reconverted ultrasonic echoes produce an electric impulse when they reach the transducer crystal. This impulse is transmitted as an amplified radio frequency (RF) (18,21) signal into the system. The RF mode appears as a series of signals above and below the baseline of the oscilloscope (Fig. 1.16a and b). Amplification increases the size of the signal without changing the information and is manually adjustable (gain control). Further modification depends on specific clinical use. Generally, after amplification, the waveform is rectified to remove all negative components so that only the upper half of the signal is presented. Further modification can be accomplished so that only the outline or boundary of the upper half of the electric signal is presented as an envelope detection (Fig. 1.16c).

FIGURE 1.14
Beam width and crystal size. (a) Wide crystal with long near field. (b) Medium crystal with shorter near field. (c) Narrow crystal with short near field and great beam divergence in the far field. T, transducer.

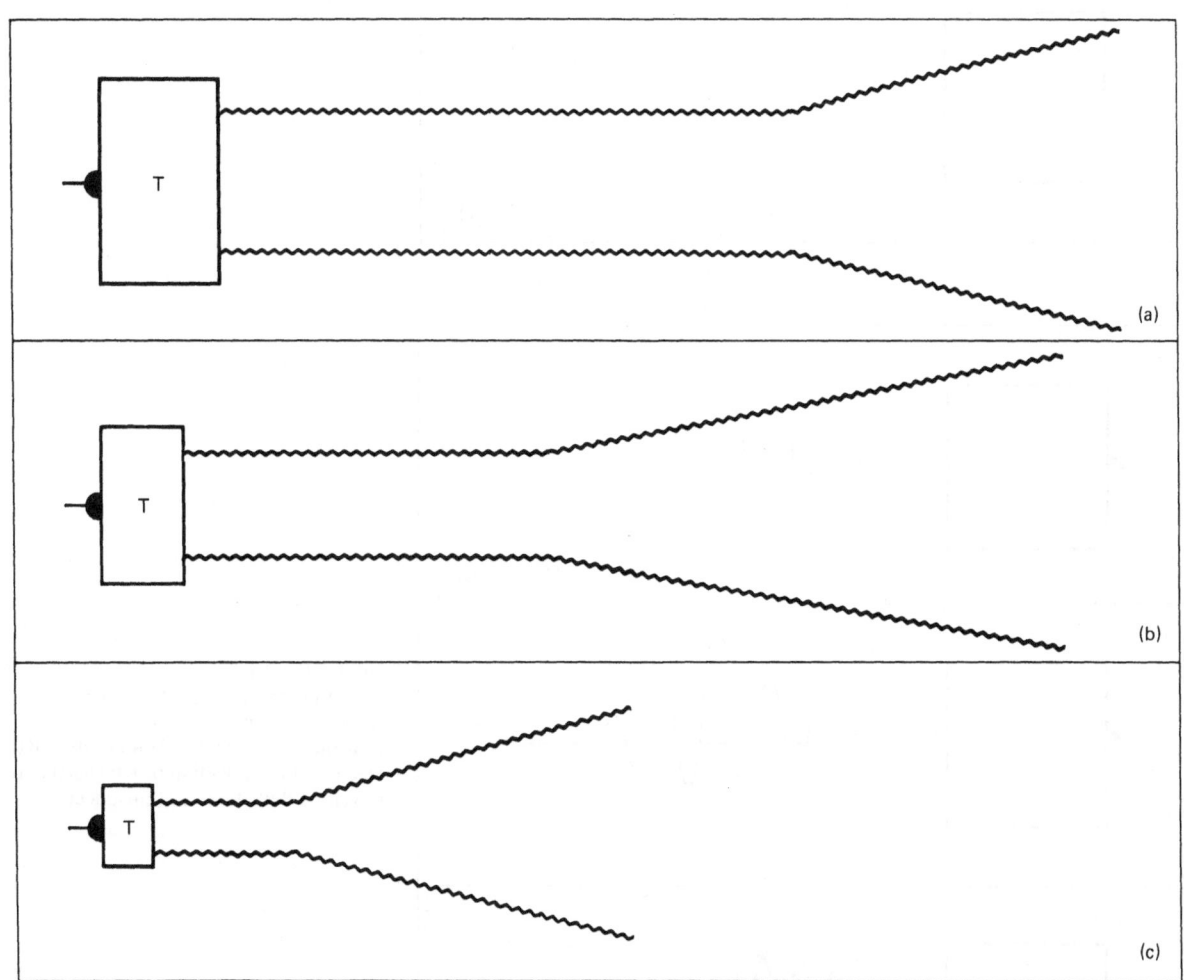

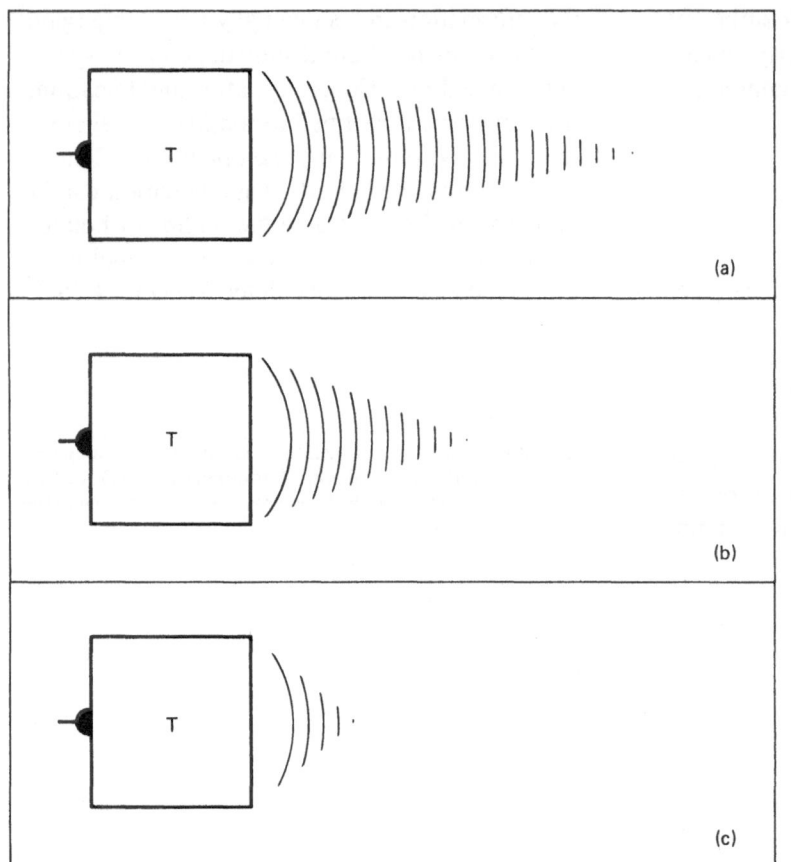

FIGURE 1.15
Damping effect. (a) Underdamping resulting in multiple oscillations of transducer crystal. (b) Proper damping producing optimal spatial pulse length. (c) Overdamping with insufficient pulse cycles. T. transducer.

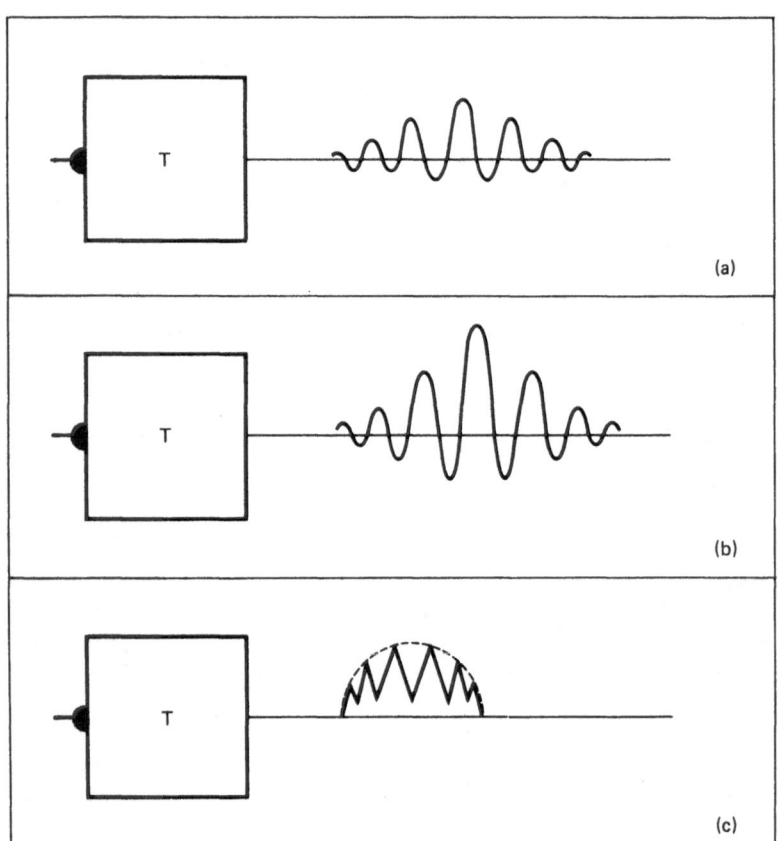

FIGURE 1.16
Signal processing. (a) RF signal produced by incoming echo on transducer crystal. (b) Amplification RF signal. (c) Rectification of RF signal and envelope detection. T. transducer.

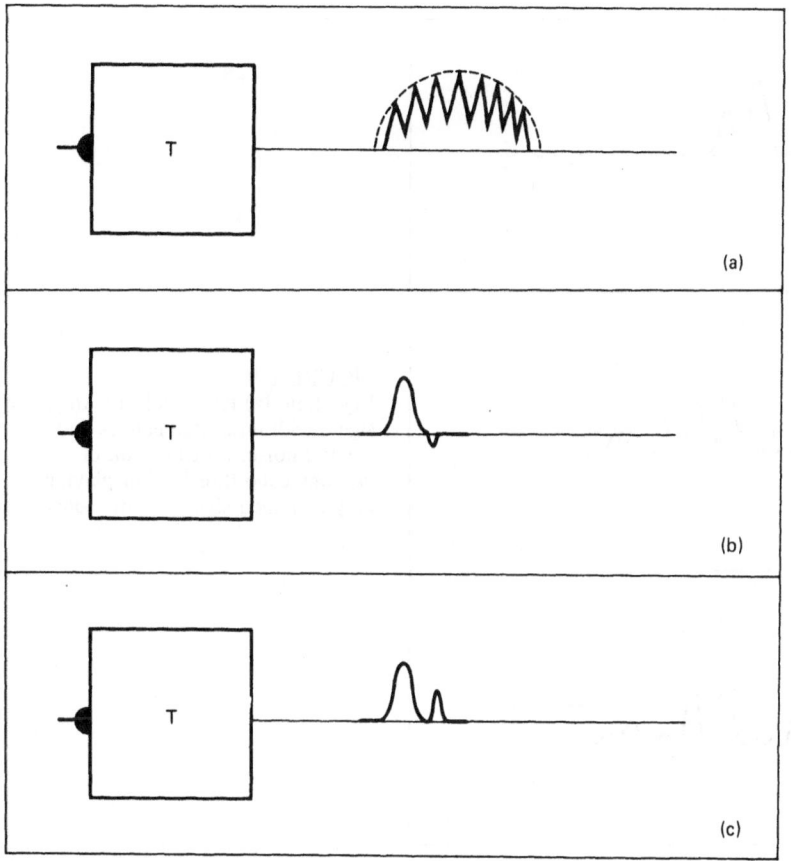

FIGURE 1.17
Signal processing. (a) Envelope detection of rectified RF signal. (b) Leading edge display or differentiation of signal. (c) Rectification and amplification of signal for oscilloscope display. T. transducer.

This presentation is called video display. Envelope detection or video display with its multiple peaks can be converted into a smooth, single, large peak called the video signal (Fig. 1.17a). This signal may be further amplified or modified by accentuating the leading edge of the signal (Fig. 1.17b) by taking the first derivative of the video signal that produces a thin echo. The small negative phase (Fig. 1.17b and c) following the initial signal further accentuates the leading edge of the echo by rectification, giving finer echoes and enhancing the resolution of the system. Another step in processing the video is to add a reject level so that only large-amplitude echoes above a certain threshold will be detected (Fig. 1.18a,b, and c). Rejection is very important to eliminate unnecessary echoes (Fig. 1.18b) and electric noise or "grass" (Fig. 1.18b and c). However, certain low-level echoes are required for optimal information. The sonographer should

adjust the rejection level, as needed, for proper ultrasonic examination.

MAIN SYSTEM CONTROL

POWER SWITCH

An on-off switch is connected to a standard 110-volt outlet. The line is grounded to prevent an electric hazard.

REJECT

The reject control varies the amplitude threshold required to record an echo. It discriminates against low-level echoes and is used to remove "grass"-like interference at higher gain settings.

GAIN

The gain control amplifies the electronic signal of the received echo. Some units employ an attenuation system to achieve this effect. Two

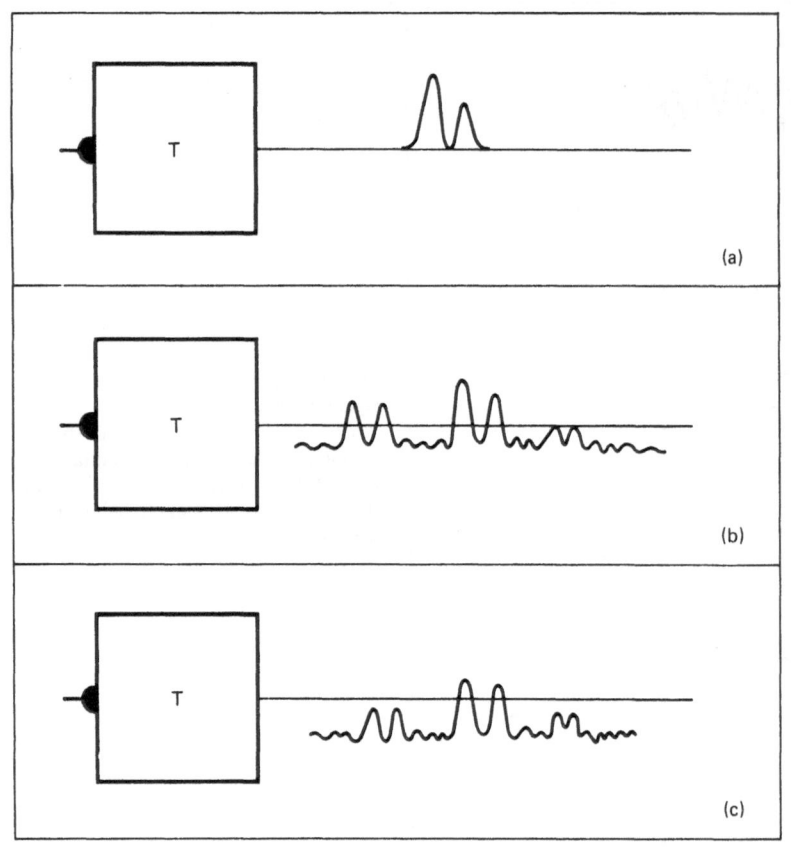

FIGURE 1.18
Rejection. (a) RF signal. (b) Amplified signal with unwanted echoes and electric noise. (c) Elevation of baseline echo threshold displaying only amplified signal. T, transducer.

types of gain are available: near gain and total gain. Near gain increases the amplitude of echoes in the near field. Total or coarse gain produces a uniform increase in size of all displayed signals, and sets the overall gain of the receiver, which is independent of range.

TGC

Time gain compensation (TGC) or depth compensation control is an adjustable amplitude correction to increase or decrease the echo intensity in any given region of the field. It was originally designed to compensate for the loss of sound energy with increasing distance due to tissue attenuation. Newer systems make it possible to selectively enhance or depress any part of the field.

DAMPING

The damping control regulates the oscillation of the transducer. By reducing or damping transducer ringing from the excitation pulse, it adjusts the cycles of sound available from each pulse. A shorter pulse increases resolution; however, a beam too highly damped lacks sufficient penetrating ability and sensitivity. Increasing the damping decreases the amplitude of all recorded echoes and is similar to decreasing the total gain.

DELAY

Delay adjusts the starting point of the oscilloscope display, and the crystal artifact as well as other near field echoes can be moved out of the visual display. Selected segments of tissue may be displayed in the far field. Delay actually helps to determine where the TGC curve starts.

DEPTH

The amount of tissue or field represented on the oscilloscope or television face can be varied from 5 to 40 cm in most commercially available systems.

INTENSITY

Brightness of the trace for all display modes may be adjusted manually.

FOCUS

The beam can be focused for optimal display. Focusing should be performed after intensity is adjusted.

ASTIGMATISM

Astigmatism may be incorporated into the focus system so that the focusing process can be refined further.

GRATICULE

A reference scale for measurements, the graticule's illumination can be adjusted. Parallel transverse and longitudinal lines form a pattern of squares.

SCALE

The field may be varied in increments of 0.5 to 3 cm per square, which is valuable for examining smaller organs.

MAGNIFICATION

The echoes displayed can be magnified by either rescanning on a smaller scale per unit square or by electronically "zooming" the image presented on the television monitor.

CONTRAST ENHANCEMENT

Newer gray-scale units offer scan converter tubes that make it possible to emphasize various shades of gray to maximize the information display.

ERASE

An erase switch clears the oscilloscope or television tube so that a new scan can be started.

CENTER

The scanning beam must be centered over the oscilloscope field, either manually or automatically.

DIGITAL READ-OUT

A computer types patient information and scan identification which can be introduced directly onto the television display, and may then be photographed. Electronic calipers measure dimensions instantaneously on the monitor.

RECORDING

A permanent record can be obtained on photographic film of the 35-mm, 70-mm, or Polaroid type. X-ray film can also be used. Videotape systems and multi-imagers may be adapted for permanent displays.

ARTIFACTS IN ULTRASONOGRAPHY

Difficulties in scanning due to bone, gas, and radiographic contrast will be discussed in this section. Echoes from internal structures vary according to acoustic impedance, organ size and shape, tissue attenuation from overlying structures, and organ depth. Artifacts may result when the ultrasound beam is not perpendicular to the skin surface, and from organ contour and image distortion due to beam width. Echoes in the near field, close to the transducer, may be lost in the "dead zone" of the beam due to continued oscillation of the crystal during the receiving phase. Newly designed low–pulse-voltage units with effective damping systems compensate for this problem.

Reverberation artifacts are recognized by their periodicity and decreasing echo amplitude on the A-mode and B-mode. These occur when sound encounters a highly reflecting interface, such as bone or air. The loud-echo artifact, distal to a strongly reflecting surface and appearing as an echo-free region immediately following the strong echo, is due to crystal reverberation. It is noted on the A-mode as echoes elevated from the baseline (22). This artifact is frequently noted when the gallbladder and edematous renal transplants are scanned. Lowering the sensitivity permits the echoes to return to the baseline and the echo-free artifact disappears.

Distortion caused by misalignment of

potentiometers in the scanning arm and changes in the preset determination of acoustic velocity may be detected by frequent calibration with an acoustic phantom.

BIOPHYSICAL EFFECTS OF ULTRASOUND

The unexpected and tragic experiences resulting from the early applications of diagnostic radiology and the great physical and psychologic trauma produced by uncontrolled use of X rays have alerted the ultrasonographer to extreme caution in the use of ultrasonic investigation in human beings. Ultrasonographers have carefully attempted to maximize their efforts to obtain diagnostic interpretations with minimal ultrasonic energy input into the adult and fetal organ systems.

During clinical applications, the possible genetic and somatic changes have been constantly monitored throughout the short- and long-term periods. Many carefully controlled experimental studies have been performed to determine the various parameters of safe ultrasonic exposure. Even at this stage of the development of ultrasound, we have had limited experience with the long-range effects. Whether the ultrasonographer's fingers will fall off in 20 years from excessive handling of ultrasonic equipment or whether he will show no detectable physical damage or definite chromosomal changes is totally unpredictable at present. However, according to the latest experimental reports and worldwide correlation of data on ultrasonic side effects, there is no substantiation of any harmful effects due to use of ultrasound at the energy levels encountered in current diagnostic scanning units. The collected data of many investigators have revealed that there is an extremely large margin of safety at acoustic energy levels used in diagnostic ultrasound. Numerous publications based on clinical and laboratory findings have documented that to date there is no evidence that this level of ultrasonic energy has any deleterious effects, whether genetic or physical (23–27).

Widely differing energy and power outputs are used in therapeutic ultrasound as compared with diagnostic insonation. In diagnostic work, the power of ultrasound is on the order of mW/cm². The energy levels used in physiotherapy are thousands of times greater and are sufficient to produce measurable heat in biologic tissues (28). Still greater power is used in such surgical applications as ablation of nerve endings and destruction of normal and abnormal areas of the brain for neurosurgical therapy (29).

Tissue damage may occur at ultrasonic power levels many thousands of times greater than currently used diagnostic beam intensities. Simple agitation may cause cellular membranes to rupture at high frequency. Elevation of tissue temperature and cavitation occur during prolonged exposure to high-energy sonic waves. Chemical changes include a change in pH caused by the release of radicals and increased tissue oxidation rates. Also noted are increased membrane permeability and greater enzymatic activity. Since ultrasound is nonionizing, cumulative effects are not to be expected (30).

Ultrasonic waves with very high energy levels are used in cleaning mechanical devices, polishing metals, and drilling.

As mentioned, the damaging effect of ultrasound depends upon the energy range and physical characteristics of the sonic beam. The ultrasonic energy is the product of the measured radiation and the sonic beam velocity, which is translated into watts. The intensity of the beam is the power per unit of specific cross-sectional area or, actually, watts per square centimeter (W/cm²). The intensity of power of an ultrasonic beam usually is calculated from the electric input to the corresponding transducer. This measurement is an estimated value because the sound intensity suffers from complex variations of the pulse shape and spatial distribution of the beam energy.

There are many reports regarding the biologic effects of ultrasound in clinical application (31–33). The work of Hellman et al (34) has revealed no evidence of fetal or maternal damage. In our experience over the past five years with a large number of patients who have undergone a variety of ultrasonic examinations involving such areas as eye, thyroid, heart, brain, abdominal organs, and pregnant uterus, we have not found any deleterious effects thus far. However, we are still following our data.

Macintosh and Davey (35), in 1970, reported an increased number of chromosomal aberrations after exposing human leukocyte cultures to low-level diagnostic ultrasound; but in their second study (36) they reported that chromosomal aberrations did not occur below the level of 8.2 mW/cm^2 intensity.

At present we conclude, on the basis of all existing evidence, that there are most likely no significant somatic changes produced by the energy level of the diagnostic range of ultrasound. The possibility of delayed genetic effects remains questionable.

GENETIC EFFECTS OF ULTRASOUND

The increased use of ultrasound in fetal and maternal disorders and its recent application to the male testis requires investigation into the potential genetic hazards of clinical ultrasonography. An excellent in vivo study (30) of mouse gonads insonated at levels up to 20 times the intensity of currently used ultrasound energy revealed no evidence that dominant lethal mutations or sterility are induced in male mice. Follow-up for 8 weeks demonstrated no drop in testis weight or sperm count and no induction of translocations or chromosome fragments in spermatocytes (30). Although the risk of genetic derangement from ultrasound appears to be slight, its carcinogenic effect may not have been fully evaluated in humans at this early stage in the widespread application of ultrasonography to the general population.

PRACTICAL ASPECTS OF SONOLAPAROTOMY

In sonolaparotomy proper direction of the beam toward a specific organ is essential. Familiarity with ultrasonic sectional anatomy and a knowledge of anatomic pathology and surface topography are extremely important. Comprehension of organ relationships and their normal ultrasonic patterns is necessary to evaluate the extent of disease and the involvement of adjacent structures by pathologic processes. Two-dimensional ultrasonic imaging uses pulses which have a frequency of 2 to 3.5 MHz. At this frequency the beam has physical characteristics which allow the sound to be concentrated into a narrow beam and easily manipulated in a directed column of waves capable of penetrating the body to a depth of approximately of 20 to 30 cm of soft tissue.

PATIENT PREPARATION

In most instances there is no need for patient preparation. In obstetric and gynecologic examinations the bladder should be distended to delineate pelvic organs and to increase the penetration of the ultrasonic beam. To study the pancreas, it is preferable that the patient be NPO (nothing per mouth, or fasting state) since it may be necessary to insert a nasogastric tube to suction out gastric air or instill gasless water to distend the stomach and outline the duodenal contour.

Scanning causes no discomfort for the patient and in many situations is similar to fluoroscopy, in that the patient must be positioned properly and the image on the screen monitored constantly. After the area to be scanned is exposed, mineral oil is usually applied to the skin surface to prevent an air gap, which would markedly reflect sound between the transducer and the area involved. Complete contact between the surface of the applicator of the real-time scanner and the skin surface is obtained by using an ultrasonic gel.

DUTIES OF THE TECHNOLOGIST

The ultrasonographer should clearly understand the various methods of examination and proper control settings of the scanning machine used.

Patience and search are basic to good ultrasonography. The method of study changes the quality of echo display. Each type of commercially available instrument has its characteristic image production. For this reason, each unit functions with its own criteria, and the art of ultrasonography is to extract maximum information from a specific unit.

However, certain techniques and criteria are essential for basic studies. These include the ultrasonographer's familiarity with the following technical considerations.

1. Arrangement of a proper TGC curve on the oscilloscope for the study of a specific organ

2. Selection of the proper transducer

3. Familiarity with a system of identification

4. Changing the gain setting as needed

5. Selection of the rate of sectoring

6. Knowledge of the types of scanning (eg, linear, compound, arc, or sector)

7. Study of the patient in multiple positions

8. Maintenance of a minimum of eight shades of gray in gray-scale units

9. Familiarity with the use of real-time scanning

10. Knowledge of the ultrasonic limitations of sonography

11. Detection of through transmission pattern in combined A-mode and B-mode for better evaluation of pathology

PHYSICIAN PARTICIPATION

Ultrasonography is similar to creating a painting. The task of the operator is to display the echoes from a lesion and demonstrate its shape, location, and texture. Ultrasonography is far more delicate than fluoroscopy in that pathology detection and physician performance are more de-

manding. The examiner must make a final interpretation before the procedure is terminated. A specifically trained nurse-technician can perform the study; however, the physician-in-charge should be in constant attendance for consultation and interpretation of specific findings shown on the Polaroid. For example, during a routine study of the liver for metastases from an unknown source, a hypernephroma of the upper pole of the right kidney may be incidentally discovered.

POSITIONING THE TRANSDUCER

The transducer acts as a transmitter and receiver and the time between sonic emission and returned echo is a measure of the depth of the reflecting surface. Maximum reflection is achieved when the organ of interest lies perpendicularly to the sonic beam. Any degree of tilt of the transducer or reflector diminishes the intensity of the echo, and the signal may even be lost. In certain cases, difficulty in positioning the transducer and factors such as obesity can attenuate the returned ultrasound.

One aspect of the art of ultrasonography is to be aware of target displacement from the transducer and make corrections. Selection of a proper scanning speed is important if every echo produced is to be recorded (37). If the scanning speed is too fast, many reflected echoes will be missed by the receiving transducer. If the speed is too slow, artifactual echoes may be produced because the reflected sound will have a higher signal concentration in specific areas at a given period of time. The rate of transducer motion should be constant regardless of the scanning speed. When a normal technique is not applicable, other variations must be devised. Changes may be made in the transducer, patient position, scanning plane, or scanning mode. For example, a 1-MHz transducer may salvage a study in which a 2.25-MHz transducer cannot penetrate excess subcutaneous fat; in renal scanning hyperextension of the patient may permit better delineation of the kidney; multiple scanning

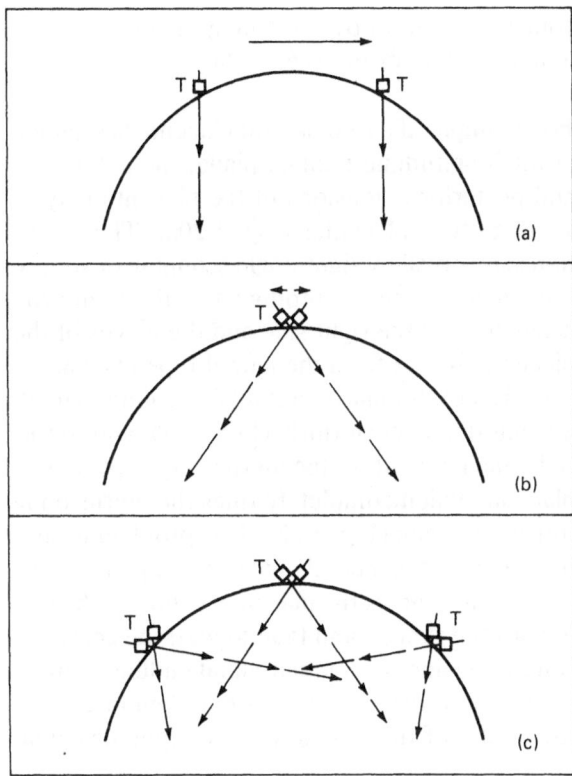

FIGURE 1.19
Types of scanning. (a) Linear scan. Sound beam
perpendicular to the skin surface. (b) Sector scan.
Transducer rotated about a fixed axis. (c) Compound scan.
Combination of linear and sector scan. T, transducer.

planes are generally necessary to visualize the
entire placenta; and minimal ascites may not be
detected on routine supine B-scanning but application of the A-mode transducer to the dependent anterior abdominal wall will demonstrate as
little as 100 ml of free fluid. M-mode and real-
time scanners may be used to verify the pulsation of a vascular structure.

TYPES OF SCANNING

There are several types of scanning, as follows.

1. Manual B-scanning
   a. Linear scan (Fig. 1.19a)
   b. Sector scan (Fig. 1.19b)
   c. Compound scan (Fig. 1.19c)
   d. Arc scan
2. Automated B-scanning
3. Real-time scanning

THREE-DIMENSIONAL
CONCEPTUALIZATION

In ultrasonography the examination of the organ
is performed in various specific planes. These
include the transverse and longitudinal planes,
but may also include oblique and decubitus or
erect scanning positions. The area of pathology
must be confirmed in at least two planes. The
shape, location, and configuration of the lesion
should be evaluated by right-angle scanning to
produce a three-dimensional representation of
the region of pathologic interest. In order to
produce complete mental integration of the scan
data, the examiner should continually
concentrate on the images appearing upon the
oscilloscope and link them together in his mind
as they are produced and erased. In this way, the
ultrasonographer has a mental image of the area
scanned which is formed from two right-angle
scan planes to produce a total three-dimensional
summation of the two-dimensional pictures.
Thus, two Polaroids at perpendicular scan
planes can document the lesion which is
extrapolated to a three-dimensional

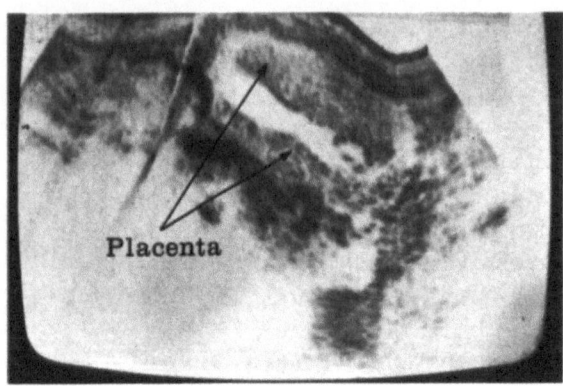

FIGURE 1.20(a)
Supine longitudinal scan. Finely stippled echo patterns of both an anterior and a posterior segment of the placenta is demonstrated. The anterior and posterior extensions of the placenta may simulate twin gestation. To avoid this problem multiple sectional studies are needed.

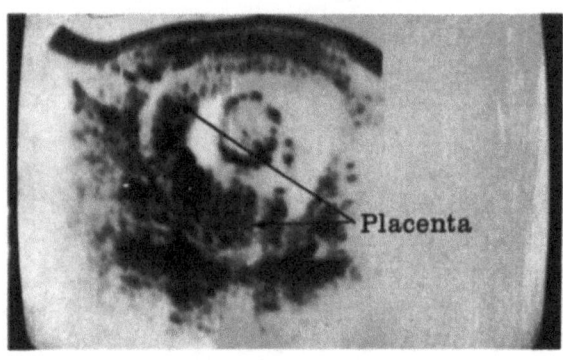

FIGURE 1.20(b)
Supine transverse scan. Gray scale. The right and left leaves of the placenta fuse to form the lateral-type placenta.

FIGURE 1.21
Supine longitudinal scan. Gray scale. A midline scan shows the placenta covering practically the entire uterine cavity. A small portion of the uterus near the internal os is free of placental echoes.

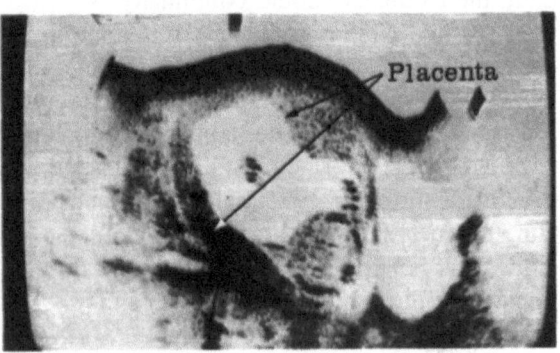

conceptualization by the sonographer's understanding of the scan data.

For example, if a right lateral placenta is scanned in the longitudinal midline plane, the anterior and posterior extensions of the placenta may simulate twin placentas (Fig. 1.20a). This situation is resolved by right-angle scanning or simply following the images produced as the scan proceeds toward the right side and the leaves of the placenta fuse to form the lateral-type placenta (Fig. 1.20b). Similarly, a fundal placenta extending anteriorly, posteriorly (Fig. 1.21), and to the right and left walls of the uterus may appear as a placenta which completely rings the uterus on a transverse scan (Fig. 1.22). This problem is corrected when the mental image of complete transverse scans shows the placental echoes to fuse toward the fundus and fade toward the cervix (Fig. 1.23a and b). A longitudinal midline scan would serve the same purpose to demonstrate the nature of the basically fundal-type placenta.

A similar problem exists when the echogenic wall of the gestational sac is sectioned tangentially, producing a dense area of echoes within the uterine cavity. Confusion is generally quickly resolved when more information is obtained by multiple sequential scans in combination with right-angle sectioning for further clarification.

It is important in ultrasonic scanning that areas of abnormal echoes must be reproducible in multiple scan planes. This double check prevents the diagnosis of pathologic conditions when confusing echo patterns are produced as either normal variants or artifacts due to motion (Fig. 1.24).

ULTRASONIC IDENTIFICATION:
PRINCIPLE OF SECTIONAL SCANNING

Evaluation of ultrasonic studies requires a complete three-dimensional representation of organs and areas of pathologic significance. As the application of ultrasound in medicine increases, more information can be obtained. A

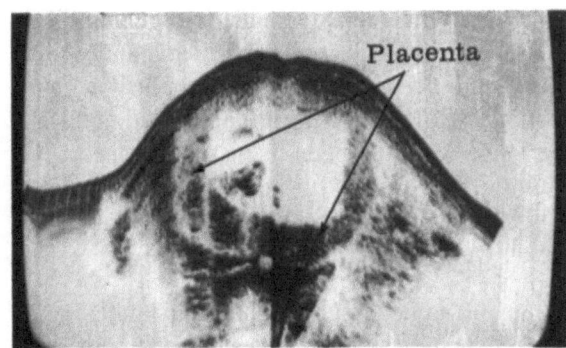

FIGURE 1-22

FIGURE 1-23a

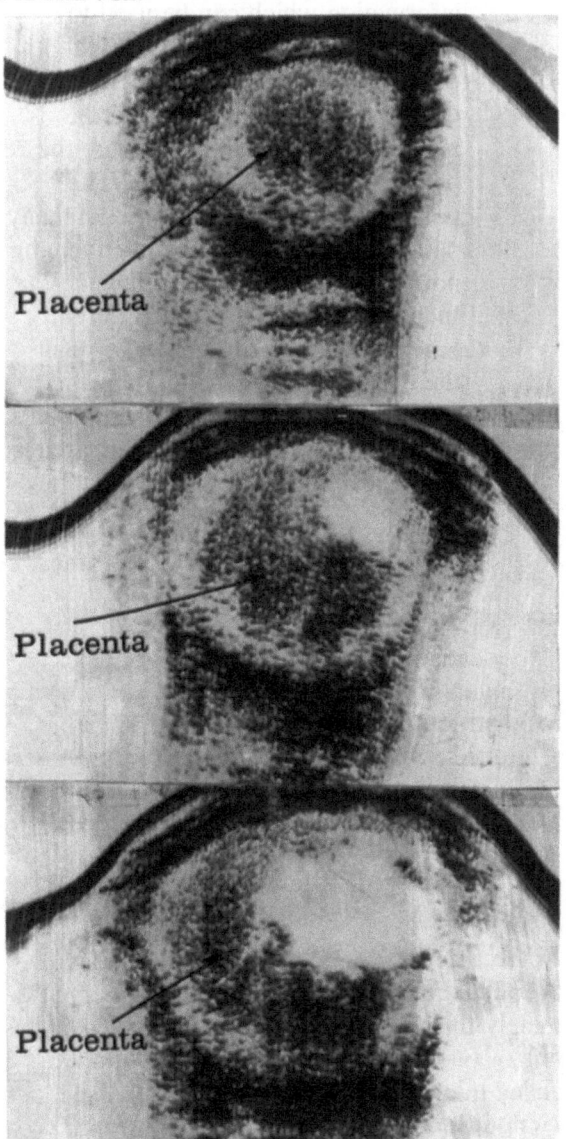

...recise and accurate identification system makes

... easier to interpret an echogram. For this

...eason special scanning planes are needed to

...erform the study and to obtain a corresponding

...onic pattern to compare with routine

...adiographs. The system of identification in

...ome ultrasound departments uses the umbilicus

...s a reference point. In supine positions

...ectional scanning (transverse and longitudinal)

FIGURE 1.22
Supine transverse scan in case shown in Fig. 1.21. Gray
scale. Scan in this plane shows the placenta to completely
...ne the visualized uterine cavity.

FIGURE 1.23(a)
Supine transverse scan. A serial complete transverse scan
...hows the placental echoes to fuse toward the fundus.

FIGURE 1.23(b)
Supine longitudinal scan. A serial complete longitudinal scan
...hows the placental echoes to fuse toward the fundus.

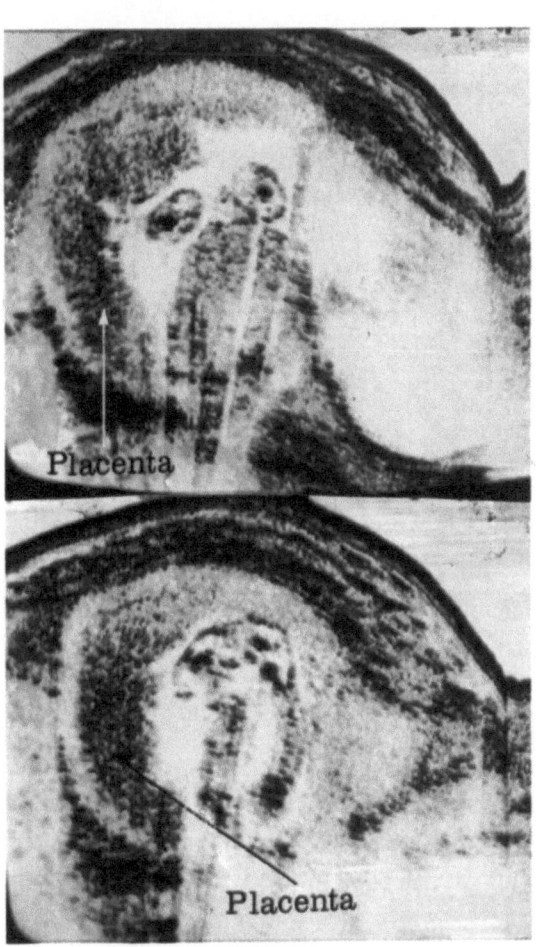

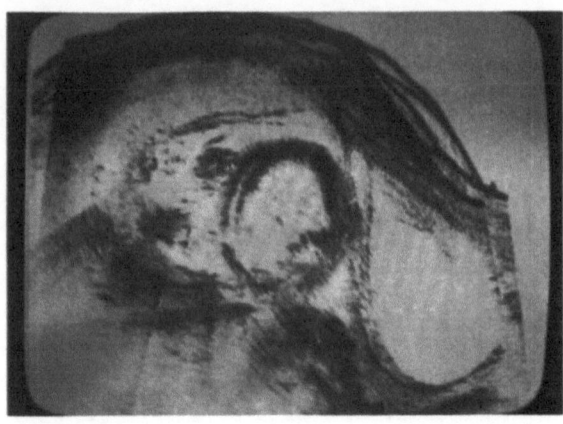

FIGURE 1.24
Supine longitudinal scan. A longitudinal midline scan
demonstrates the motion artifacts in the chorionic plate, fetal
head, and posterior wall of the bladder.

planes are obtained by considering the umbilicus as the zero point. Sections above and to the right of the umbilicus are designated as plus cuts and sections below and to the left are called minus sections. We have been using a different identification system for upper abdominal and pelvic ultrasonography to avoid disadvantages of the above system, which are as follows.

1. It is necessary in many instances (especially in studies of the upper abdomen) to compare ultrasonic photographs with corresponding radiographs. When the umbilicus is used as a topographic reference point, information which can be used to compare radiographic studies with ultrasonic sectoral scanning is not obtained, unless a lead marker is attached to the umbilicus before the patient is exposed to X rays. The position of the umbilicus varies in many pathologic conditions and even among normal young and old individuals. Indeed, it may be surgically absent. Since it is not a fixed reference point, the exact echogram cannot be reproduced on repeat examination in many pathologic conditions (eg, ascites, abdominal mass) after a lapse of time.

2. Absence of use of prone, decubitus, angled, and oblique scanning planes.

REFERENCE POINTS

Experience has shown that many obstacles present in previous studies would be avoided if a fixed structure in the body was used as a reference point (38). We use the xiphoid process of the sternum, symphysis pubis, and crest of the ilium as reference points.

ANTERIOR PROJECTION

ATC series
In the anterior projection, if a line is drawn between the two iliac crests, it will pass approximately through the plane of the umbilicus. This line or plane represents the zero point and is called the ATC (anterior transcrestal) plane. All sections above this plane are known as ATC-

plus (eg, ATC+1, +2, +3), and all sections below this plane are called ATC-minus (eg, ATC−1, −2, −3), Each number corresponds to the distance in centimeters from the ATC plane. In scanning the pancreas, the hilum of the right kidney is localized and oblique sections are made between the hilum of the right kidney and the spleen. These slices are called KP (kidney-pancreas) sections.

LXP series

The line or plane between the xiphoid process and symphysis pubis in normal individuals also crosses the umbilicus and is called the LXP line or plane. The LXP plane transecting the midportion of the body is designated as LXP-0 and all the sections toward the patient's right side are known as LXP-plus (eg, LXP+1, +2, +3), while sections toward the patient's left side are called LXP-minus (eg, LXP−1, −2, −3).

POSTERIOR PROJECTION

PTC series

In the posterior projection the transcrestal line or plane represents the zero point and is called the PTC (posterior transcrestal) plane. The transcrestal plane is PTC-0 and all sections above this plane are known as PTC-plus (eg, PTC+1, +2, +3).

PLS series

The spine is also used as a reference point for posterior views and sections, and is called the PLS (posterior longitudinal spine) line or plane. PLS-0 indicates a midline scan. Sections toward the right side of the spine are called PLS-plus sections (eg, PLS+1, +2, +3), and those toward the left are called PLS-minus sections (eg, PLS−1, −2, −3).

DECUBITUS PROJECTION

Transverse decubitus

In the lateral projection, with the patient lying on his side, the crest of the ilium is the zero point and all planes above it are plus cuts. If the patient's right side is up he is said to be lying in the right lateral decubitus (RDC) position, and if his left side is up he is in the left lateral decubitus (LDC) position (right decubitus crest or left decubitus crest). The term decubitus in

ultrasound refers to the side of the examination closest to the sonic beam. Sections above the iliac crest are called RDC- LDC-plus.

Longitudinal decubitus

In longitudinal sections the axillary line becomes the reference point. Therefore, all sections anterior to the right (RDA) or left (LDA) decubitus axillary line are plus sections, and all sections posterior to the axillary lines are minus sections.

ERECT PROJECTION

If the patient is sitting, instead of the term decubitus (D) we use the term erect (E), and abbreviations such as REC or LEC and REA or LEA are used.

These views are specifically used to study the chest wall, as for pleural effusion, and to evaluate the effect of gravity on abdominal structures, ptotic organs, or positional changes of organ relationships in normal and abnormal conditions in the supine, semierect, and erect positions.

ANGULATION

If the transducer is pointing toward the head or the right side, the degree of angulation relative to the perpendicular body section is designated as plus. If the transducer is pointing toward the feet or the left side it is designated as minus. For example, ATC+2+15° is the section 2 cm above the transcrestal line in anterior projection with a 15° angulation toward the head.

SUBCOSTAL AND INTERCOSTAL SECTIONS

Subcostal sectional study starts at the xiphoid process and runs parallel to the ribs from the xiphoid. Intercostal section is similar to subcostal section. On the right side it is called right subcostal (RSC) section, and on the left side it is called left subcostal (LSC) section. The rib itself is the zero point. Thus, RSC-0 is meaningless because the rib produces a sonic shadow. The sections below the pertinent rib are numbered accordingly. For example, RSC-11 is a section below the 11th rib on the right side, and LSC-11 is the section below the 11th rib on the left side.

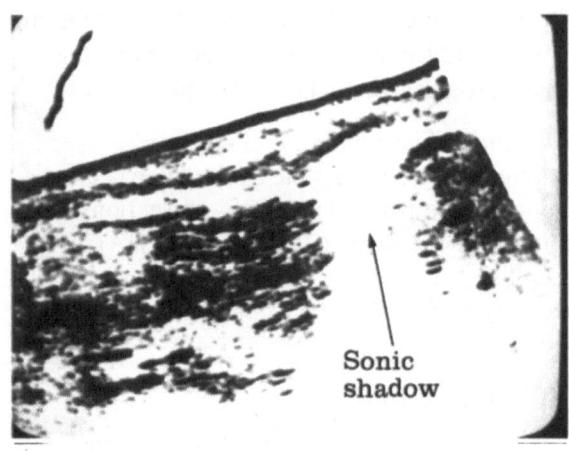

Sonic
shadow

FIGURE 1.25
Supine longitudinal scan. Gray scale. Scan shows an echo-dence linear structure in the deep subcutaneous tissues which casts a sonic shadow. Calcified scar due to 20-year-old incision.

TRANSDUCER CONTACT

Various scanning planes are utilized during a routine study. If the plane of interest does not lie perpendicularly to the body surface, acoustic contact may be impaired. As a result a large number of echoes are lost during scanning if sectional planes are perpendicular to the table rather than to the patient. To prevent loss of contact at curved areas of the body, the examiner must direct the transducer perpendicularly to the body contour to achieve maximum beam intensity.

In scanning over scar tissue sonic shadow (Fig. 1.25) may prevent the obtaining of adequate information, and the best maneuver would be to scan obliquely at the edge of the scar tissue. This may occur after scarring of C-section (Cesarean section).

SENSITIVITY SETTING OR ATTENUATION STUDIES

As in routine EKG tracings, the ultrasonographer should establish a standard baseline sensitivity setting for each organ to avoid confusion in interpretation. After each study or section, the attenuation may be changed to differentiate various components of an organ, or cystic from solid masses.

The frequency of ultrasound determines the average attenuation beam pattern (12). Using a higher frequency and a shorter sonic pulse a narrower beam may be obtained, which increases resolution. By lowering the frequency, however, deep structures can be visualized better. At higher frequency, deep structures reflect weak echoes (12). These produce serious problems in diagnosis, and can be corrected by adjusting the time gain compensation (TGC) control. The TGC corrects for higher average absorption (39). This adjustment must be made when an organ returns echoes at a certain frequency but does not return them at another frequency. In this case the pattern of the beam from the transducer has changed or the receiver is not properly compensating for average attenuation loss.

GAIN SETTING OR TGC CHANGE DURING STUDY

Opinions vary regarding changing TGC settings during scanning. One group is in favor of changing the TGC during the study if it is necessary (40), because the attenuation of sonic waves varies in different organs. Consequently, it is difficult to outline the entire organ in one plane with a fixed attenuation. On the other hand, changing the attenuation control during the examination may produce artifacts. These problems are avoided with gray-scale systems.

COMPARATIVE STUDIES AND SHIFTING METHOD

When difficulties exist in distinguishing a purely cystic lesion from a complex mass or solid mass with few internal echoes, comparative studies with the contact scanner or use of the shifting method with the real-time scanner may help to eliminate the uncertainty. A known fluid-filled body cavity such as the distended bladder may be taken as a cystic reference standard during scanning. The gray-scale unit or real-time scanner is adjusted for the known cystic structure so that it is displayed on the oscilloscope as an echo-free area with distinct borders. Comparison between the bladder and the suspected mass lesion is then made while scanning to obtain both in the same slice. This is most easily performed with the contact scanner when using a real-time scanner. The comparison method may not be easily done if the suspected cystic pathology is at a great distance from the bladder, since many real-time transducer heads or applicators are of limited length.

The shifting method is a form of sonofluoroscopy where the applicator of the unit is first placed over the pelvic region with the bladder as a baseline, and then moved over the area of pathologic interest for further evaluation. In this fashion, confirmation of a cystic lesion is readily made and the nature of the mass can be determined. In addition to its use in pelvic disorders, this method may be used in many other areas of the body. The differential diagnosis of a thyroid cyst from a solid tumor is made with certainty when the cystic lesion is compared to the cystic cavity of the globe of the eye as the transducer is shifted over the closed eyelid. Similarly, the gallbladder is used as a cystic reference point in upper abdominal scanning if it is distended.

FACTORS ALTERING NORMAL ACOUSTIC IMAGE

There are certain limitations to, and problems inherent in, each study. Some can easily be avoided; others, which are extremely difficult to prevent, include the following.

1. Respiratory motion.
2. Marked dehydration, which can be avoided by proper hydration.
3. Gas in the bowel. Gas interferes with sound transmission and the deep abdominal and retroperitoneal regions cannot be properly evaluated. Therefore, the study should be repeated after the patient has been given a laxative and a cleansing enema. When excessive gas is present in the stomach, the semierect position allows the gas to rise to the fundus where it will not interfere with the scan of abdominal organs. As previously described, bone effectively blocks the ultrasonic beam and no information is gained distal to a bony structure.
4. Presence of radiographic contrast material in the gastrointestinal tract. Water-soluble contrast in the

gastrointestinal tract does not alter gross anatomy nor the transmission of ultrasonic waves through the abdomen. With barium in the gastrointestinal tract, however, even with a high-gain setting, only the anterior aspect of the bowel is detectable for imaging (41). Barium blocks the passage of ultrasound to organs located behind barium-filled bowel loops. This problem can be detected by a plain film of the abdomen and a history of contrast examination.

5. Deep mediastinal area and lung pathology cannot be evaluated by ultrasonography because the air-containing lung transmits ultrasound poorly.

6. The pelvic bone prevents evaluation of structures deep in the pelvic cavity. Evaluation of this area can be improved by using an internal transducer.

7. Resolution of systems. At present, commercially available ultrasonographic units have limited resolution, and deep intraabdominal structures, smaller than 1 cm in diameter, cannot be evaluated by conventional presentation or gray scale.

ORIENTATION

TOPOGRAPHIC MARKING OF SUSPICIOUS AREA

In any ultrasound department, a water-soluble dye or grease pencil should be available so that an organ or area of interest can be marked upon the skin. Multiple markings of suspected pathology will allow this area to be scanned in the plane delineated on the skin. If the area is constant in this plane and also demonstrated in a perpendicular plane, then it is a true area of disease as opposed to artifact (37).

ORIENTATION OF SCAN

The ultrasonographer can find the true orientation of an organ or area of pathology by making appropriate markings on the skin and

scanning in this plane. Three-dimensional visualization is obtained when the area perpendicular to the markings is scanned.

MARKING THE BODY WITH THE TRANSDUCER

By convention, the symphysis pubis is marked with an angle and the umbilicus or transcrestal plane is designated by a perpendicular line.

MARKING THE POLAROID PICTURE

For complete information (as in X-ray techniques) each Polaroid should have at least two figures on the front. The first figure represents distance from reference points (either transversely or longitudinally) in centimeters. The second figure is used to show the gain setting, sensitivity setting, or attenuation. A third number may be used to designate the angle of tilt. The name, date, age, and sex of the patient will appear on the back of the Polaroid, or these data may be digitized onto the scan by a computer. After each Polaroid is labeled, it is good practice to string each in sequence on a strip of masking tape.

VISUAL ORIENTATION OF POLAROID PRINTS

Anterior abdominal transverse scans are viewed from below. Longitudinal scans are viewed from the left side of the patient in the supine, and from the right side of the patient in the prone position.

SIMULTANEOUS DISPLAY OF A-MODE WITH B-SCAN

During the course of B-scanning, any anechoic or echo-free area can be verified by A-mode. For example, the aorta is detected and identified by a narrow, echo-free area between two high spikes that exhibit a characteristic "to-and-fro" motion on the A-scope.

Because of the nature of the electronic threshold of the B-scan, an echo of low intensity will not be registered; hence, a mass with few internal echoes may be considered cystic in the B-mode. On the other hand, the small internal echoes

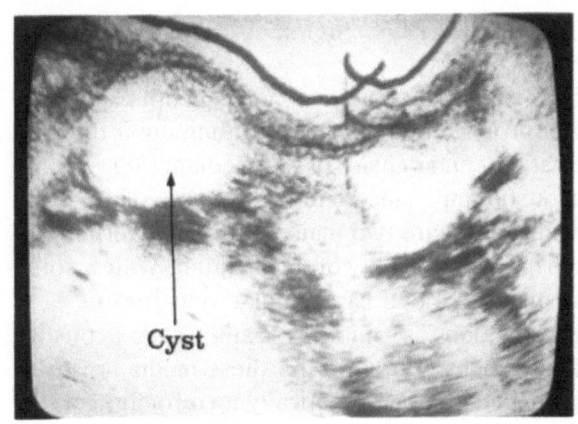

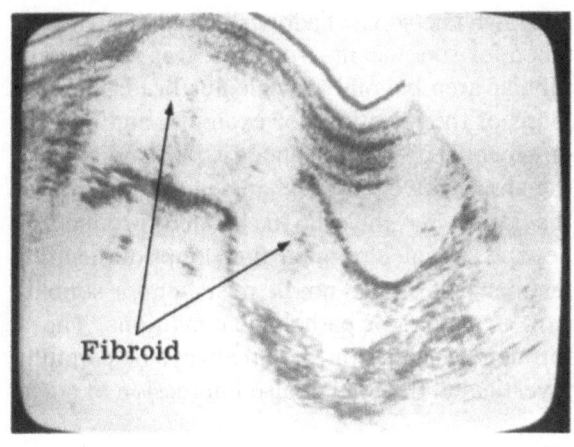

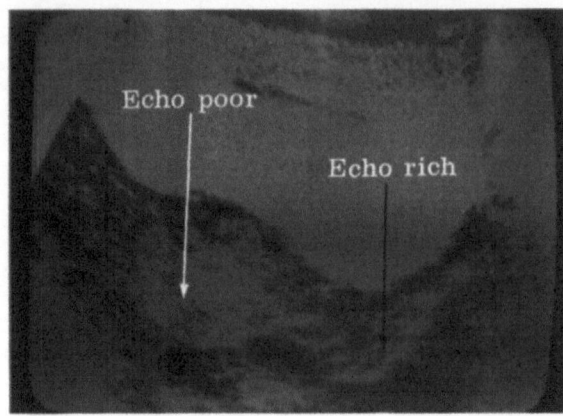

FIGURE 1.28
Supine longitudinal scan. Gray scale. This fibroid uterus is rounded with a low- and high-level internal echo pattern. Compare the area of poor echoes with the area of rich echoes. Echo-rich areas are found in many solid tumors.

FIGURE 1.29
Supine transverse scan. Gray scale. The echo-free ovarian cyst is well circumscribed and the posterior wall is sharp with high through transmission. Adjacent to it is an irregular fibroid uterus, where the sonic beam is attenuated. Areas of high through transmission are echo dense.

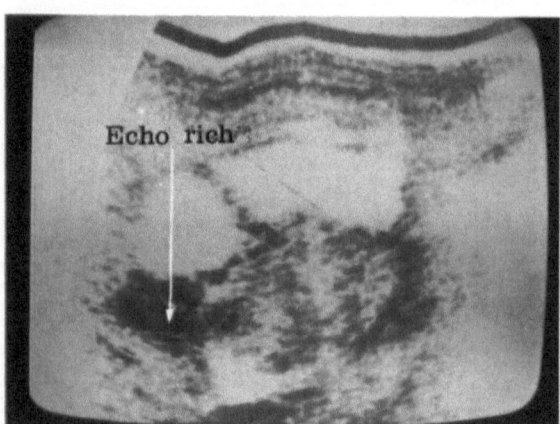

SONIC SHADOW SIGN

Ultrasonic waves are mechanical entities, and will propagate at a rate depending upon the elasticity and density of the medium (38). The acoustic impedance and the velocity of propagation are two main factors in determining the nature or density of the medium. Water, soft tissue, and blood have similar velocities of propagation for sonic waves and similar acoustic impedances (38). Grossly, these media are homogeneous and practically no refraction of the beam will occur during passage through these media.

The velocity of ultrasonic waves in bone and their acoustic impedance therein is high. Thus, a large amount of refraction of the beam in a new direction will occur. There is a high absorption of sonic waves in bone. Similar conditions are also noticeable in heavily calcified organs or organs containing calculus. As a result of high absorption of the ultrasonic beam in bone, heavily calcified organs, or calculus, there are no sonic waves beyond these structures. The acoustic impedance of air is low and as a result there is no propagation of ultrasonic waves in an air-fluid interface. This dominant interface causes complete reflection, or bounces back all ultrasonic waves. Thus, air, bone, heavily calcified organs, and calculus are barriers to ultrasound.

The absorption of osseous structures, calculus, and heavily calcified organs, or the complete reflection of sonic waves at an air-fluid interface, causes a sonolucent area which is called a sonic shadow. The sonic shadow should not be mistaken for sonolucent structures. It is usually a tubular area beyond the calculus or air-filled loops of the intestine, for example, and extends downward, if the transducer is perpendicular to the area. However, by changing the position of the transducer, the echo itself can be produced beyond the calculus or air-fluid loops of the intestine. This should not be mistaken for sonolucent structures or pathologic conditions. The through transmission should always be carefully investigated to avoid a false impression of sonic

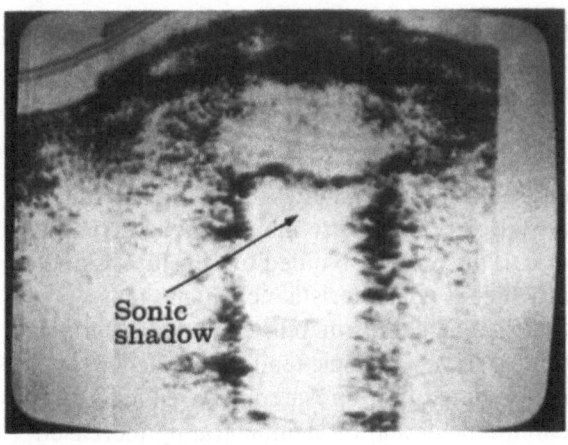

FIGURE 1.30(a)
Supine transverse scan. Gray scale. Below the echoes of the distal bladder wall–uterus interface is a total sonic shadow. Air or calcium will produce a total acoustic shadow. Gas gangrene of the uterus is demonstrated.

FIGURE 1.30(b)
Prone longitudinal scan. Gray scale. Scan over the spine in the midline shows the vertebral spinous processes and parts of the dural covering of the spinal canal. This is a PLS-0 section.

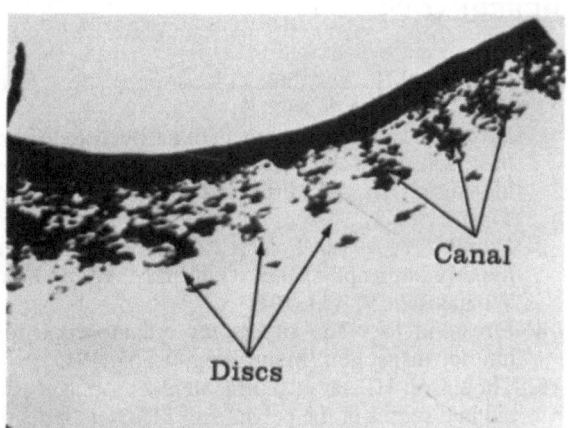

shadow, especially during angulation of the transducer.

In summary, the sonic shadow will occur when the ultrasonic beam hits bone, calculus, heavily calcified organs, or an air-fluid interface (Fig. 1.30a and b), thus causing a sonolucent area behind these structures. It should not be mistaken for a pathologic condition. For better evaluation of this false impression, the transducer should be moved perpendicularly to the area of interest to investigate the through transmission.

DETECTION OF THROUGH TRANSMISSION PATTERN

Through transmission is the sound energy that passes through a structure and is then recorded by the receiving transducer. It is inversely proportional to the attenuating properties of the medium and is registered on the oscilloscope as the number of echoes and their amplitudes at the distal interface of the region insonated.

We designate through transmission for the purposes of abdominal scanning to mean the echo density of the reflections distal to the organ or region under ultrasonic investigation. Characteristically, cysts have posterior multiple echoes of high amplitude. We term this high through transmission. Large, solid tumors such as fibroids tend to absorb significant sound energy, and have few posterior echoes which are generally of low amplitude. This phenomenon is called low through transmission. In between these extremes, other levels of echo density will be appropriately defined as moderate through transmission. The echo density noted is related to the effect of the TGC and reverberation characteristics of the medium. Since the sound is not attenuated by a cyst, the TGC is overcompensating when echoes are produced at the distal interface. These high-amplitude echoes are associated with significant reverberation effects. The combination produces the flood of echoes which we refer to as through transmission.

To evaluate transmission characteristics of a structure, the posterior border of that structure must be identified. The distal border is visualized at low-sensitivity settings when the medium is highly transonic, as in fluid structures and parenchymatous glands, such as the liver and spleen. When the medium is poorly transonic, the sound beam is attenuated significantly and sensitivity must be increased to amplify distal echoes. This is particularly true for solid, acoustically homogeneous tumors such as leiomyomata and lymphomas. Indeed, maximum gain settings may be necessary to faintly image the distal wall. These masses may not contain sufficient internal interfaces to produce echoes and may appear as sonolucent lesions. In these cases, the echo-free region is differentiated from a cyst by a poorly delineated posterior wall, indicating poor through transmission.

Through transmission does not occur when scanning over bone, barium, or air. Air interfaces reflect, bony interfaces absorb, and heavy metals tend to scatter sound. The net effect is a lack of penetration of the ultrasonic beam. During the scan, a sonic shadow is noted when the transducer is passed over bone, barium, or air. If the incident sonic energy is sufficient, reflection artifacts may be noted over air and bone. The artifacts appear as a series of echoes spaced at equal intervals, gradually diminishing in amplitude. These electronic artifacts must not be confused with echoes from deep interfaces.

Sonic shadowing is best appreciated during linear scanning with B-mode and by simultaneously noting the abrupt termination of A-scope echoes in a single high-amplitude echo. During compound scanning the posterior border of an ultrasonically shadowed region may be filled in with echoes, spuriously creating a distal interface. The examiner must exercise great caution when scanning over bone or bowel so as not to "create" an echo-free lesion.

Tumors with internal degeneration permit better through transmission than do architecturally intact masses of the same histologic type. The presence of fluid-filled necrotic spaces within a tumor increases beam transmission and the tumor appears on the oscilloscope as a lesion with multiple posterior echoes. At low sensitivity, anterior and posterior borders of a degenerating tumor may be outlined and the high posterior echo density may simulate a simple cyst. This error is avoided by sensitivity studies in which a characteristic echogenic mass is revealed as gain is increased. Indeed, certain tumors have a biologic tendency to degenerate (eg, leiomyomas, liposarcomas, renal cell carcinomas), and by demonstrating increased through transmission in a previously poorly transmitting tumor internal degeneration can be documented, which may aid in histosonographic tissue typing.

A highly transonic structure may exhibit a low posterior echo density when the distal interface lies adjacent to bone or air. Known as a reverse sonic shadow, this occurs when a lesion's distal wall lies next to a gas-containing viscus (eg, a renal cyst whose posterior wall lies over the air-filled colon) or bony surface (eg, an ovarian cyst lying over the spine). The presence of a sharply outlined distal wall will alert the ultrasonographer to the possibility of such acoustic damping, and the area should be rescanned in multiple projections to demonstrate the intrinsic, high through transmission of the transonic structure.

REFERENCES

1. Langevin MP: Les ondes ultrasonores. Rev Gen Elect 23:626, 1928
2. Dussik KT: Uber die moglichkeit hochfrequente mechanische schwingungen als diagnostisches hilfsmittel zu verwerten. Z Neurol Psychiat 174:153, 1942
3. Dussik KT, Dussik F, Wyt L: Aufdem Wege zur hyperphonographie des Gehirnes. Wien Med Wochenschr 97:425, 1947
4. Firestone FA: The supersonic reflectoscope for interior inspection. Metal Prog 48:505, 1945
5. Thompson HE, et al: Ultrasound as a diagnostic aid in diseases of the pelvis. Am J Obstet Gynecol 98:472, 1967

6. Gottesfeld KR, et al: Ultrasonic placentography. A new method for placental localization. Am J Obstet Gynecol 96:538, 1966

7. Wild JJ, Neal D: Use of high frequency ultrasonic waves for detecting changes in texture in living tissue. Lancet 1:655, 1951

8. Baum G, Greenwood I: The application of ultrasonic locating techniques to ophthalmology. Arch Ophthalmal 60:263, 1958

9. Hertz CH, Edler I: Die regrstrierung von herzwanbewegungen mit hilfe des ultraschallimpulsverfahrens. Acustica 6:361, 1956

10. Carlsen EN: Ultrasound physics for the physician. A brief review. J Clin Ultrasound 3:69, 1975

11. Wells PNT: Physical Principles of Ultrasonic Diagnosis. New York, Academic Press, 1969

12. Garrett WJ, Robinson DE: Ultrasound in Clinical Obstetrics. Springfield, Ill, Thomas, 1970

13. Kossoff G: Display techniques in ultrasound pulse echo investigation. A review. J Clin Ultrasound 1:61, 1974

14. Carlsen EN: Gray scale ultrasound. J Clin Ultrasound 1:190, 1973

15. Marich KW, Zatz LM, Green PS, et al: Real time imaging with a new ultrasonic camera. I. In vitro experimental studies on transmission imaging of biological structures. J Clin Ultrasound 3:5, 1975

16. Weill F, Elsenschar A, Aucent D, et al: Ultrasonic study of venous patterns in the right hypochondrium. An anatomical approach to differential diagnosis of obstructive jaundice. J Clin Ultrasound 3:23, 1975

17. Zatz LM, Marich KW, Green PS, et al: Real time imaging with a new ultrasonic camera. II. Preliminary studies in normal adults. J Clin Ultrasound 3:17, 1975

18. Goldberg BB: Diagnostic Ultrasound in Clinical Medicine. New York, Grune & Stratton, 1975

19. Ballantine HT, Bolt RH, Hueter TF, et al: On the detection of intracranial pathology by ultrasound. Science 112:525, 1950

20. Ballantine HT, Hueter TF, Nauta WJH, et al: Focal destruction of nervous tissue by focused ultrasound. Biophysical factors influencing its application. J Med (Basel) 104:337, 1956

21. Feigenbaum H, Chang S: Echocardiography. Philadelphia, Lea and Febiger, 1972

22. Bartrum RJ: Practical considerations in abdominal ultrasonic scanning. N Engl J Med 291:1068, 1974

23. Buckton K, Baker N: An investigation into possible chromosome damaging effects of ultrasound on human blood cells. Br J Radiol 45:340, 1972

24. Curzen P: The safety of diagnostic ultrasound. Practitioner 209:822, 1972

25. Hellman L, Duffus GM, Donald I, et al: Safety of diagnostic ultrasound in obstetrics. Lancet 7:1133, 1970

26. Mannor S, Serr D, Isaschar T, et al: The safety of ultrasound in fetal monitoring. Am J Obstet Gynecol 113:653, 1972

27. Watts P, Hall A, Fleming J: Ultrasound and chromosome damage. Br J Radiol 45:335, 1972

28. Lehmann JF, and Guy AW: Ultrasound therapy. In Reid JM, Sikov MR (eds): Interaction of Ultrasound and Biological Tissues. Workshop Proceedings. US Department of Health, Education, and Welfare Publication FDA 73-8008, BRH/DBE 73-1. Washington, DC, USGPO, 1973, pp 121–128

29. Pennington CL, Stevens EL, Griffin WL: The use of ultrasound in the treatment of Meniere's disease. Laryngoscope 80:578, 1970

30. Lyon MF, Simpson GM: An investigation into the possible genetic hazards of ultrasound. Br J Radiol 47:712, 1974

31. Wells PNT: Physical principles of ultrasonic diagnosis. London, Academic Press, 1969, pp. 53–72

32. Hill CR: The possibility of hazard in medical and industrial applications of ultrasound. Br J Radiol 41:561, 1968

33. Freimanis AK: The biological effects of medically applied ultrasound and their causes. CRC Crit Rev Radiol Sci 1:639, 1970

34. Hellman LM, et al: Safety of diagnostic ultrasound in obstetrics. Lancet 1:1133, 1970

35. Macintosh IJC, Davey DA: Chromosome aberrations inducted by an ultrasonic fetal pulse detector. Br Med J 4:92, 1970

36. Macintosh IJC, Davey DA: Relationship between intensity of ultrasound and induction of chromosome aberrations. Br J Radiol 45:320, 1972

37. Hassani N: Method and usage of ultrasound in clinical medicine. J Natl Med Assoc 67:41, 1974

38. Hassani N: Ultrasonic appearance of pedunculated uterine fibroids and ovarian cysts. J Natl Med Assoc 66:432, 1974

39. Holm HH: Ultrasonic scanning in the diagnosis of space-occupying lesions of the upper abdomen. Br J Radiol 44:24, 1971

40. Holm HH, Rasmussen SN, Kristensen JK: Errors and pitfalls in ultrasonic scanning of the abdomen. Br J Radiol 45:835, 1972

41. Holmes JH: Urologic ultrasonography. In King DL (ed): Ultrasound Diagnosis. St Louis, Mosby, 1974

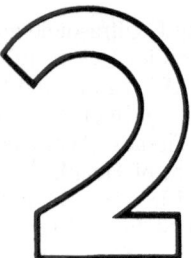

gynecologic ultrasound

GENERAL INTRODUCTION

Evaluation of gynecologic disease by pelvic scanning has proven to be highly rewarding with the new high-resolution gray-scale units and real-time scanners. However, adequate scanning of pelvic organs in the nonpregnant female can only be accomplished with adequate distension of the bladder, because the sound-reflecting bowel loops of the colon and small intestine produce a barrier to proper examination of the pelvic organs. The bowel loops must be displaced out of the pelvic area by the distended urinary bladder. Failure to produce this sonic window results in incomplete demonstration of pathology and the creation of artifacts.

The pelvic structures are physiologically related organs in close physical proximity. Because of this anatomic arrangement, there may be difficulty in distinguishing ovarian from uterine masses, since these organs generally approximate one another. Also, completely different pathologic entities may have similar ultrasonic appearances.

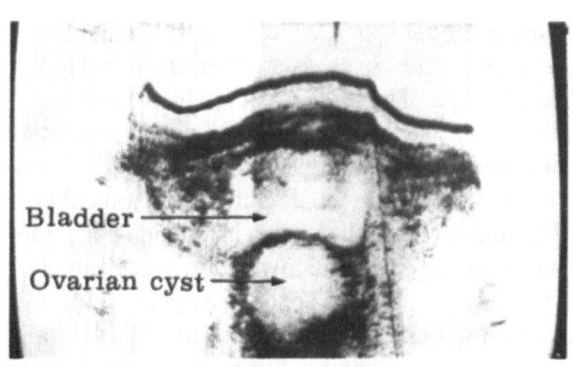

FIGURE 2.1(a)
Supine transverse scan. Gray scale. An echo-free cystic mass with irregular posterior borders is distal to the bladder. This midline mass simulates a degenerating fibroid. However, in this patient the uterus was totally removed. This illustrates the importance of considering history in ultrasonographic diagnosis. Irregular outline in this ovarian cyst is due to pericystic fibrosis.

FIGURE 2.1(b)
Supine transverse scan. Gray scale. An echo-free cystic mass with irregular posterior borders is distal to the bladder. This midline cystic structure developed following hysterosalpingo-oophorectomy. Diagnosis was localized hematoma.

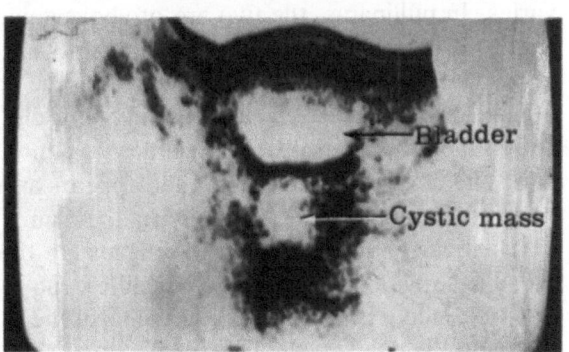

Analysis of altered morphology must be modified by the internal echo pattern of the lesion, through transmission characteristics, and clinical and palpatory findings. A thorough appreciation of the gross pathology of the ovaries and uterus is necessary to fully assess the restructured anatomy and variable echo pattern of pelvic diseases.

Using this multifaceted approach, a nonspecific pelvic mass may be reliably given a histologic diagnosis. Although it may be impossible with present equipment to differentiate a solid ovarian tumor plastered to the uterus from a myomatous fibroid nodule, or a focal area of marked cystic internal degeneration of a fibroid uterus from an adjacent ovarian cyst, many specific diagnoses are now available to the clinician. Degenerative changes and inflammatory conditions may be evaluated and the relationship of the mass to the regional organs and its effect on the surrounding structures may be studied.

It must be emphasized that accurate history is essential for proper ultrasonic diagnosis. If a complete history is not available, or if the person performing the examination is not present during final analysis of the scans, gross errors may be made (Fig. 2.1a and b). Also, the examiner must be familiar with the limitations of ultrasound described in Chapter 1.

ANATOMY

VAGINA

The vagina is a musculomembranous structure arising from the vulva and extending to the uterus, and is located between the bladder and rectum.

Anteriorly, the vagina is in contact with the bladder wall and urethra, this portion being called the vesicovaginal septum. Approximately one-fourth of the vagina is separated from the rectum, which is called the cul-de-sac of Douglas or rectouterine pouch. The anterior and posterior walls of the vagina lie in close apposition

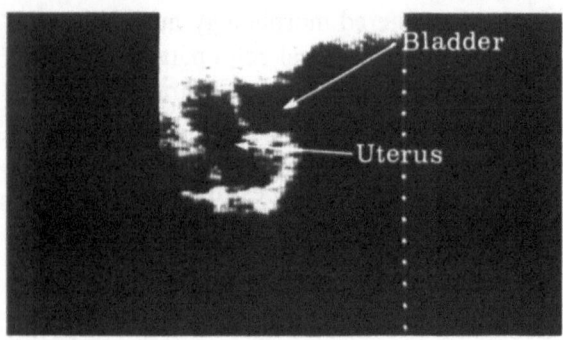

FIGURE 2.2(a)
Supine longitudinal scan. Real-time scanner. In the nongravid state, the uterus is located between the bladder and rectum. The uterus has a flattened pear-shaped configuration.

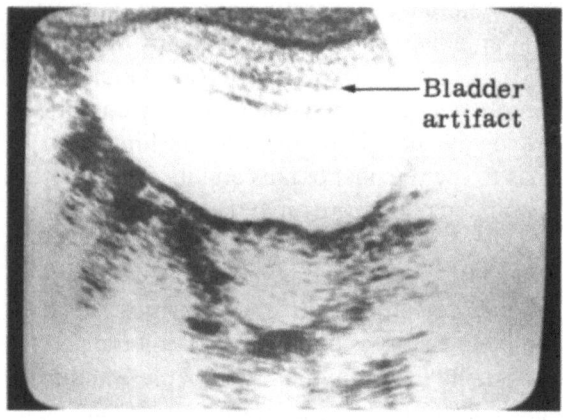

FIGURE 2.2(b)
Supine longitudinal scan. Gray scale. Bladder artifact is common and appears as a multilayered linear echo pattern interspersed with amorphous dots. This disappears with reduced gain settings.

FIGURE 2.2(c)
Supine longitudinal scan. Gray scale. The cephalic portion of the bladder may produce echogenic artifacts when scanned while incompletely filled. Further distension generally clears these artifacts.

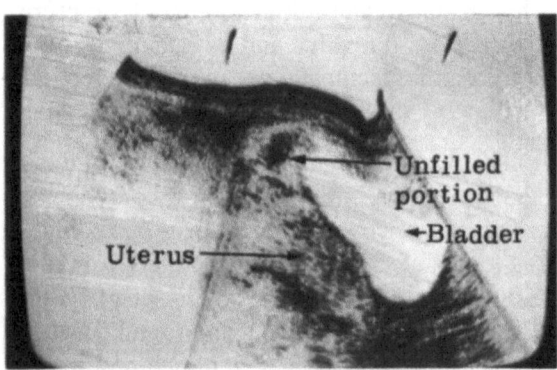

with potential space which lies transversely, and, as a result, in cross-section, the canal has an H-shape. The vagina is capable of marked distension, such as occurs with an accumulation of blood behind an imperforate hymen. This pathology may easily be detected ultrasonically. The upper end of the vagina is a blind space into which is projected the lower portion of the uterine cervix. The blind space or vaginal vault is subdivided into anterior, posterior, and lateral fornices. The posterior fornix is longer than the anterior one. The vagina joins the uterus at an acute angle; as a result its anterior wall is shorter than its posterior wall.

UTERUS

The uterus is a muscular organ partially covered by peritoneum. In the nongravid state, the uterus is located between the bladder and rectum. It has a flattened, pear-shaped configuration (Fig. 2.2a) and consists of two parts, eg, an upper triangular part or corpus, and a lower cylindrical part or cervix. The posterior surface of the corpus is slightly convex, while the anterior surface of the corpus is flat. The fallopian tubes originate from the cornua at the junction of the superior and lateral margins. The upper segment of the uterus, having a convex configuration, is called the fundus. From the lateral margins on either side are attached the broad ligaments. In the adult the uterus measures grossly 6 × 4 × 3 cm, in greatest dimension longitudinally, transversely, and anteroposteriorly, respectively. It is slightly larger in multiparous women. The relation between the lengths of the corpus and cervix varies. In nulliparas, the two are of about equal length. In multiparas, the cervix represents approximately one-third of the total length of the organ. The bulk of the uterus consists of muscle, and the anteroposterior walls lie almost in contact. The cavity between them then appears as a narrow slit. The cervix has an internal and an external os. The ligaments of the uterus are the broad ligaments, which are two winglike structures extending from the lateral margins of the uterus to the pelvic wall. This divides the pelvic cavity into anterior and posterior compartments. A fallopian tube is attached to the inner two-thirds of the superior margin from the mesosalpinx. The other ligaments are the round and uterosacral ligaments.

The usual position of the uterus is slightly anteflexed. In examining the patient in the upright position ultrasonically, the uterus is almost horizontal and somewhat flexed anteriorly, the fundus resting upon the bladder. The cervix is directed backward toward the sacrum. The uterine artery, which is a main branch of the hypogastric artery, can be easily detected by the real-time scanner.

The fallopian tubes extend from the uterine cornua toward the ovaries. They measure approximately 8 to 14 cm in length. Each tube has an interstitial portion, isthmus, ampulla, and infundibulum. The infundibulum or fimbriated extremity is the funnel-shaped opening of the distal end of the tube, which opens into the abdominal cavity. Diverticula may sometimes extend from the lumen of the tube for a variable distance into its muscular wall and reach almost to its serosa. These may play a role in the development of ectopic pregnancy.

OVARIES

The ovaries are almond-shaped and, in the adult, they measure 2.5 to 5 cm in thickness. After menopause they diminish markedly in size. The ovaries are situated in the upper part of the pelvic cavity, located in the slight depression on the lateral wall of the pelvis between the divergent external iliac and hypogastric vessels known as the ovarian fossa of Waldeyer. The ovary is attached to the broad ligament by the mesovarium. The ovarian ligament extends from the lateral and posterior portion of the uterus to beneath the insertion of the fallopian tube at the uterus. The major part of the ovary is located in the abdominal cavity and is free of a peritoneal covering except near the hilum, where there is a narrow band toward the peritoneum covering the mesosalpinx.

SONOANATOMY

Detection of gynecologic pathology necessitates a thorough knowledge of the normal pelvic ultrasonic anatomy as well as the age- and hormone-dependent physiologic normal variants. The size of the uterus and ovaries varies with the patient's age, menstrual cycle, and hormonal therapy.

The normal distended bladder is echo free, sharply outlined, and smoothly contoured, with high through transmission characteristics. It is situated immediately below the anterior abdominal musculature. Linear artifacts are commonly noted along the ventral portion of the bladder paralleling the muscle planes of the abdominal wall (Fig. 2.2b). When the bladder is incompletely filled, the cephalic border will be sliced tangential to the ultrasonic beam and may simulate a solid echogenic lesion (Fig. 2.2c). Further filling of the bladder will produce an echo-free center in this area as the bladder distends cephalically. The vagina and uterus form the dorsal boundaries of the bladder (Fig. 2.3). Superiorly and cranially, reflections of the small bowel are noted. The acoustic configuration of the bladder varies according to the degree of distention of the bladder as well as the size and position of the normal and pathologic pelvic structures. The overdistended bladder may produce difficulties in the proper examination of the pelvic organs. For example, an ovarian cyst may not be ultrasonically separable from the bladder (Fig. 2.4). For this reason, we study the pelvis with the bladder initially greatly distended to search as much of the lower abdomen as possible. The bladder is then partly emptied to a moderate size to visualize the pelvic organs without the mass effect of the full bladder or to separate the bladder from surrounding cystic structures (Fig. 2.5).

The bladder is finally emptied to distinguished this echo-free structure from any other adjacent echo-free zone such as an ovarian cyst or bladder diverticulum.

The vagina presents as a set of parallel lines dorsal to the lower bladder wall. This double line

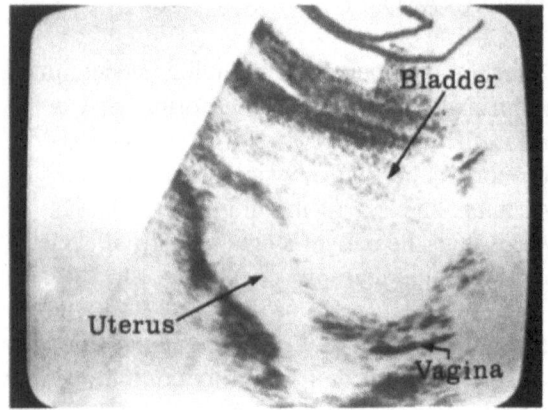

FIGURE 2-3

represents the ventral and dorsal walls of the vagina, which diverge as the region of the cervix is encountered. A bulge in the dorsal vaginal wall is the posterior fornix (Fig. 2.6). Sufficient fluid may accumulate in this potential space to simulate an echo-free cyst. Aspiration of the secretions in this area will remove the cystic space.

The uterus appears on B-scan systems as an echo-free, pear-shaped organ at low sensitivity. Gray-scale imaging shows the tissue of the normal uterus as a low-amplitude, diffuse reflector contained within the dark gray echoes of the outer margins. The fundus of the uterus

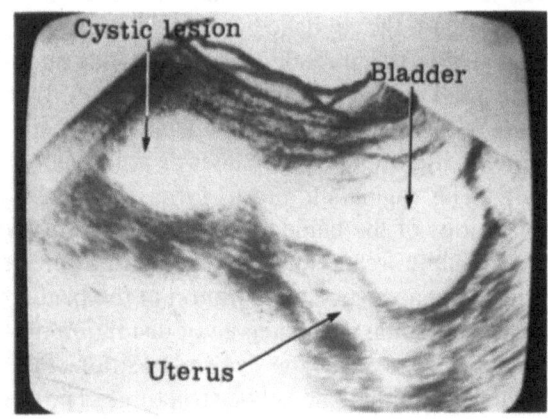

FIGURE 2-4

FIGURE 2.3
Supine longitudinal scan. Gray scale. The normal uterus may produce a slight impression against the bladder wall. Note the typical echo pattern of the vagina projecting from the region of the fornix.

FIGURE 2.4
Supine longitudinal scan. Gray scale. The presence of an overdistended bladder may produce difficulty in the imaging of a distinct interface between the bladder and a cephalically located ovarian cyst.

FIGURE 2.5
Supine longitudinal scan. Gray scale. Same patient as in Fig. 2.4. The bladder is now partially emptied. Note the echogenic area separating the ovarian cyst from the bladder. We routinely empty the bladder in all patients with pelvic cystic lesions.

FIGURE 2.6
Supine longitudinal scan. Gray scale. The normal uterus may produce a slight impression against the bladder wall. The posterior fornix appears as an echo-free area when fluid filled. Note the typical echo pattern of the vagina projecting from the region of the fornix.

FIGURE 2-5

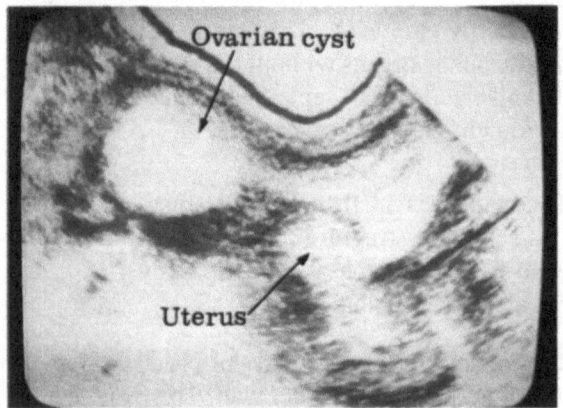

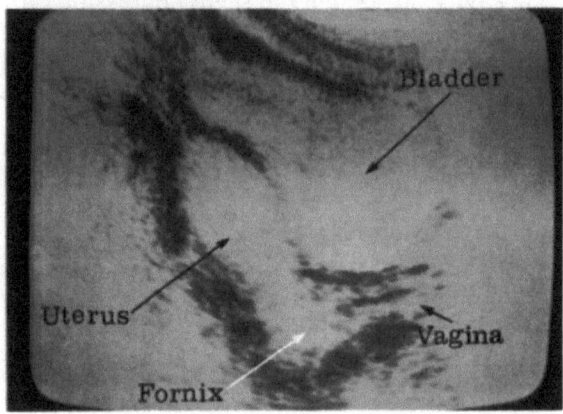

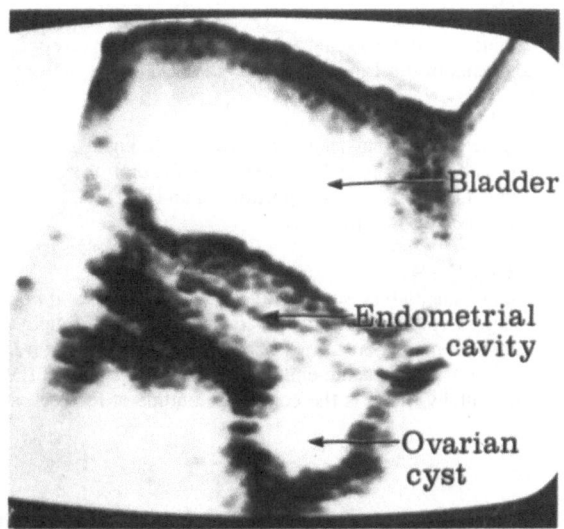

FIGURE 2-7 (a)

will normally produce only a slight impression on the dorsal bladder wall (Fig. 2.6). The uterus usually forms a variable angle with the vagina since it assumes an anteverted position in most women. The endometrial cavity is frequently seen as a central, linear echo, running along the craniocaudal axis of the uterus (Fig. 2.7a), and it is heavier in postpartum patients (Fig. 2.7b). This linear type of echo should not be confused with the echo of an intrauterine contraceptive device (IUCD) (Fig. 2.8). These echoes disappear at low sensitivities and thus are distinguished from an IUCD echo which may appear identical in shape (Fig. 2.9a,b, and c). Since the uterus has moderate through transmission characteristics, structures such as

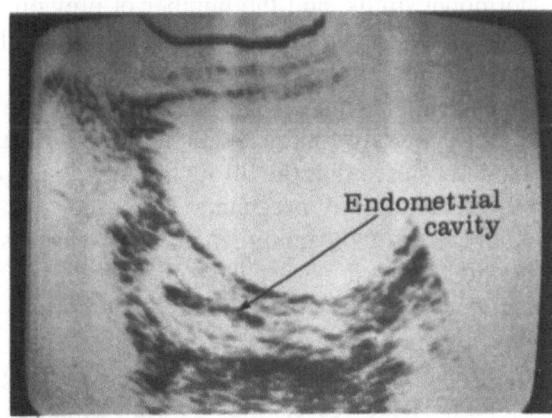

FIGURE 2-7 (b)

FIGURE 2.7(a)
Supine longitudinal scan. Gray scale. The endometrial cavity is frequently seen as a central linear echo running along the craniocaudal axis of the uterus. Note ovarian cyst.

FIGURE 2.7(b)
Supine longitudinal scan. Gray scale. The echo pattern of the endometrial cavity is heavier during menstruation.

FIGURE 2.7(c)
Supine longitudinal scan. Gray scale. Scattered low-amplitude echoes may be noted within the uterus corresponding to the endometrial canal. These frequently disappear at low gain settings, which distinguishes this entity from an IUCD of similar ultrasonographic appearance. The echo pattern of the endometrial cavity is heavier in postpartum patients.

FIGURE 2.8
Supine longitudinal scan. Gray scale. The echo pattern of an IUCD is usually stepladder-shaped and does not disappear by changing the sensitivity setting.

FIGURE 2-7 (c)

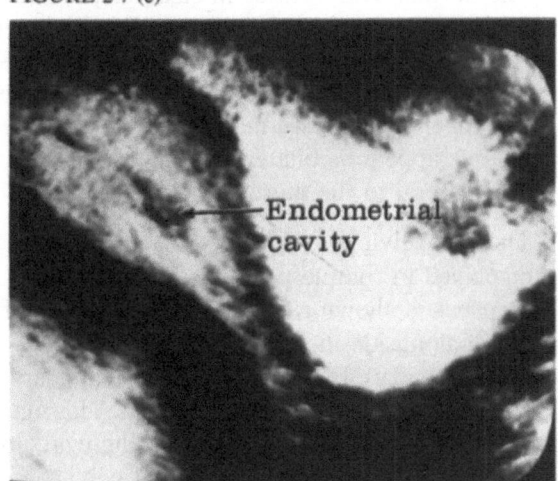

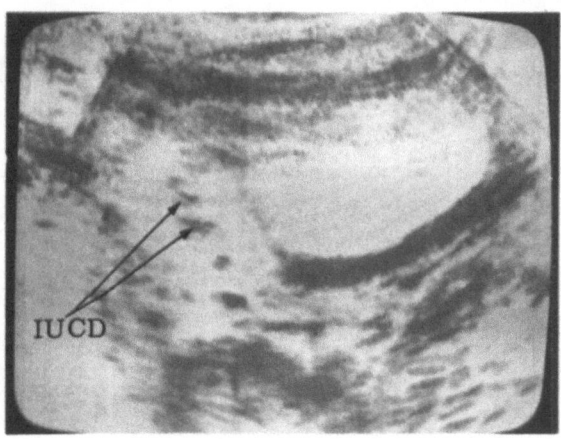

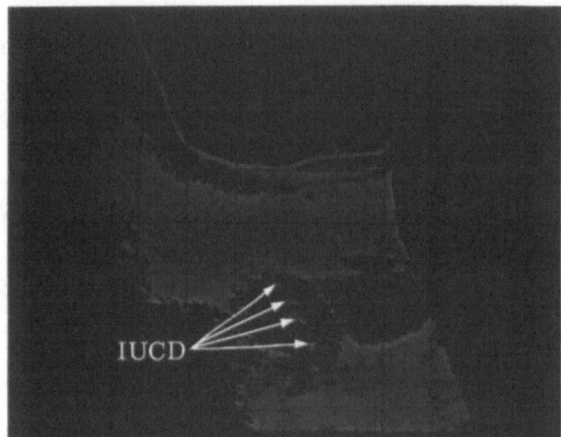

FIGURE 2-9 (a)

FIGURE 2.9(a)
Supine longitudinal scan. B-mode. This is a scan through four segments of the Lippes loop.

FIGURE 2.9(b)
Supine longitudinal scan. Gray scale. The linear stepladder-type echoes of Lippes loop are seen in the uterine cavity. A number of echo-reflecting portions of an IUCD related to the beam axis during the study.

FIGURE 2.9(c)
Supine longitudinal scan. Gray scale. A halo of echo-poor tissue surrounds the centrally located IUCD. Through transmission is increased. Localized bulging of the uterus at this site is due to acute endometritis secondary to the IUCD. Incidentally noted is the echo-poor outline of the rectum.

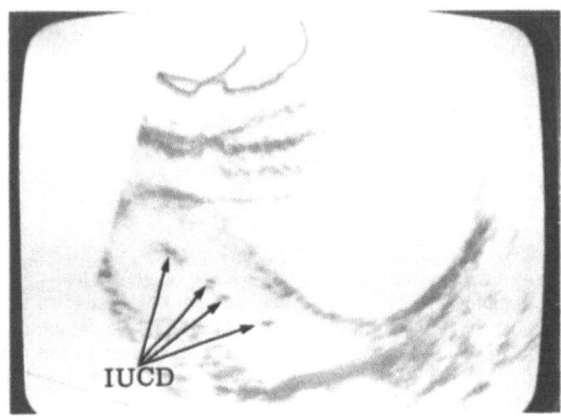

FIGURE 2-9 (b)

FIGURE 2-9 (c)

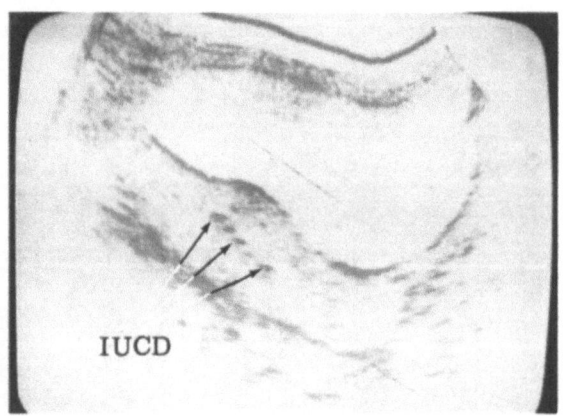

the rectum and the sacral curvature are generally observed. The size, shape, and position of the uterus depend on the age of the patient, hormonal status, and the number of previous pregnancies. The fundus of the uterus is smaller in premenarchal and postmenopausal patients than in patients in the child-bearing years. The uterus generally enlarges with increasing parity. We have noted that the through transmission of the uterus of early pregnancy increased compared with the nonpregnant uterus. This is presumably due to vascular enlargement which is noted clinically at this time. The uterine arteries may be imaged if a high-frequency transducer is used with the real-time scanning system. These vessels may be seen as paired pulsatile structures lateral to the body of the uterus.

The normal ovary varies in size, shape, and position. It may vary from 2.5 to 5 cm in length (1). The normal ovary may be demonstrated as a relatively sonolucent area if its size approaches the upper limits of normal. When visible, the ovaries appear as bilateral ovoid masses dorsolateral to the uterus.

The parapelvic musculature is frequently displayed in routine pelvic scanning. The iliopsoas is shown as a broad echo-free band noted alongside the pelvic sidewalls (Fig. 2.10a,b, and c). In transverse scans it appears as an elliptical, bilateral, anechoic area. This may simulate a renal outline; however, there are no echoes corresponding to the renal pelvic

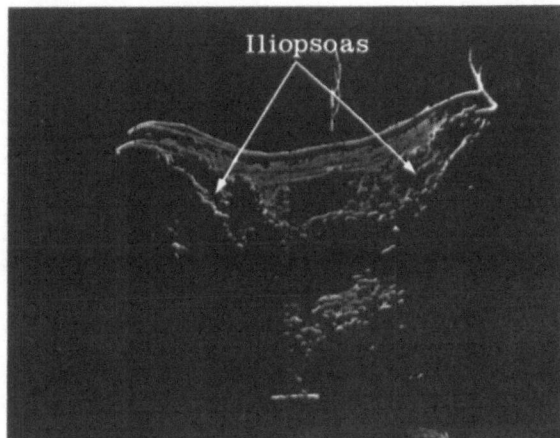

FIGURE 2-10 (a)

FIGURE 2.10(a)
Supine transverse scan. B-mode. The echo-free, winglike iliopsoas is symmetrically located at the pelvic sidewalls.

FIGURE 2.10(b)
Supine transverse scan. Gray scale. The iliopsoas lines the ventral sidewalls of the pelvis with a winglike pattern.

FIGURE 2.10(c)
Supine longitudinal scan. Gray scale. A triangle of echo-free fluid is noted during scanning over the pelvic sidewalls. Beneath the ascitic fluid is the bandlike configuration of the iliopsoas.

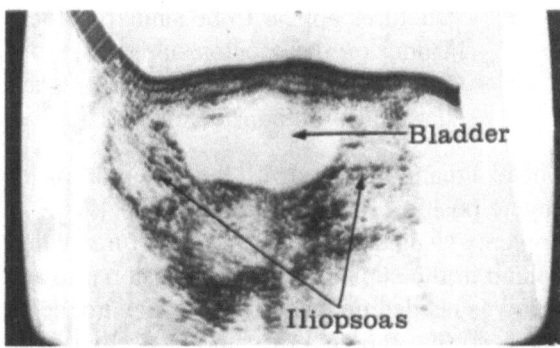

FIGURE 2-10 (b)

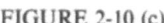

FIGURE 2-10 (c)

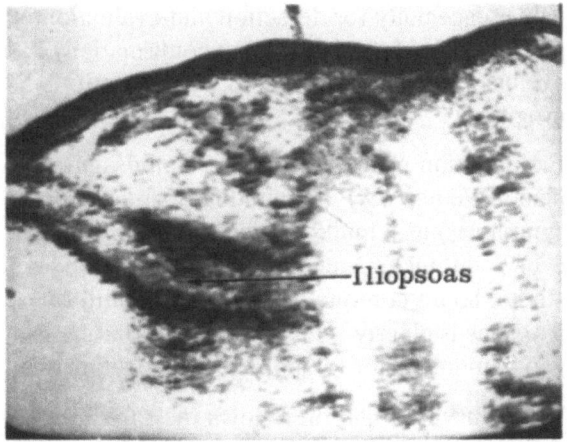

collecting system. The muscle will fill in with echoes at high sensitivity, distinguishing this structure from a cystic lesion. In longitudinal scans a parallel set of interfaces demarcates this muscle as it passes anteriorly upon entering the pelvis. This is generally seen between 5 and 8 cm lateral to the midline longitudinal scan plane. Further caudally in the pelvis the iliacus lines the lateral pelvic walls as a saucer-shaped, echo-free band beyond which no sound passes due to the attenuation of the pelvis. Laterally and anteriorly, the external iliac artery and vein are often noted as echo-free, tubular or rounded structures, depending upon the scan plane. They are easily distinguished as to the artery or vein by the distinctive pulsations shown with the real-time scanner.

Scanning of the anterior abdominal wall is very rewarding in evaluating diseases of the subcutaneous tissues and ventral musculature. Areas of fibrosis due to scarring will distort the ultrasonic beam while the presence of calcified scar tissue produces a sonic shadow (Fig. 2.11). An abdominal wall hematoma may be noted as an echo-free area within the muscle echoes, and is most often due to violent coughing or trauma (Fig. 2.12). Abscess formation in the abdominal wall may be noted in diabetic patients or patients with regional enteritis (Fig. 2.13).

SONOLAPAROTOMY

The full bladder as described is essential to pelvic ultrasonography. Gynecologic examination of a patient without a distended bladder does not yield information for diagnosis.

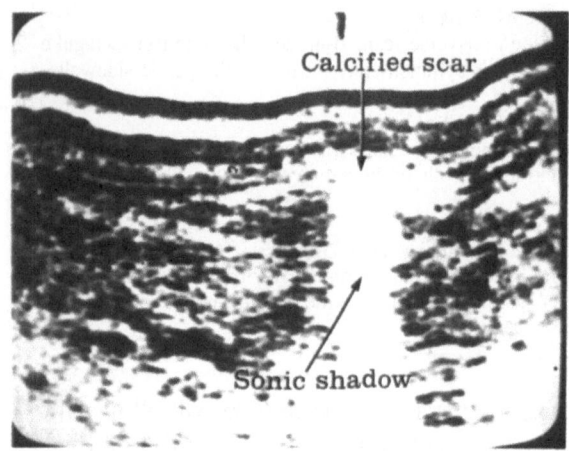

FIGURE 2.11
Supine longitudinal scan. Gray scale. Scan shows an echo-dense linear structure in the deep subcutaneous tissues which casts a sonic shadow. Calcified scar due to 20-year-old incision.

On the other hand, a distended bladder has several advantages.

1. The distended bladder is a good transmitting medium, and as a result the examination of deep-seated pelvic lesions is easier.

2. The distended bladder displaces the bowel loops upward, which otherwise would prevent proper ultrasonic examination.

3. The distended bladder can be used as a reference standard for "cystic" and other areas, which are compared with the bladder for tissue signature. For example, echogenic masses at standard sensitivity fill in with echoes as the sensitivity is increased, while cystic structures appear to be similar to the bladder on the oscilloscope screen. Other criteria described in Chapter 1 should also be considered.

The examination starts with the patient in the supine position. Basically, the bony pelvis prevents visualization of pelvic structure from behind in the supine position; occasionally, a pillow is needed under the hips to elevate the pelvis so that the area of pathology remains perpendicular to the sonic beam. On other occasions, it may be necessary to elevate the table top so that an abdominal mass descends and its relationship with the pelvic organs can be evaluated.

Other positions, such as the oblique, are of great value, especially for detection and evaluation of peritoneal fluid and adhesions; confirmation or exclusion of adhesions could alter the entire prognosis.

Examination usually starts in the midsagittal plane. We use LXP (longitudinal, xiphoid, pubic symphysis) as a midline reference. Sectioning in every centimeter yields excellent results. The study should continue longitudinally until the iliopsoas is clearly seen, since this structure is a good landmark for the border of the true pelvis.

The transverse section follows the sagittal examination. We use the transcrestal line as a

FIGURE 2.12
Supine transverse scan. B-mode. Abdominal wall hematoma may be noted as an echo-free area within the muscle. Note a few scattered echos within the echo-free zone.

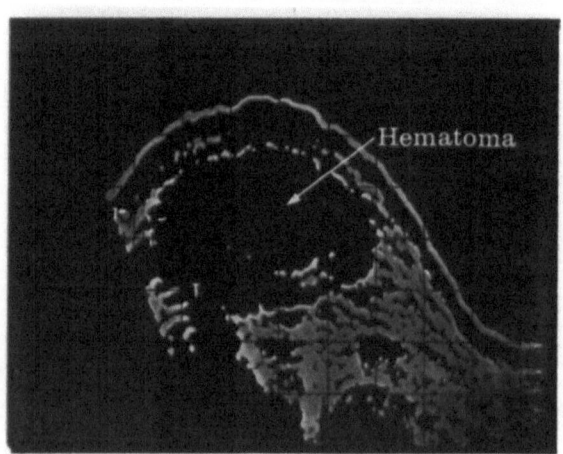

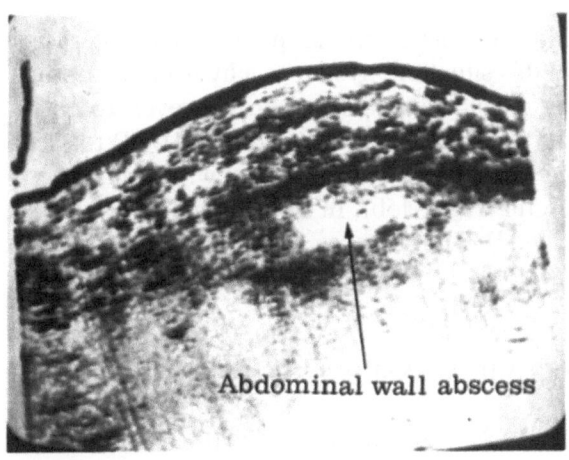

FIGURE 2.13
Supine transverse scan. Gray scale. The patient is obese and diabetic. Beneath the thick subcutaneous fat layer is an echo-free zone with a few internal echoes. The margins are slightly irregular. Abdominal wall abscess.

FIGURE 2.14
Supine longitudinal scan. Gray scale. At moderate gain the IUCD stands out in sharp contrast to the normally echo-poor uterus.

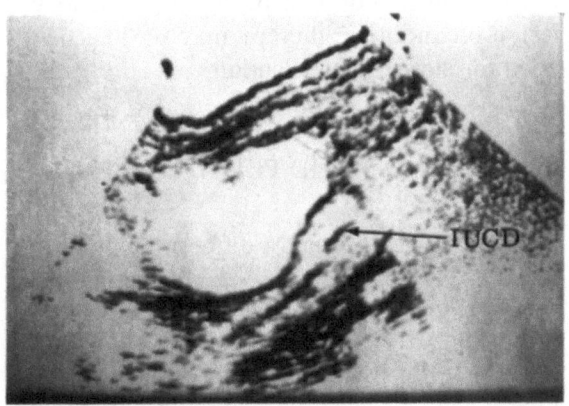

reference point (ATC-0). Usually it is a matter of choice as to whether the scan is performed in an ascending maneuver from the pubic bone or in a descending maneuver from the transcrestal line (the line passing through both iliac crests usually traversing the umbilicus in a normal individual). Additional examination may include oblique and angled scanning.

LOCALIZATION OF IUCDs

Most of the commonly used intrauterine contraceptive devices (IUCD) are strongly echogenic and have a characteristic configuration. They are readily identified in both cross-sectional and longitudinal scans at low sensitivity by their specific shapes. The linear echoes of the endometrial cavity may simulate an IUCD (Fig. 2.14) but disappear at low sensitivity. In our experience, the small Dalkin shield may be more difficult to image at present due to its size and shape; however, this device may be better imaged with the higher resolution of gray-scale units. The IUCD is optimally located when it lies centrally within the uterine cavity near the fundus. It has proven valuable to study the position of the IUCD immediately after insertion rather than at a later date, since an abnormally placed device may be replaced at once.

When the string of the IUCD cannot be identified by vaginal examination, uterine perforation of the device must be ruled out. Our experience shows that ultrasonography is sufficiently sensitive for intrauterine detection of IUCDs (Fig. 2.15a). It has been stated that in the case of a Lippe's loop, if the plain film reveals the loop to be closed the IUCD is located inside the uterus, and if the loop is open the IUCD is in an extrauterine location. Ultrasonographically, if the strong echoes of the IUCD are not demonstrated within the uterus, then the IUCD is located outside the uterus. The extrauterine IUCD is difficult to image since it is masked by the surrounding bowel echoes. The appearance of the radiographic image of the IUCD on plain X-ray film with evidence that no intrauterine echoes were observed during ultrasonic scanning indi-

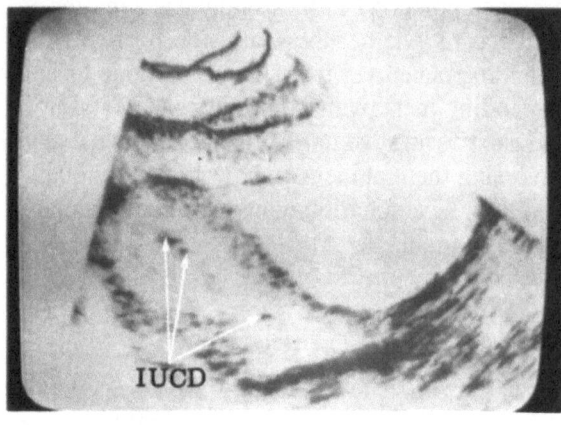

FIGURE 2.15(a)
Supine longitudinal scan. Gray scale. Intraluminal echoes of strong amplitude within the uterus are aligned with regularity. IUCD in position.

FIGURE 2.15(b)
Hysterosalpingogram. When the IUCD is located within the uterus it is easily imaged by ultrasound. When it is outside the uterus, as in this case, no intrauterine echoes will be noted and X rays must be taken to demonstrate the IUCD within the pelvis. This hysterosalpingogram shows the IUCD in relation to the uterine cavity.

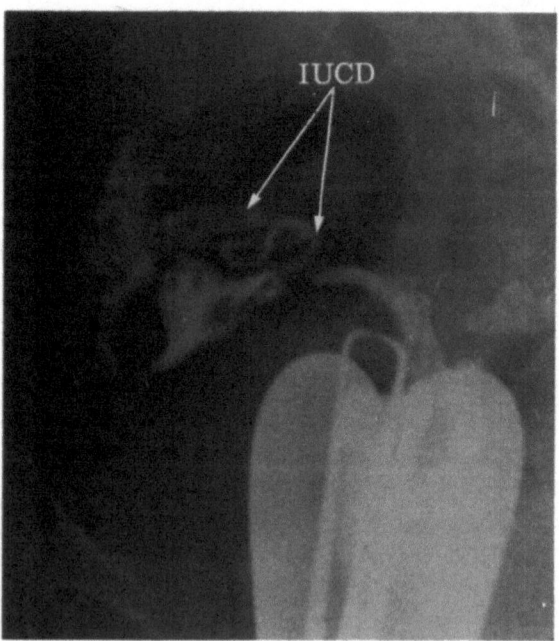

cates that the device has perforated the uterus. In this situation, hysterography is not necessary for diagnostic confirmation. However, to obtain the relationship of the perforated IUCD to the uterine cavity, hysterography with contrast is useful (Fig. 2.15b). In spite of an optimally located IUCD, however, intrauterine pregnancy may still occur (Fig. 2.16).

PELVIC MASSES

The most frequent request in the ultrasound laboratory is to evaluate a clinically evident pelvic mass or confirm the existence of such a mass in patients who are difficult to examine. Frequently, due to excess obesity, poor patient cooperation during pelvic examination, or reflex guarding due to pelvic disease, ultrasound is the only method of establishing the diagnosis of a pelvic tumor of inflammatory process.

Ultrasonography may not only document the presence of questionable palpatory findings, but may also offer the clinician a differential diagnosis of the most likely possibilities. Ultrasonography provides an undistorted, three-dimensional spatial representation of the pelvic mass under study. The biologic history of the pathology may be studied by evaluating the changing ultrasonic appearance of the lesion with serial sonograms. Such findings as increase in tumor size, appearance of lymph node masses, and cystic internal necrosis may be documented. These further data sharply narrow the differential diagnostic possibilities to that of a malignant process. Satisfactory sequential decrease in size of a suspected inflammatory lesion on antibiotic therapy may obviate the need for surgical intervention.

CYSTIC AND SOLID PELVIC LESIONS

The ultrasonic criteria for differentiation of cystic and solid lesions have been presented earlier. A brief review is useful to classify the gynecologic tumors in a practical manner. Typically, cysts have a lack of internal echoes at low and high sensitivity and remain the same size as the

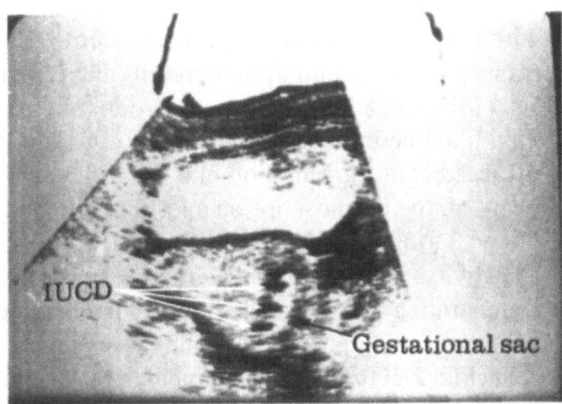

FIGURE 2-16

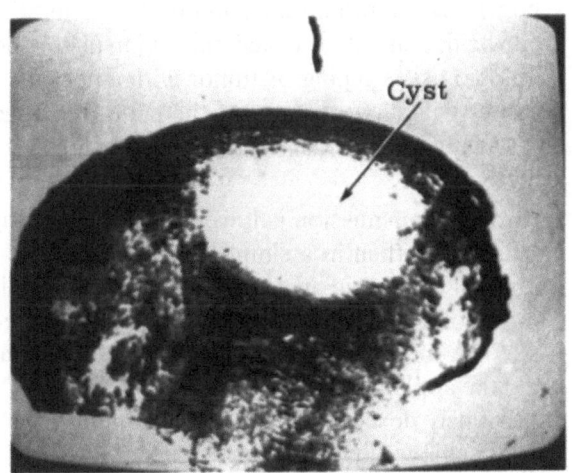

FIGURE 2-17

FIGURE 2-18

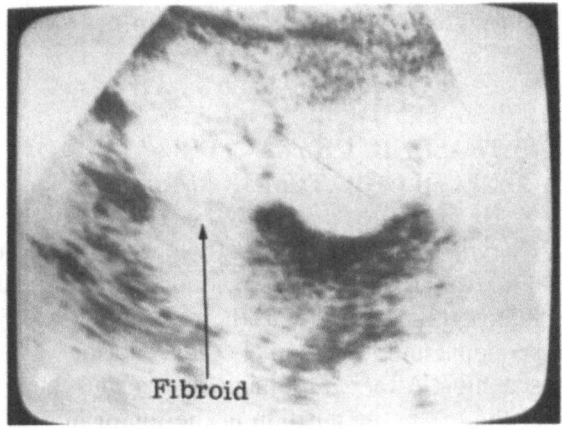

FIGURE 2.16
Supine longitudinal scan. Gray scale. The bulbous uterine fundus contains a gestational sac with medium-amplitude echoes characteristic of the pregnancy ring. Within the sac are stepladder-shaped high-amplitude echoes typical of a Lippes loop. Coexistent intrauterine pregnancy with IUCD.

FIGURE 2.17
Supine transverse scan. Patient with epigastric mass. Liver and kidney noted on right. Echo-free area extended from pelvis to xiphoid process. Paraovarian cyst at surgery.

FIGURE 2.18
Supine longitudinal scan. Gray scale. The uterus is enlarged with an irregular outline. It is generally echo poor. Areas of high and low through transmission are noted, consistent with the diagnosis of a fibroid uterus.

sensitivity is increased. The procedure by which the sensitivity is increased, wherein cysts are noted to remain echo free while solid lesions fill in echoes, is known as an attenuation study. The attenuation study is used to differentiate cystic from solid masses and aid in the detection of cystic internal degeneration in solid masses. It may also be termed a sensitivity study. The principle of measuring the sonic through transmission or sonic attenuation of a lesion is extremely useful in the differential diagnosis of pelvic tumors.

Echoes are usually obtained from the anterior and posterior walls of cystic, complex, or solid lesions. As the attenuation is decreased or the sensitivity increased, the cystic lesion remains echo free. This is because the ultrasonic beam is minimally attenuated by the homogeneous fluid (Fig. 2.17). Due to this lack of attenuation, an echo-dense area occurs behind the distal wall of the cyst which is due to reverberation-type echoes and is amplified by the effect of the TGC curve upon the amplitude of the received echoes.

Lymphomas and certain lymph node masses may simulate a cystic lesion. Solid tumors fill in with echoes at high sensitivity. At low gain settings the distal border is imaged when the substance of the mass is highly transonic or poorly attenuating. If the tumor is highly attenuating, the distal border may not be imaged even at maximum gain setting. This is especially true of solid, acoustically homogeneous masses such as lymphomas and leiomyomas (Fig. 2.18). Tumors

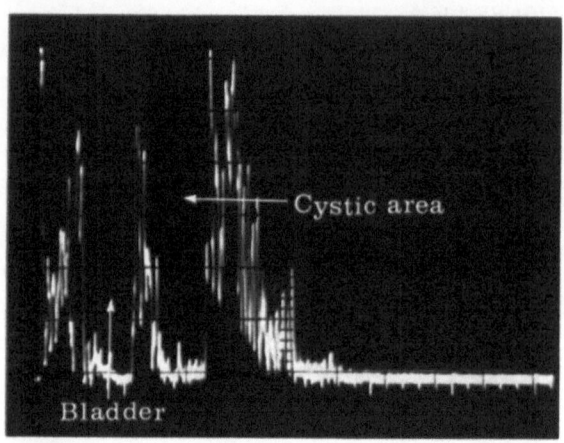

FIGURE 2.19
A-mode confirmation of cystic structure with echo-free space followed by high-amplitude echoes of distal wall.

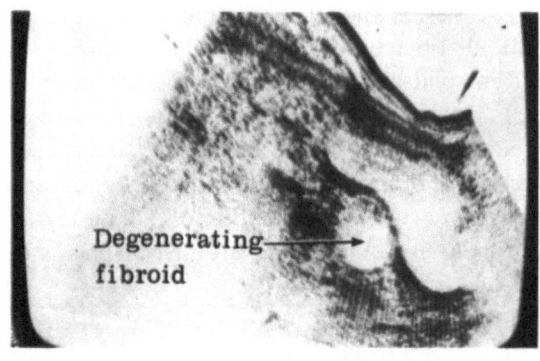

FIGURE 2.20
Supine longitudinal scan. Degenerating fibroid uterus simulating ovarian cyst. Solid portion of fibroid uterus seen in video-display (not included in this book).

FIGURE 2.21
Supine longitudinal scan. Gray scale. Complete separation of a cyst from the uterus is documented when no part of the lesion is noted to be in continuity with the uterus or vagina. Diagnosis of ovarian cyst.

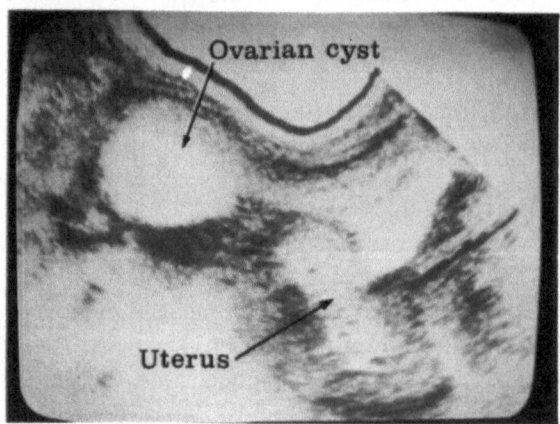

with internal degeneration permit better through transmission than do architecturally intact masses of the same histologic type. Production of fluid-filled necrotic spaces within a tumor increases beam transmission and the tumor appears on the oscilloscope as a lesion with multiple posterior echoes (Fig. 2.19). At low sensitivity, anterior and posterior borders of a degenerating tumor may be outlined and the high posterior echo density may simulate a simple cyst (Fig. 2.20). This error is avoided by sensitivity studies in which a characteristic echogenic mass is revealed as gain is increased. Indeed, certain tumors have a biologic tendency to degenerate (leiomyomas,) and by demonstrating increased through transmission in a previously poorly transmitting tumor internal degeneration can be documented, which may aid in histosonographic tissue typing. A tumor with a necrotic center will show the size of the echo-free space to visibly decrease as the gain setting is increased.

Through transmission is lower in a degenerating solid tumor than in a simple cystic lesion. Optimal ultrasonic analysis of the cystic or solid nature of a lesion is obtained with the combined use of A-mode, B-mode, and gray-scale imaging and the application of the attenuation study as previously described. With this technique, we have achieved over 96 percent accuracy in evaluating cystic and solid lesions. Other solid tumors of the pelvis which may appear echo free are seen with the frozen pelvis of advanced ovarian or cervical carcinoma. In this case, the internal texture of the lesion remains echo free, but the distal border has a lower through transmission pattern than does a simple cystic lesion.

ULTRASONIC CHARACTERIZATION OF GYNECOLOGIC TUMOR MASSES

Knowledge of the gross pathology of the uterus and ovaries allows the ultrasonographer to easily interpret these entities as they appear in cross-sectional and longitudinal studies during scanning. After determining the size and shape of the mass, the position of the tumor in

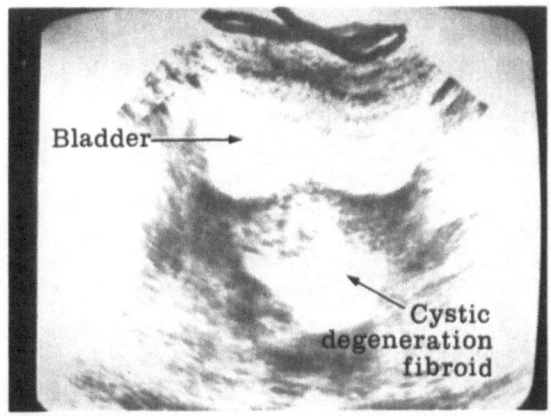

FIGURE 2-22 (a)

FIGURE 2.22(a)
Supine transverse scan. Gray scale. There is an echo-free space with high through transmission. The anterior margin of this zone is irregular and is in connection with the uterine cavity. Fibroid with massive cystic degeneration.

FIGURE 2.22(b)
Supine longitudinal scan. Gray scale. The echoes of the outline of the tumor are quite useful to the ultrasonographer. Cystic structures have a sharp anterior and posterior interface. Diagnosis in the cystic lesion shown in Fig. 2.22a using multiple sectional studies was compatible with ovarian cyst, which was later proven at surgery.

FIGURE 2.22(c)
Supine longitudinal scan. B-mode. Same case as in Fig. 2.22a and b. Demonstration of well-defined ovarian cyst.

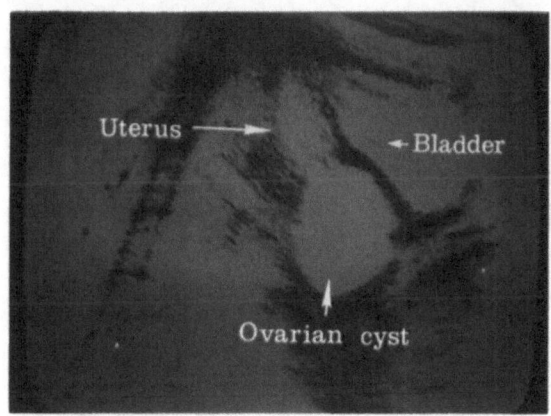

FIGURE 2-22 (b)

FIGURE 2-22 (c)

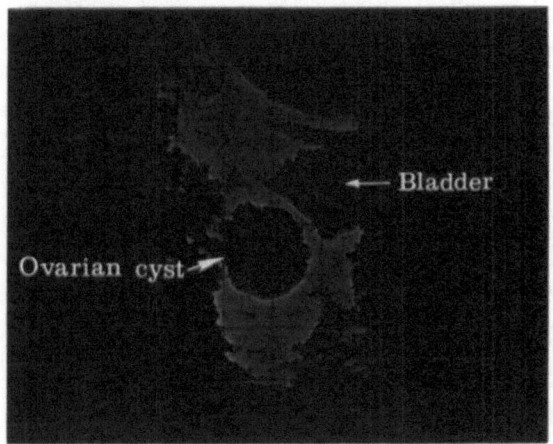

topographic relation to the uterus is evaluated. Complete separation of a mass from the uterus is documented when no part of the mass is noted to be in continuity with the uterus or vagina (Fig. 2.21). Thus, the lack of a separating interface between a tumor and the uterus implies that it is in continuity with and may be part of the uterus (Fig. 2.20). This necessitates that the normal uterus be positively identified in all scans and that the absence of a separating interface be inferred only after multiple cuts in many different scan planes are performed.

The echoes of the outlines of the tumor are quite useful to the ultrasonographer. Cystic structures have a sharp anterior and posterior interface. The amplitude of the distal wall echoes is stronger than that of the anterior wall echoes due in part to the concave reflecting surface of the distal wall returning a large portion of the transmitted sound energy (Fig. 2.22a,b, and c). Solid lesions tend to have poorly defined margins. The anterior wall echo amplitude is generally higher than that of the distal wall due to the attenuation properties of the solid tumor tissue (Fig. 2.23a). These characteristics of the margins of cystic and solid tumors must be demonstrated by scanning the lesion in many planes for total evaluation. Similarly, the wall-contents interface of the tumor is smooth and sharp in cystic lesions while, in contrast, it is poorly demarcated in solid tumors. Echoes from the borders are best imaged by linear or sector scanning maneuvers.

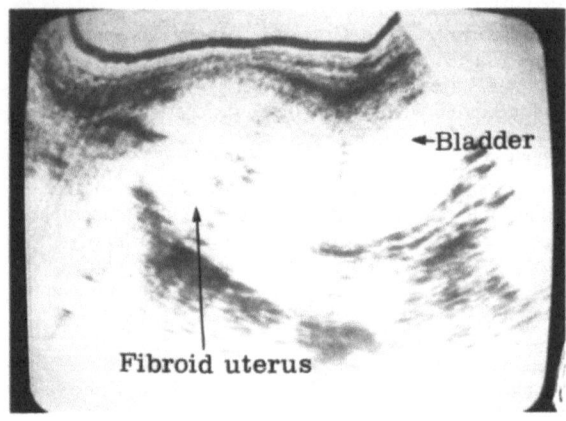

FIGURE 2.23(a)
Supine longitudinal scan. Gray scale. The vaginal walls appear echo poor. At the point of contact between the anterior and posterior aspect is an echogenic interface. The cervix is enlarged; the huge mass that represents the enlarged uterus is due to fibroid uterus.

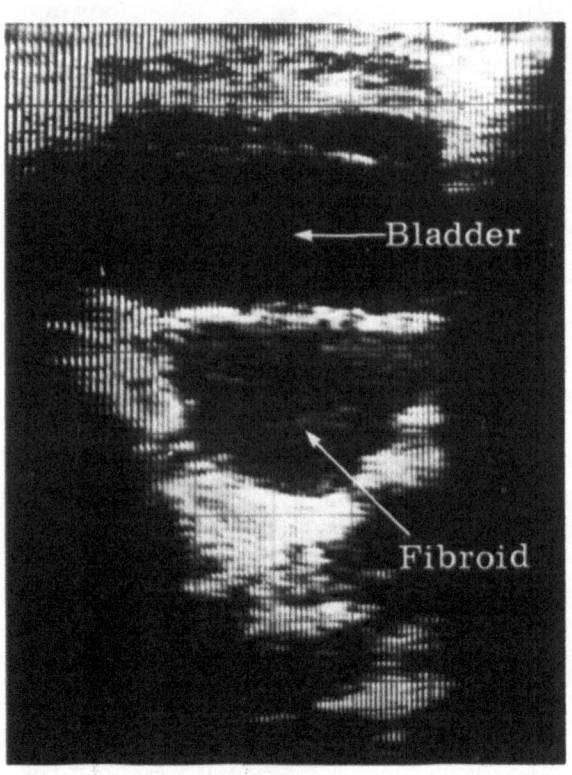

FIGURE 2.23(c)
Supine transverse scan. Real-time scanner. The body of the uterus is enlarged with a diffuse low-level echo pattern. Through transmission is high in this example of a fibroid uterus.

FIGURE 2.23(b)
Supine longitudinal scan. Gray scale. The bladder is incompletely filled. The uterus is massively enlarged with an echo-poor pattern. High through transmission is noted in the degenerating portion of the superior fibroid uterus. The poor through transmission of the lower fibroid portion signifies lack of cystic changes.

FIGURE 2.23(d)
Supine longitudinal scan. Gray scale. The uterus is enlarged with a distinctly nodular outline. An irregular echo pattern and the presence of a variable through transmission pattern confirm the diagnosis of fibroid uterus.

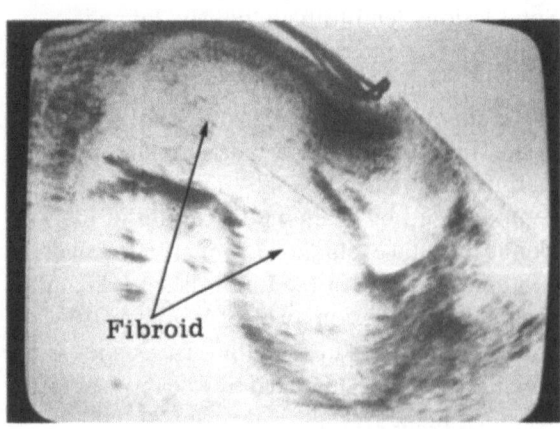

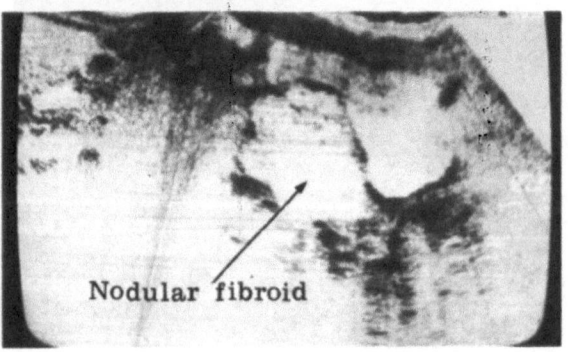

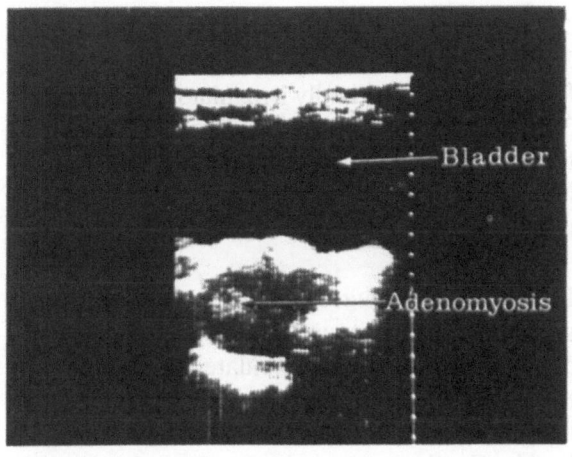

FIGURE 2.24
Supine transverse scan. Real-time scanner. The echo-free
bladder is above a diffusely enlarged smooth uterine outline.
Centrally located echoes are noted. This pattern is typical of
adenomyosis, although it may occur in fibroids of the small
intramural type.

FIGURE 2.25
Supine transverse scan. Gray scale. Uterine enlargement
with a nonhomogeneous echo-poor internal texture.
Endometrial carcinoma. Note lateral echo-free iliopsoas.

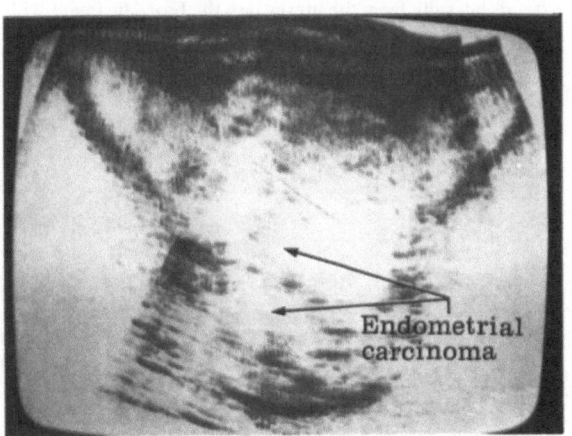

The internal texture of the mass is best studied
with compound scanning techniques, since the
parenchyma of tumors are diffuse reflectors.
Cysts are echo free except for occasional linear
echoes due to clearly delineated septa. Anterior
compartment echo artifacts may be noted in
cysts at higher gain settings. Through
transmission is high in cysts except when the
mass sits adjacent to a highly attenuating
surface. In this case a very high amplitude echo
marks the distal wall. Solid tumors have poor
through transmission except when there is cystic
internal degeneration. It is not uncommon to find
a massively degenerated fibroid nodule
appearing as an ovarian cyst.

UTERUS

ENLARGED UTERUS

The commonest finding in the field of obstetrics
and gynecology is an enlarged uterus. Pregnancy
is the most probable common cause, because the
fluid content of the pregnant uterus is high at 5
weeks. Posterior echo-rich areas may be demonstrated ultrasonically, along with the presence of
a gestational sac. After delivery the uterus remains enlarged for a period of time. Ultrasonographic findings related to threatened and missed
abortions will be described in detail.

Inflammatory conditions are another cause of
enlarged uterus. A hematometra may present a
cystic appearance in an enlarged uterus. Uterine
tumors are an additional cause of uterine enlargement and will be discussed in detail.

UTERINE MASSES

The most common pathologic cause for an
enlarged uterus is leiomyoma uteri (Fig.
2.23a,b,c, and d). Other conditions enlarging the
uterus include polyps, endometriosis,
endometrial hyperplasia, adenomyosis (Fig.
2.24), idiopathic uterine enlargement, and
malignant tumors of the uterus (Fig. 2.25).

The majority of uterine fibroids occur in the
myometrium as intramural fibroids. The submu-
cus variety tend to bulge into the endometrial

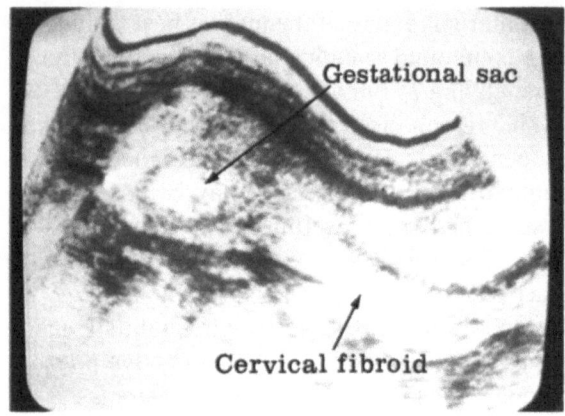

FIGURE 2-26

Gestational sac

Cervical fibroid

cavity and produce spontaneous abortion (Fig. 2.26). The subserous type distorts the outer surface creating a markedly irregular outline (Fig. 2.27). The cervical fibroid is generally solitary in this site and may easily complicate labor if enlarged (Fig. 2.28). Intraligamentous (Fig. 2.29) and pedunculated fibroids are rare.

Degenerative changes are more common in the submucous, subserous types (Fig. 2.30a,b, and c), ligamentous and pedunculated fibroids due to the poorer blood supply. Various degrees of hyaline degeneration are noted in all types of fibroids. Cystic degeneration is a sequel to hyaline changes and increases with the size of the tumor and the age of the growth (Fig. 2.30d). Torsion is

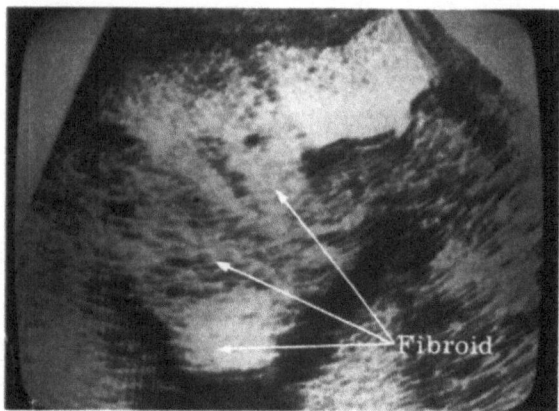

FIGURE 2-27

Fibroid

FIGURE 2.26
Supine transverse scan. Gray scale. Massive elongation of the cervix which is also echo-free due to fibroid tumor. The gestational sac is eccentric with opening of the caudal sac and multiple irregular echoes. Spontaneous abortion soon followed.

FIGURE 2.27
Supine longitudinal scan. Gray scale. Massive protrusion of myoma from the dorsal uterine outline characteristic of subserous myoma.

FIGURE 2.28
Supine transverse scan. Real-time scanner. A moderately echogenic mass with variable through transmission patterns is noted adjacent to the uterine cervix. Patient is 4 months pregnant and the amniotic fluid of the uterus is noted as an echo-free area. Pedunculated cervix fibroid.

FIGURE 2.29
Supine transverse scan. Gray scale. Solid tumor mass extends laterally from the uterus into the broad ligament with an echo-poor internal echo pattern. Intraligamentous fibroid.

FIGURE 2-28

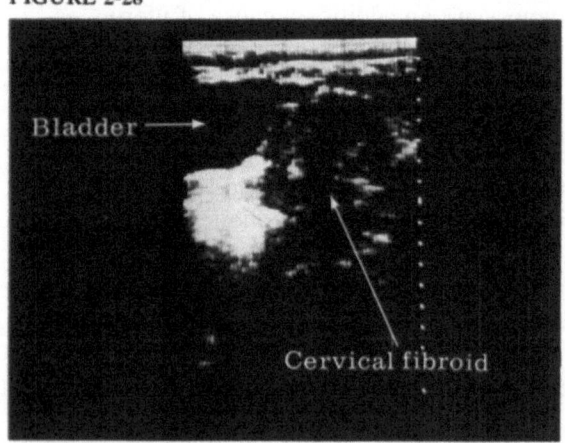

Bladder

Cervical fibroid

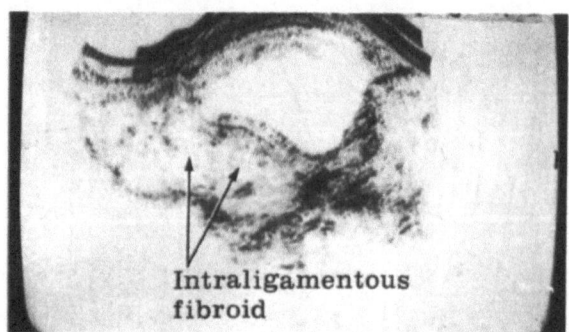

Intraligamentous fibroid

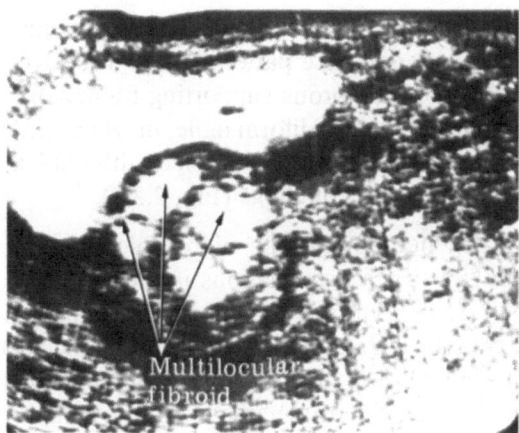

FIGURE 2-30 (a)

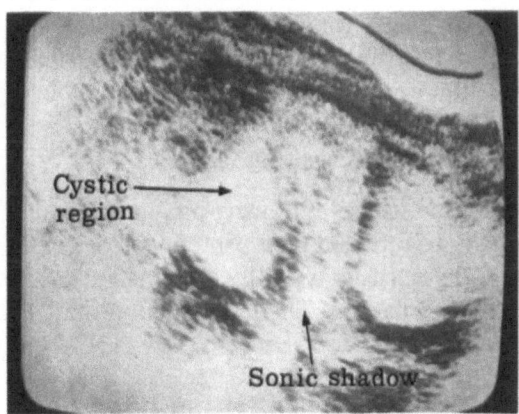

FIGURE 2-30 (b)

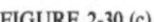
FIGURE 2-30 (c)

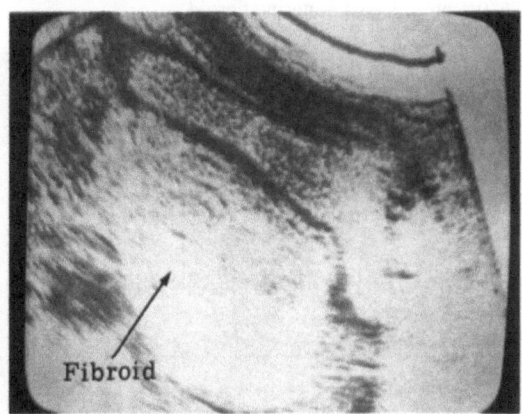

common in pedunculated fibroids (Fig. 2.30e). Calcification often occurs, but is rare in the submucous growths. Occasionally, frank bone formation may be noted. Infection and suppuration are most common in the submucous type due to the effects of local ulceration and its relation to the uterine cavity. Sarcomatous changes occur in less than 1 percent of cases.

The ultrasonic appearance of fibroids varies with the gross pathologic process. The usual presentation is that of a large, irregular uterine outline, with a nodular architecture and poor margin properties. The solid and undegenerated fibroid markedly attenuates the sound so that the distal margin is poorly imaged. The coarseness of the echo pattern is related to the cellularity of

FIGURE 2.30(a)
Supine longitudinal scan. Rounded lesion with sharp septations simulates ovarian cyst of multilocular type. This is a degenerating portion of a large fibroid uterus.

FIGURE 2.30(b)
Supine longitudinal scan. Gray scale. Inferior portion of fibroid uterus produces sonic shadow due to great attenuation of sonic beam. Superior myoma has completely degenerated with cystic changes and high through transmission.

FIGURE 2.30(c)
Supine longitudinal scan. Gray scale. Bulbous, irregular outline to this fibroid uterus. Note that internal degeneration is best demonstrated by observing areas of high through transmission.

FIGURE 2.30(d)
Supine longitudinal scan. Gray scale. Cystic degeneration is a sequel to hyaline changes and increases with the size of the tumor and the age of the growth. Note focal area of cystic degeneration.

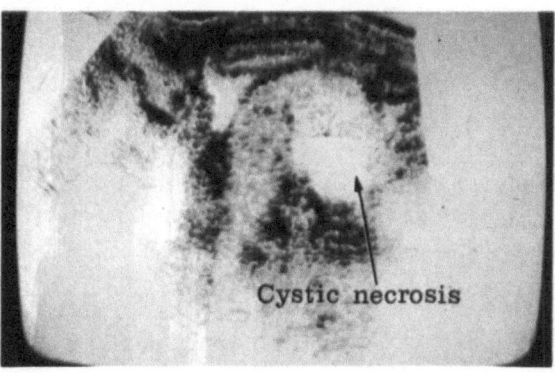

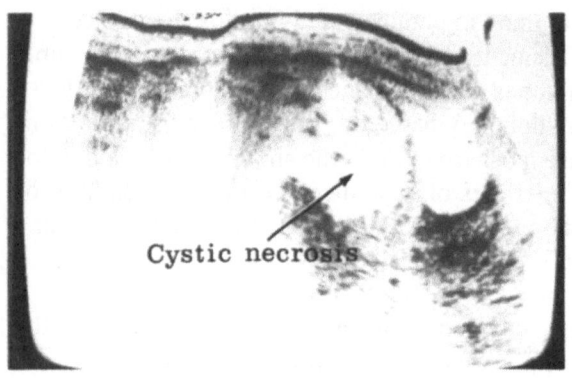

FIGURE 2.30(e)
Supine longitudinal scan. Gray scale. Cystic degeneration of the pedunculated fibroid uterus due to torsion.

the tumor parenchyma. Very cellular leiomyomas may show a snowflake pattern due to wide separation of the fibrous supporting framework, and may mimic hydatidiform mole, in which case ultrasonography should be coupled with clinical data and laboratory findings (Fig. 2.30f).

Cystic degeneration may be microsopic or gross. The tiny cystic transformations in the fibroid appear as areas of greater echogenicity and increased through transmission. The presence of echoes in a fibroid previously not noted to have echoes signifies internal necrosis. Large echo-free spaces may occur when cystic changes are massive and confluent. Calcification may be amorphous or ring shaped (Fig. 2.31a and b). Amorphous calcium deposits produce high-amplitude echoes and attenuate the sound beam (Fig. 2.32a and b). Ring-shaped calcification may simulate a fetal head. In spite of all diagnostic studies, the origin of the mass may never be determined and laparotomy may be necessary for definitive diagnosis (Fig. 2.33a).

Endometritis occurs following pregnancy and is secondary to retained fetal contents or placental tissue. The uterus is typically involuted at this time and is enlarged. The inflammation may

FIGURE 2.30(f)
Supine longitudinal scan. Gray scale. Very cellular leiomyomas may show a snowflake pattern due to wide separation of the fibroid supporting framework, and may mimic hydatidiform mole. Note the echo pattern of the uterus. Compact fibroid tissue in the cervix and snowflake pattern in the fundus are observed.

FIGURE 2.31(a)
Supine transverse scan. Gray scale. A rounded echogenic structure is seen in the echo-poor uterus. This calcific fibroid mimics a fetal head outline. Another calcific fibroid might mimic the body. Absence of fetal motion and fetal heartbeat signifies the presence of a uterine fibroid.

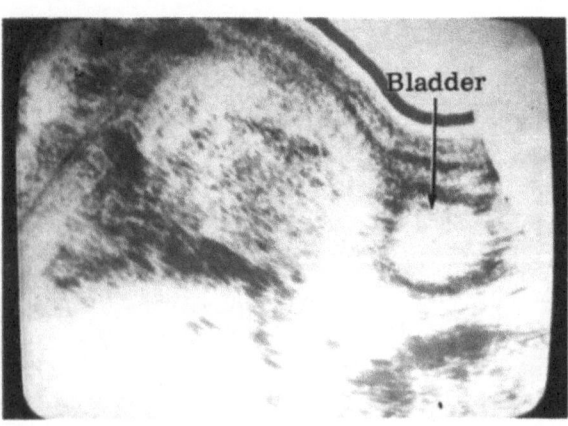

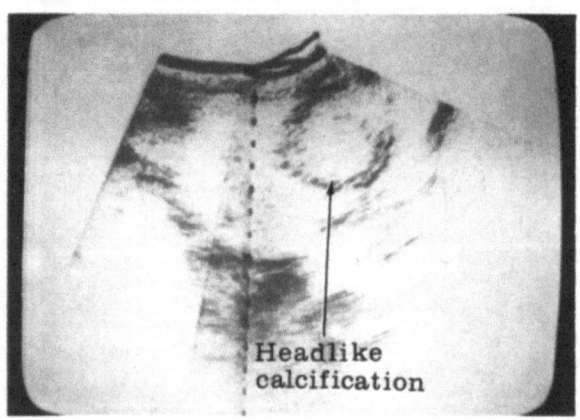

extend to the myometrium and is depicted by the sonogram as generalized anechoic areas in the affected portions of the uterus. If severe, associated changes of salpingitis and pelvic abscess formation may be observed (2).

Small intramural fibroids may simulate adenomyosis of the uterus. However, in adenomyosis, due to endometrial tissue of the uterine cavity projecting into the myometrium, the uterine enlargement is generally symmetric and smooth with little gross distortion of the

pear-shaped appearance (Fig. 2.33b). These endometrial inroads have a tendency to be echo poor and located near the endometrial canal, in our experience. Others have described an echogenic pattern (3).

Uterine polyps or endometrial polypoid hyperplasia may simulate adenomyosis, since the uterus may be diffusely enlarged with echoes in the region of the endometrial cavity. A widened endometrial cavity with internal echoes is more characteristic of polypoid disease.

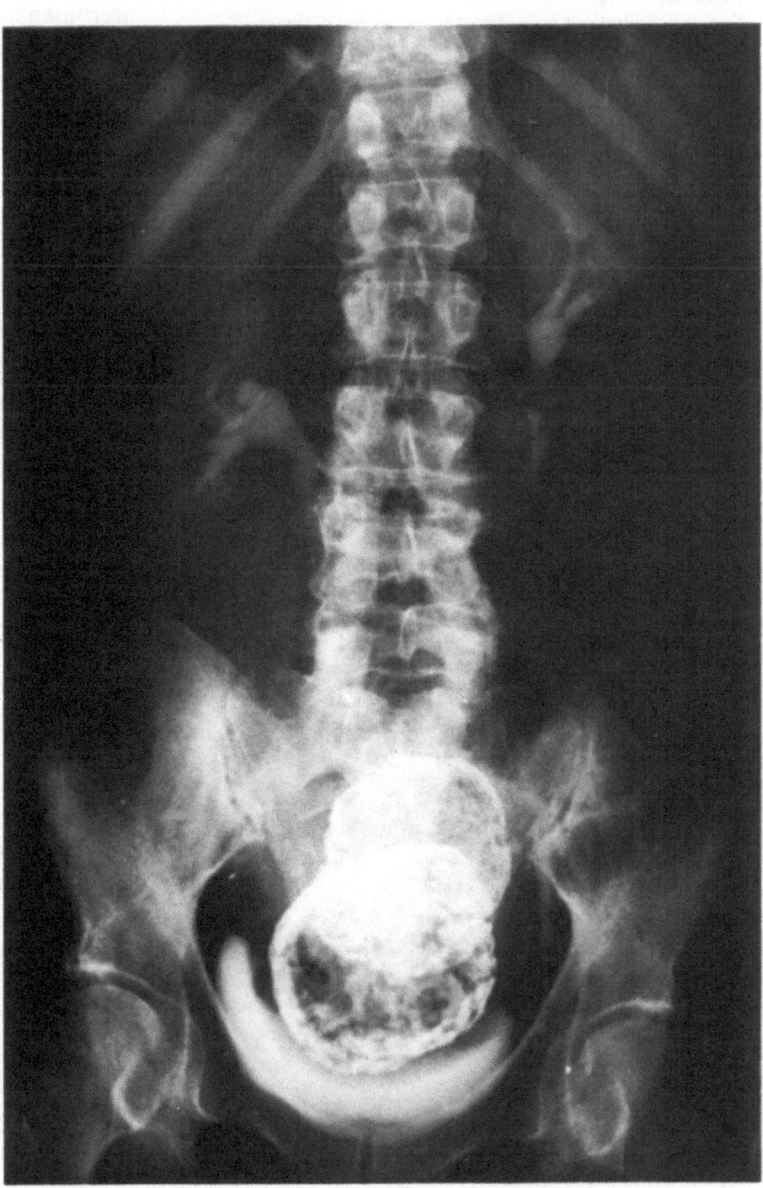

FIGURE 2.31(b)
Supine film from IVP (Intervenous Pyelogram). Double ringlike shadows of calcific fibroids are noted in the pelvis. These films are useful in evaluating a heavily calcified pelvic mass when sonic shadowing prevents optimal ultrasonic imaging.

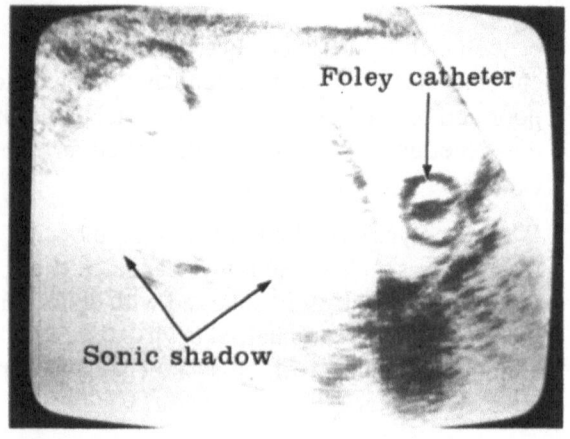

FIGURE 2.32(a)
Supine longitudinal scan. Gray scale. Foley catheter in bladder. High-amplitude echoes anteriorly with sonic shadow represent clusters of amorphous calcification.

FIGURE 2.32(b)
Supine longitudinal scan. Gray scale. An irregularly outlined mass in the pelvis is noted with multiple sonic shadows. Distal wall reverberation artifacts are noted. Sonic shadowing may prevent effective imaging of the distal boundaries of the mass. Roentgen analysis is necessary for certain calcific masses.

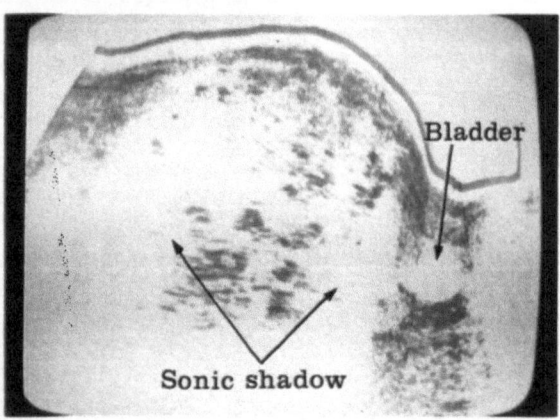

Endometriosis is caused by ectopic endometrium in various locations in the pelvis and abdomen. Cystic or solid lesions may be noted in various combinations. The cystic lesions contain dark, unclotted blood surrounded by a thick cyst wall due to the marked fibrotic reaction in this disease process. The solid lesions cause irregularity of the uterine echo pattern and the frequent intense desmoplastic changes tend to fuse the neighboring organs together.

Our experience with uterine cancer or sarcoma has shown an enlarged uterus that could not be definitively distinguished from other causes of uteromegaly.

OVARY

In our experience, with the application of various ultrasonic techniques, positional maneuvers, and multiple frequency scanning, we have been unable to visualize the normal-sized ovary within the pelvis. In most instances the ovaries are hidden in the soft tissues of the pelvis and the resulting returned echoes must merge and interphase with the echoes of the surrounding soft tissues and bony pelvic walls. Occasionally, in routine study normal ovaries can be seen (Fig 2.34a). As the ovaries enlarge there is a better chance of recording the image of this structure by scanning since it occupies more space within the pelvic cavity (Fig. 2.34b).

The detection of early enlargement of the ovaries depends upon the nature of the expansile process. A simple cystic lesion projecting from the ovary rather than being within the stroma of the ovarian tissue may be detected easily at a rather small size. Small cysts within the ovarian structure, such as the multiple cysts of the Stein-Leventhal syndrome with surrounding thick fibrous septa, are detectable when of moderate size and appear as a complex mass on the oscilloscope. Complex masses that are more solid than cystic, such as the dermoid cyst, may be extremely large and still be very difficult to detect ultrasonically. Thus, the nature of the lesion and its geometry with respect to the

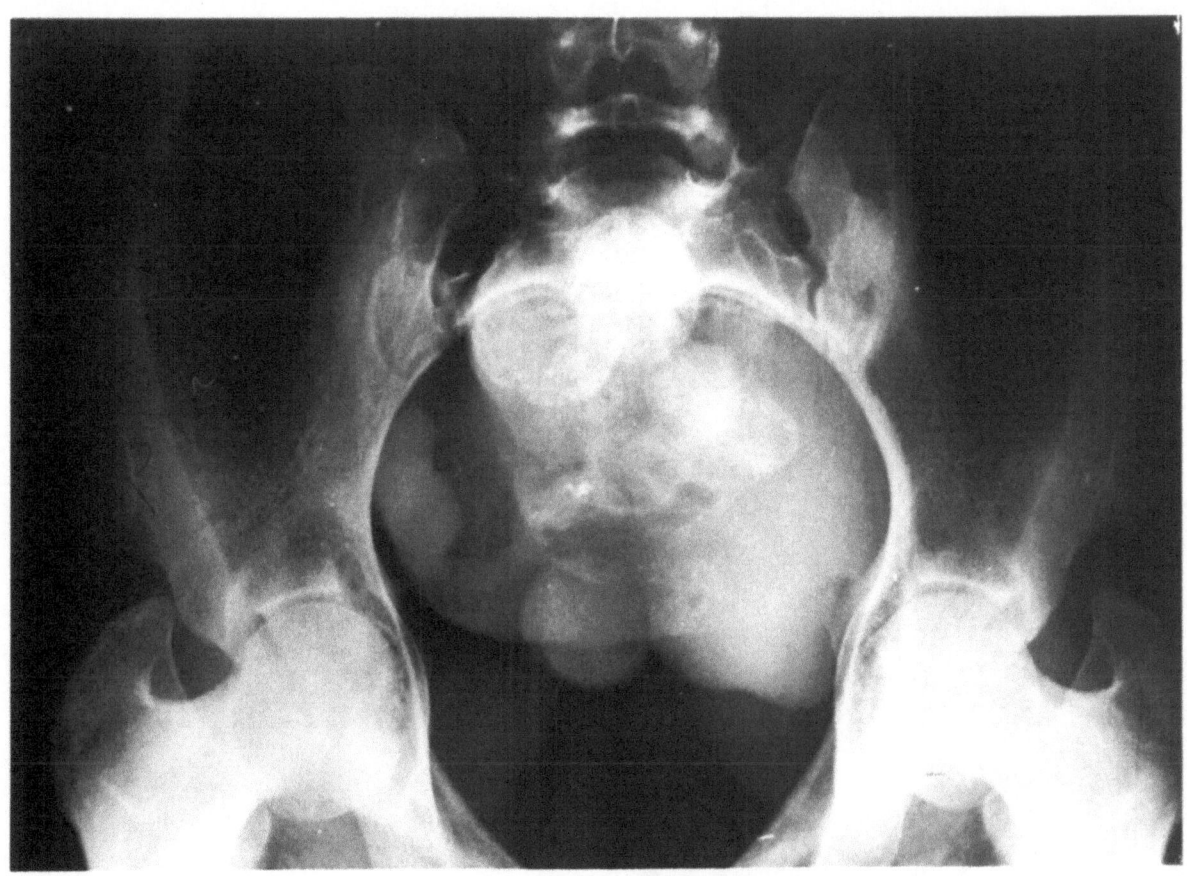

FIGURE 2.33(a)
Air contrast gynecogram. Pelvic mass with multiple discrete nodules projecting from the tumor. With this complicated lesion it is virtually impossible to distinguish the boundaries between the uterus and the ovaries. Similarly, ultrasound may not be able to separate adherent ovarian and uterine masses.

FIGURE 2.33(b)
Supine transverse scan. Gray scale. Adenomyosis simulates fibroid uterus. Adenomyosis was demonstrated at operation. Adenomyosis

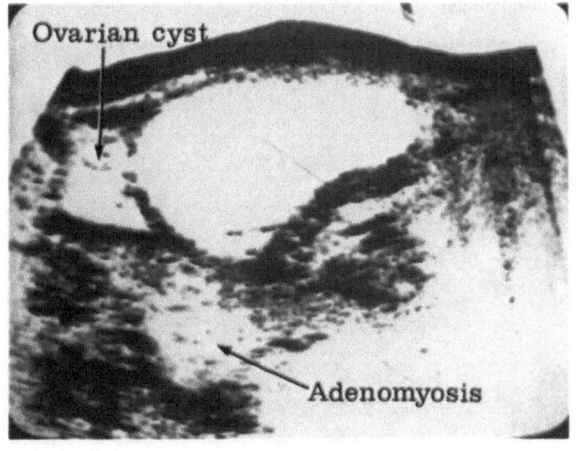

perpendicularity of the scanning beam are extremely important in the imaging of ovarian lesions. A simple ovarian cyst has an echo-free lumen with a sharp posterior wall, and an echo-rich reverberation pattern is noted distal to the posterior interface at high sensitivity settings. Ovarian cysts with internal septations may be easily demonstrated if the walls of the septa are perpendicular to the interrogating ultrasonic beam. Internal septa may also be visualized by compound scanning techniques with high gain

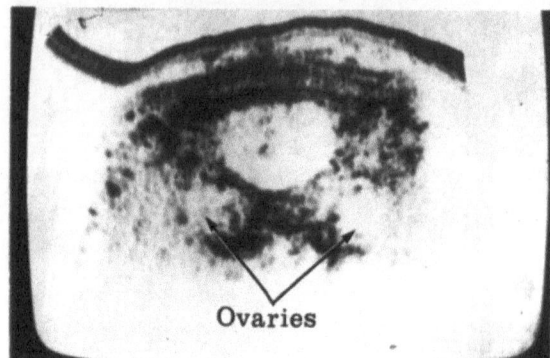

FIGURE 2-34 (a)

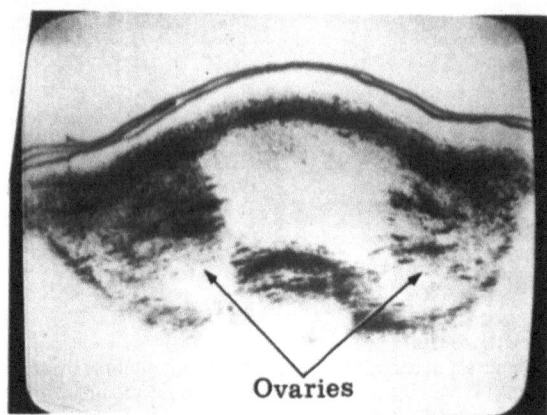

FIGURE 2-34 (b)

FIGURE 2-35 (a)

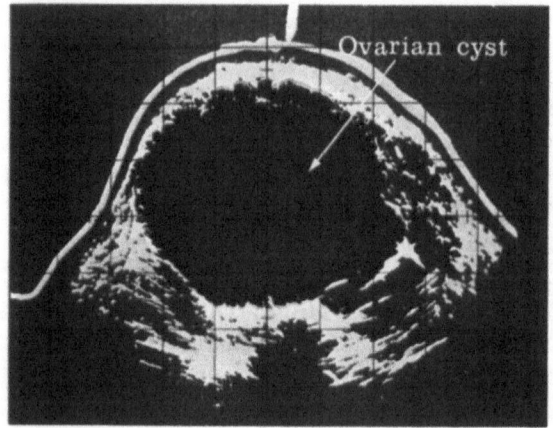

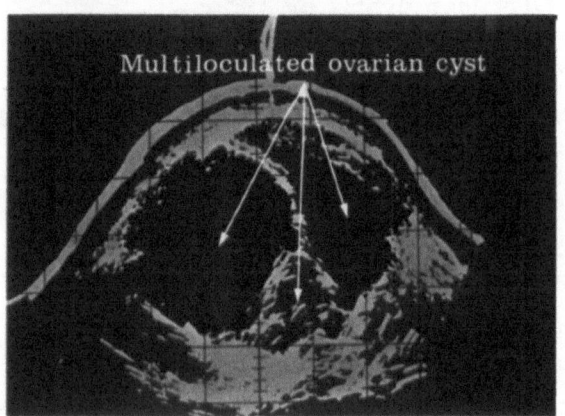

settings to image the diffuse reflections of the portions of the septa that are nonperpendicular to the sound beam.

OVARIAN MASS

The gross morphology, internal architecture, and consistency of ovarian tumors are subject to wide variation. Follicular cysts and serous cystadenomas present as unilocular echo-free lesions. Mucinous cystadenomas are multilocular, so that the echo-free picture is broken by multiple septa usually with thin walls (Fig. 2.35a and b). Ovarian cysts may present with various shapes, positions, and contours and may be located anywhere in the pelvic cavity (Fig. 2.36a and b) or may occupy the entire abdomen (Fig. 2.36c). Ovarian cysts may regress and completely disappear. This is the usual biologic history of thecal lutein cysts associated with pregnancy.

FIGURE 2.34(a)
Supine transverse scan. Gray scale. Occasionally, in routine study normal ovaries can be seen.

FIGURE 2.34(b)
Supine transverse scan. Gray scale. As the ovaries enlarge there is a better chance of recording their image by scanning since they occupy more space within the pelvic cavity.

FIGURE 2.35(a)
Supine transverse scan. B-mode. Large echo-free area with sharp boundaries and high through transmission. Simple ovarian cyst.

FIGURE 2.35(b)
Supine transverse scan. B-mode. Large echo-free area with sharp boundaries and high through transmission. Multiloculated ovarian cyst.

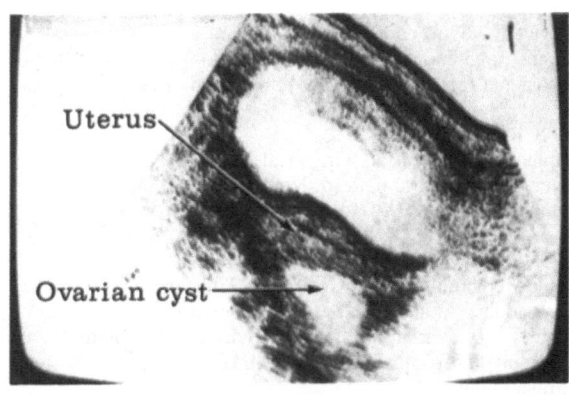

FIGURE 2.36(a)
Supine longitudinal scan. Gray scale. Small echo-free cystic space is typical of ovarian cyst.

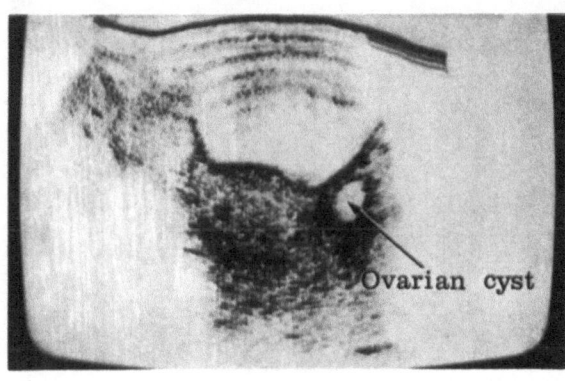

FIGURE 2.36(b)
Supine transverse scan. Gray scale. The echo-free ovarian cyst is seen in sharp contrast to the echogenic uterus. Note high through transmission pattern.

FIGURE 2.36(c)
Supine longitudinal scan. Gray scale. Ovarian cyst occupying the entire abdomen.

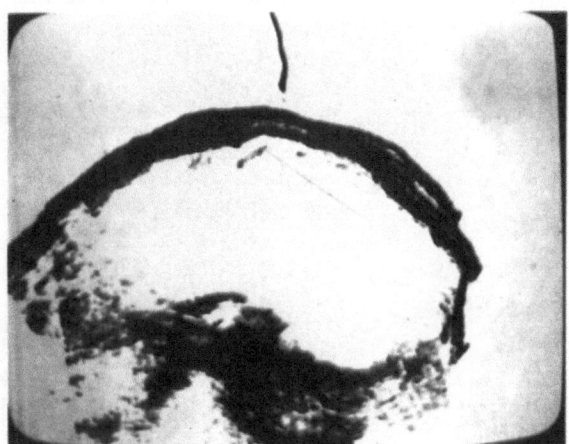

Teratomas comprise roughly 10 percent of ovarian cystic tumors. They may be cystic or solid (Fig. 2.37a and b). If the fatty contents of the tumor are in one position for a sufficient time, a fluid level may be seen in the fat interface during scanning. Cystic dermoids may present as echo-free areas of varying size at high gain. As the sensitivity is decreased, the solid portion of the tumor may be identified. Due to the irregular outline of the tumor and the multiplicity of its internal contents, the teratoma is frequently difficult to image. Often only the cystic zone can be delineated. The physical finding of a large tumor mass with the ultrasonic demonstration of a small cystic space suggest the possibility of a dermoid tumor. Areas of calcification appear as highly echogenic zones. If the calcification or ossification is sufficient, a sonic shadow will be cast.

A second pattern of the benign ovarian teratoma has been demonstrated with gray-scale units. The solid contents of the tumor may show distinctive ultrasonic findings. The most frequent sign is the presence of a highly reflecting irregular region in the vicinity of an echo-free cystic cavity. This is presumed to be related to the presence of hair and sebum which are highly echogenic (4), but not as reflective as calcium or bone. When the tumor has a predominance of hair, sebum, or calcium as opposed to the cystic components, the sonic shadow may be produced. This sonic shadowing often obscures the remainder of the mass and may simulate colonic gas or feces. When this is encountered, a flat plate of the abdomen may be performed to rule out the presence of feces or to demonstrate the suspected fat lucency or dental structure of a dermoid cyst. Alternatively, a cleansing enema may be given and the patient rescanned.

Ovarian fibromas cannot be differentiated from pedunculated fibroids. Indeed, they may show areas of focal cystic degeneration typical of longstanding fibroid tumors (Fig. 2.37c). There is no way to differentiate a solid ovarian carcinoma from a fibroma at this time (Fig. 2.38a and b). Papillary cystadenomas appear as cystic spaces with the small papillary excrescences showing as

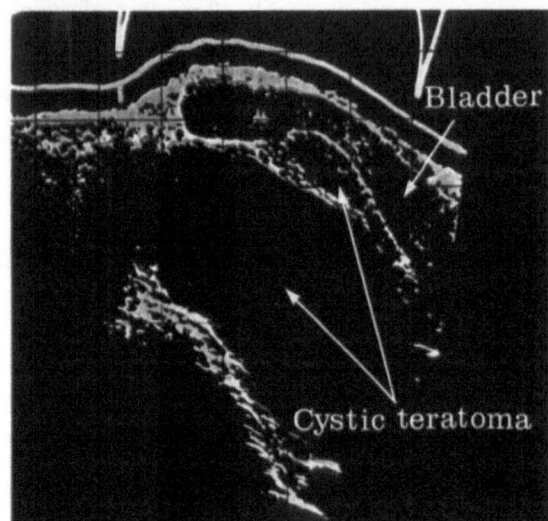
FIGURE 2-37 (a)

FIGURE 2.37(a)
Supine longitudinal scan. B-mode. Echo-free space with occasional septations noted. Predominantly cystic teratoma.

FIGURE 2.37(b)
Supine transverse scan. Gray scale. Cystic teratoma with heterogeneous echo pattern. Note cystic and solid components.

FIGURE 2.37(c)
Supine longitudinal scan. Gray scale. Huge mass posterior to the bladder is noted with cystic degeneration. Diagnosis at surgery was ovarian fibroma. Ovarian fibromas cannot be differentiated from pedunculated fibroids by ultrasonography.

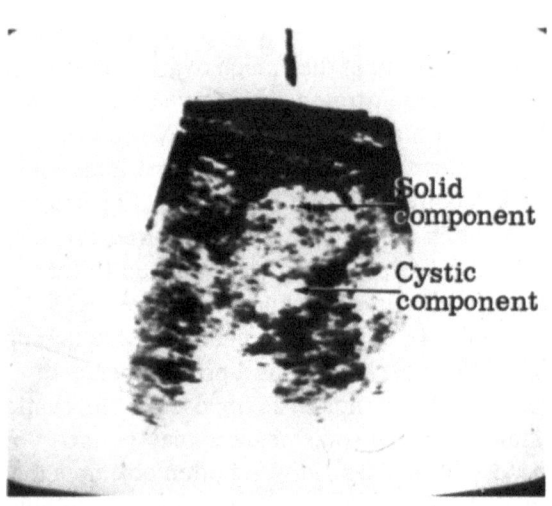
FIGURE 2-37 (b)

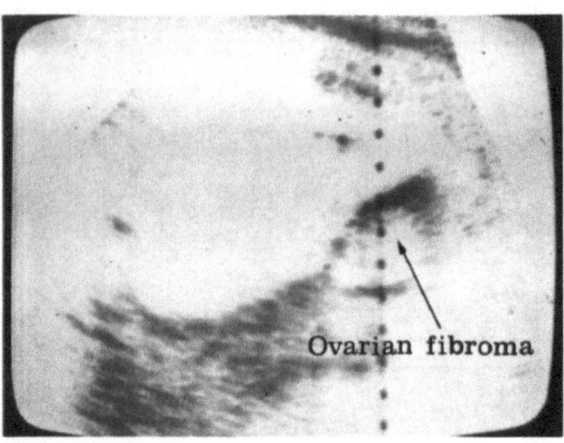

FIGURE 2.38(a)
Supine transverse scan. Gray scale. Small, sharply circumscribed lesion with scattered central echo pattern and high through transmission represents degenerating ovarian fibroma. This tumor cannot be differentiated from a pedunculated uterine fibroid.

FIGURE 2.38(b)
Supine transverse scan. An irregular solid mass with a large cystic component is fused to the uterus. Surgery showed ovarian carcinoma infiltrating the uterus and local structures.

FIGURE 2-37 (c)

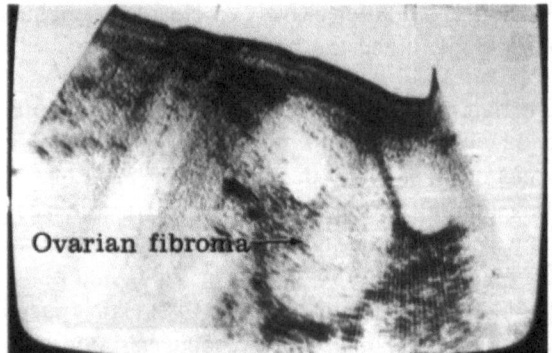

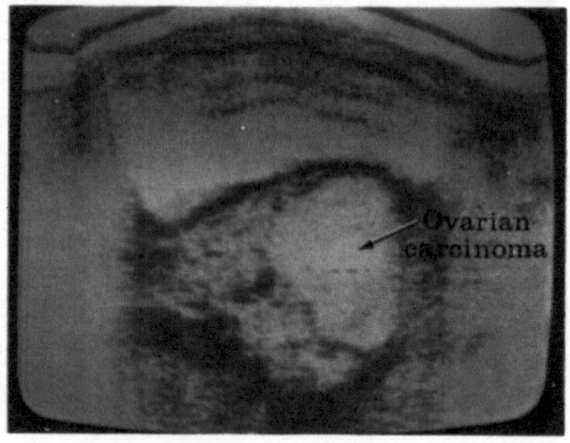

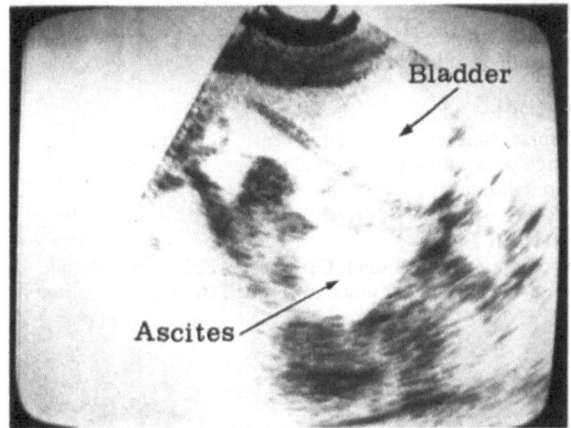

FIGURE 2-39 (a)

fine echoes projecting into the lumen. If papillations are noted outside the lumen of the cystic areas, the presence of ascites must be inferred. The fluid surrounding the outer projections permits them to be imaged as separate interfaces. The presence of loculated ascites in conjunction with a cystic papillary lesion implies malignancy (Fig. 2.39a,b,c, and d). Indeed, the serous cystadenocarcinoma is the most common type of ovarian cancer. Early in its course, this tumor may be well defined with echo-free spaces associated with fine echo speckling peripherally. However, as the tumor spreads to the omentum and peritoneum, loculated ascites develop and the pelvic organs become fixed by malignant

FIGURE 2.39(a)
Supine transverse scan. Gray scale. Area of loculated ascites may simulate an ovarian cystic tumor. Motion of bowel loops noted with real-time scanner and presence of other areas of ascites confirm the diagnosis.

FIGURE 2.39(b)
Supine longitudinal scan. Gray scale. The bladder is empty. There is an echogenic mass with irregular contours superiorly representing bowel and omentum adhesion. Anteriorly, a single bowel loop apparently "standing erect" in the ascites is noted. This is connected to the anterior abdominal wall by an adhesion which is cut by the ultrasound beam at an angle too oblique to permit registration on the oscilloscope.

FIGURE 2.39(c)
Supine transverse scan. Gray scale. The "erect" bowel loop is connected to the anterior abdominal wall by an adhesion. Adhesions are characteristic of malignant ascites. Patient had ovarian carcinoma.

FIGURE 2.39(d)
Supine transverse scan. Gray scale. The bladder has been emptied. Echo-free areas with scattered internal echoes and irregular margins were fixed and did not change position with motion. Malignant ascites from ovarian carcinoma.

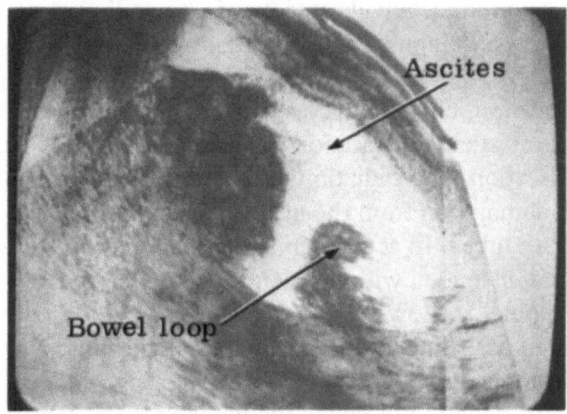

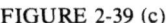

FIGURE 2-39 (b)

FIGURE 2-39 (c)

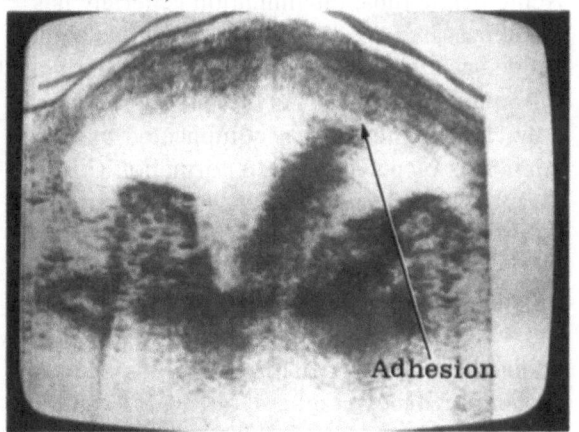

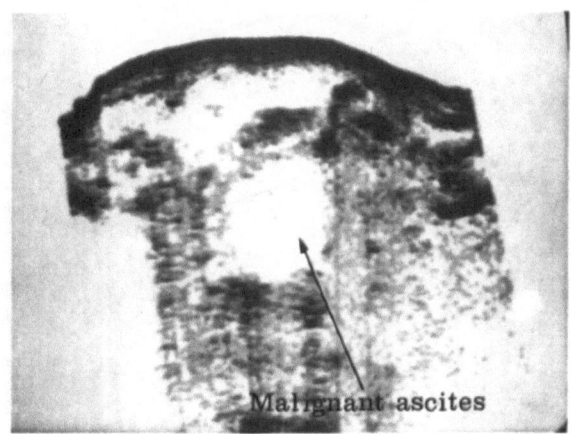

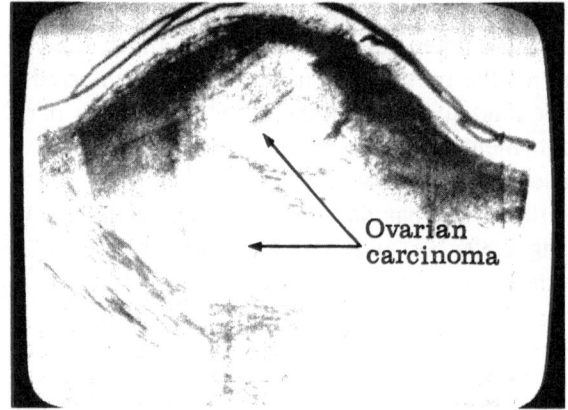

FIGURE 2-40 (a)

FIGURE 2.40(a)
Supine transverse scan. Gray scale. Echo-free ovarian
carcinoma with septation.

FIGURE 2.40(b)
Supine transverse scan. Gray scale. Echo-free ovarian
carcinoma with a few internal echoes. Note absence of
through transmission.

FIGURE 2.40(c)
Supine longitudinal scan. Gray scale. Echo-free ovarian
carcinoma. Again absence of through transmission is noted.

loculated ascites develop and the pelvic organs
become fixed by malignant adhesions or frozen
pelvis (Fig. 2.40a,b, and c).

Inflammatory lesions of the tubes and ovaries
may produce a wide variety of ultrasonic patterns. Salpingitis is the most common pathologic
condition of the tube. This infection may follow
abortion, childbirth, cervicitis, surgical procedures such as dilatation and curettage or IUCD
insertion, and radiation therapy. The ascending
inflammation from the uterus usually involves
both tubes. In acute salpingitis the tube is red
and distended with purulent exudate. Chronic
salpingitis shows variable enlargements of the
tube associated with dense local adhesions.
Complications of salpingitis include pyosalpinx
with retention of pus in the blocked tube, and
hydrosalpinx with the distended tube having a
sausage or distorted shape and thin walls. Pelvic
abscess and oophoritis are also associated with
the sequelae of salpingitis.

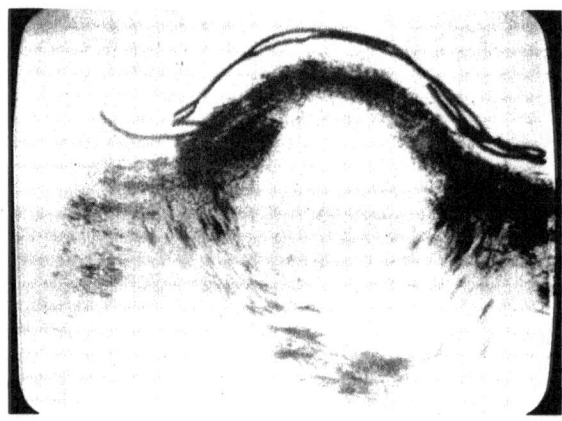

FIGURE 2-40 (b)

FIGURE 2-40 (c)

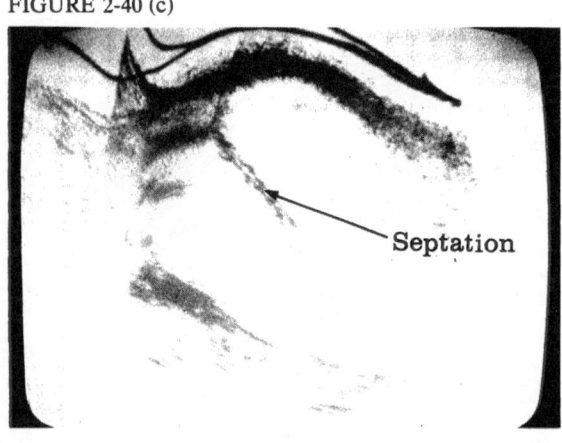

Acute pelvic tubal inflammation generally has
the appearance of a small rounded adnexal or
cul-de-sac cystic mass with regular borders, and
is frequently bilateral. As the infection produces
a much larger mass or is complicated by
oophoritis or pelvic abscess formation (Fig.
2.41a), a larger, multilocular mass with irregular
borders frequently obscuring the outline of the
uterus is apparent (5). Simple pelvic abscesses
frequently are found in the midline in the cul de
sac, while uncomplicated tuboovarian abscesses
tend to have an adnexal location or may develop
during pregnancy (Fig. 2.41b).

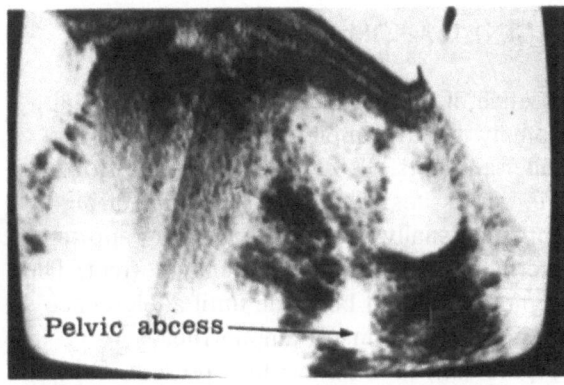

FIGURE 2.41(a)
Supine longitudinal scan. Gray scale. The pelvic tubal inflammation generally has the appearance of a small rounded adnexal or cul-de-sac cystic mass with regular borders.

FIGURE 2.41(b)
Supine longitudinal scan. Gray scale. Simple pelvic abscesses frequently are found in the midline in the cul de sac. This abscess developed during pregnancy.

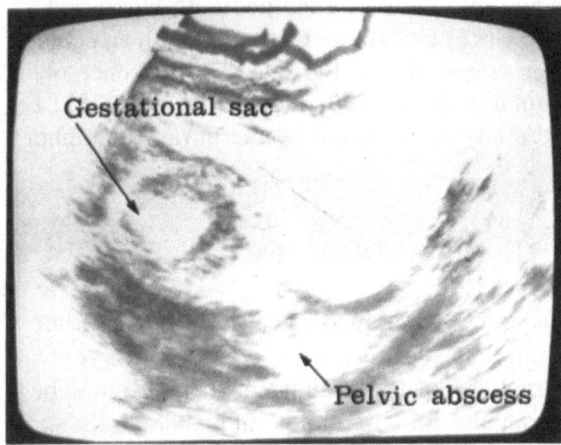

ULTRASONIC DIFFERENTIAL DIAGNOSES OF OVARIAN MASSES

The following differential diagnoses of ovarian masses may be inferred by ultrasonography.

1. Distended cecum. The cecum lies in the right iliac fossa and extends over the iliopsoas. Occasionally, the cecum hangs over the pelvic brim or lies further down in the pelvic cavity. When filled with gas, there is a sonic shadow; when filled with fluid, the cecum may simulate an ovarian cyst.

2. Redundant sigmoid colon. The sigmoid lies within the true pelvis. When a loop is filled with fluid and, especially, is redundant, it may mimic ovarian cyst or ovarian mass.

3. Appendicular abscess. When the appendix is long, it may extend into the right pelvis. If this type of appendix develops infection and finally ruptures, with or without adhesions, it may simulate ovarian mass.

4. Paraovarian cyst. Paraovarian cysts originate from the vestigial remnants of the wolffian body and are located within the broad ligament. Ultrasonographically, they cannot be distinguished from other cysts. They may bleed into the peritoneal cavity.

5. Hematocele. If hematocele is a result of ruptured ectopic pregnancy at the time of ultrasonographic examination, the following conditions should be considered.
   a. Torsion of an ovarian cyst
   b. Enlarged cystic corpus luteum
   c. Hemorrhagic corpus luteum
   d. Appendicular abscess

6. Distended bladder. Unusually distended bladder or bladder diverticulum ultrasonographically may simulate an ovarian cyst or ovarian mass most of the time. An insertion of a Foley catheter is of great assistance.

7. Hematometra. Complete obstruction below or at the level of the cervix during menstrual life can cause detectable mass. As previously described, an imperforate hymen may cause hematocolpos, hematotrachelos, hematometra, and hematosalpinx.

8. Cystic degeneration of fibroid uterus.

9. Mesenteric cyst.

10. Polycystic kidney disease.

11. Pelvic kidney.

12. Retroperitoneal pelvic neoplasia.

13. Hematoma of the rectus.

14. Adherence of omentum.

15. Carcinoma of sigmoid.

16. Tuboovarian masses.

17. Ascites.

CONGENITAL ANOMALIES

Congenital anomalies of the genital tract are related to maldevelopment of the embryonic müllerian ducts and urogenital sinus. The majority of congenital anomalies of the vagina and uterus are caused by failure of the müllerian ducts to fuse completely. The müllerian ducts in the embryo migrate caudally and midline to fuse in the formation of the rudimentary uterus, cervix, and upper vagina. Abnormalities in the development of the müllerian ducts lead to congenital absence or atresia of the vagina, double or septate vagina, double uterus, absent uterus, and uterus unicornis. These anomalies are frequently accompanied by congenital defects of the urinary tract such as absent or ectopic kidneys. Developmental defects of the urogenital sinus create the imperforate hymen and persistent urogenital sinus membrane.

The ultrasonographer must be aware of the gross pathologic changes of the internal genitalia and urinary tract associated with external anomalies of the genital organs for effective pelvic scanning.

VAGINAL ANOMALIES

Absence of the vagina is a severe congenital anomaly due to complete lack of union of the müllerian ducts. The vagina is derived from different tissues. The lower one-third of the vagina is usually unaffected and may appear externally intact and anatomically correct. The diagnosis may not be made until adolescence when the symptoms of amenorrhea, dyspareunia, or hematocolpos present. Other failures of müllerian duct fusion result in double vagina, with a complete longitudinal'septum, or a partial septate vagina with an incomplete septum. A rudimentary second vagina may fill with secretions and produce a cystic lesion bulging into the vaginal canal.

The imperforate hymen is due to developmental error of the urogenital sinus and is the most frequent genital anomaly. The hymen is located at the junction of the vagina and the vestibule. This membrane is usually thin and sheetlike, although it may be thick and fibrous. The application of ultrasonic diagnosis in this area is extremely important, and may show the echo-free appearance of retained secretions or old blood behind the hymen. The vagina and uterus may be sufficiently distended with blood to produce hematocolpos and hematometrium. This may present as amenorrhea, an abdominal mass, or the area may become secondarily infected. Ultrasonography in this case will show the fluid-filled vagina as tubular in shape and echo free. The posterior fornix will also bulge while the uterus is engorged with blood and appears as an enlarged structure with an echo-free lumen of variable size. The presence of hematosalpinx and hemoperitoneum should be carefully investigated by the ultrasonographer.

UTERINE ANOMALIES

Disorders of the müllerian ducts result either from failure of formation of these embryonic structures or from failure of their fusion. The anomalies may be unilateral or bilateral.

Unilateral absence of the duct results in uterus unicornis with a normal vagina and cervix. The uterus possesses only one cornu and fallopian tube. Bilateral absence of the ducts is associated with congenital absence of the uterus and vagina.

Imperfection of fusion causes duplication anomalies of the uterus. The double uterus may be externally intact with two internal cavities formed by a longitudinal ridge of tissue. This septation may be complete, producing two uterine cavities, or incomplete, giving partial separation of the uterine cavity. This latter is called a subseptate uterus. The uterus may be divided externally in the more severe forms of fusion defects, producing two uteri. Uterus arcuatus is a heart-shaped uterus with minimal external division. A partial fusion defect produces the bicornuate uterus. The resultant two uteri are associated with a single common cervix. The most extreme variety of fusion failure results in uterus didelphys with two completely independent uteri, each capable of sustaining normal pregnancy. This is often accompanied by a double vagina deformity.

Asymmetric duplication anomalies produce rudimentary horns which may or may not communicate with the remaining uterine cavity. Clinical problems arise when gestational implantation occurs in this type of horn or retained menstrual flow dilates the noncommunicating rudimentary horn, producing mass effect or rupture of this structure.

Septation defects may be clinically silent and never diagnosed in the preconception state or during the normal course of pregnancy. They may be incidentally detected at cesarean section after removal of the fetus and manual exploration of the uterine cavity. The most common symptoms of uterine duplication are repeated abortion, premature delivery, and difficult labor with malposition and dystocia. Ultrasonography of the uterus must be accompanied by renal ultrasonography to evaluate the presence of the frequently associated urinary tract abnormalities. Since ultrasonography is technically a laparotomy with sound waves, septations of the uterus are best revealed with scanning in multiple planes. This diagnostic ability depends upon the examiner's experience and his previous exposure to similar cases. In our experience, the transverse lie is the most common malpresentation. Our customary method is to evaluate all transverse lies, in which external version attempts have failed, by ultrasound with the specific intention of demonstrating a uterine anomaly as one of the causes of malpresentation. We find that Trendelenburg's position is often a useful maneuver in addition to routine scanning planes.

Although contrast hysterosalpingography best shows the internal uterine cavity, it does not show the external configuration of the uterus. This test also cannot safely be performed during early pregnancy and allow continuation of gestation. Hysterography is limited in that it will not show a rudimentary horn that does not communicate with the uterine cavity. Ultrasound may show the gross extent of the intrauterine septation as well as the outer shape of the uterus. The site of gestation may be evaluated and the growth and the relative position of each uterine cavity may be assessed. Serial ultrasonography may allow preliminary diagnosis of a genital tract anomaly and still permit the patient with a miscarriage history to safely deliver a viable fetus due to proper obstetric management.

INFLAMMATORY PELVIC LESIONS

Ultrasound is not only extremely valuable in the detection of inflammatory diseases of certain size such as tuboovarian abscesses, hydrosalpinx, and pelvic abscesses, but is the only tool able to aid in follow-up of these conditions, ie, final surgical intervention or medical treatment. In addition, serial studies can give excellent information regarding pelvic mass associated with inflammatory disease. With this tool, subsidance or exacerbation of disease process can easily be recorded (5).

ENDOMETRIOSIS

Endometriosis with chocolate cyst produces different echo patterns relating to the size and duration of the process. It usually is of a complex nature.

METASTATIC LESION TO PELVIS

Metastatic lesion to the pelvis may produce any pattern and should be differentiated from pelvic masses by detecting the source of metastasis.

APPENDICEAL ABSCESS

Appendiceal abscess in our experience produces an echo-free area in the right lower quadrant with irregular borders. With interval serial studies, the course of the disease can be predicted.

FREE FLUID COLLECTION

Free fluid collection in the pelvic region can be detected ultrasonically and, by changing the patient's position, can be differentiated from loculated fluid. In free fluid, ascites, or loculated fluid, if the source is unknown, special attention should be directed toward the ovary.

REFERENCES

1. Von Micsky: Gynecologic Ultrasound. In King, DL (ed.): *Diagnostic Ultrasound*. St. Louis, CV Mosby, 1974, pp. 204–240
2. Haines M, Taylor CW: Gynecologic Pathology. Edinburgh, Churchill Livingstone,·1975, p 161
3. Kobagashi S, Sekiba K, Niwa K, et al: Ultrasonic classification of uterine myomas. Presented at 1st World Federation Ultrasound in Medicine and Biology, San Francisco, 1976
4. Guttman PH: Benign ovarian teratoma. Tip of the iceberg sign. Presented at 1st World Federation Ultrasound in Medicine and Biology, San Francisco, 1976
5. Uhrich PC, Sanders RC: Ultrasonic characteristics of pelvic inflammatory masses. J Clin Ultrasound 4:199, 1976

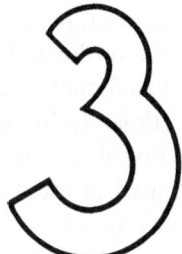

ultrasonography in obstetrics

GENERAL INTRODUCTION

The application of ultrasound in obstetrics and gynecology was first described by Donald et al in Europe in 1958 (1). In America it was described by Taylor et al in 1964 (2). Today, ultrasound is rapidly replacing the use of X-ray studies in the field of obstetrics and gynecology. Since ultrasound study is safe, atraumatic, and noninvasive, it is thus an ideal scanning procedure for the abdominal and pelvic regions. At present it is essential to the practice of modern obstetrics and gynecology.

Exploration with ultrasound proceeds with the patient placed in the supine position. After examining the abdomen, a coupling agent such as mineral oil is applied to the skin. As previously described, the umbilicus or the symphysis pubis is used as a reference point. In obstetric studies, it is better to choose the transcrestal plane and puboxiphoid line as reference points. This is of particular importance in the case of the pregnant woman with progression of conception and increasing fetal size. In pregnancy the umbilicus moves upward and comparison of earlier with later pictures is difficult. Transverse, longitudinal, and oblique scans with varying angulation are used to produce a diagnostic set of data suitable for comparison.

In obstetrics, B-mode or gray-scale two-dimensional ultrasound in combination with a real-time scanner yields the greatest diagnostic information. In scanning certain areas, such as the fetal head, the usage of A-mode adds more information and improves accuracy.

PATIENT HISTORY

The examiner's first procedure in using ultrasound is to take a proper history from the patient. All information should be recorded.

PATIENT'S AGE

The patient's age is critical in evaluating the history. For example, in the childbearing years, patients with bleeding most likely have reproductive disorders; while in adolescent females, the cause of bleeding with a normal utlrasonographic appearance has an endocrine basis. In postmenopausal females, the ultrasonographic examination of a patient with bleeding usually reveals a pelvic mass, and carcinoma of the genital tract is high in the list of differential diagnoses.

GRAVIDITY

Gravidity is synonymous with pregnancy. A primigravida is a female who is pregnant for the first time. A multigravida is a female with several previous pregnancies.

PARITY

The term parity is used when a female has given birth to an infant weighing 500 grams (g) or more, alive or dead. When the weight is not known, ultrasonography helps to estimate gestational age. A primipara is a female who has given birth

for the first time to an infant alive or dead with a minimal weight of 500 g. A multipara is a female who has given birth two or more times to infants weighing 500 g or more, alive or dead. The term grand multipara is applied to a female who has given birth seven or more times to infants weighing 500 g or more. In our history taking, we follow a scheme of recording obstetric data using four digits. The first number refers to the number of pregnancies, the second number refers to the number of premature deliveries, the third number refers to the number of abortions, and the fourth number refers to the number of living children. For example, 4-2-1-1 would mean four pregnancies, two premature deliveries, one abortion, and one living child.

PARTURIENT

A parturient is a female in the process of giving birth.

PUERPERA

A puerperal female is one who has given birth during the past 42 days.

MENSTRUATION

The date of the last normal menstrual period (LNMP) should be thoroughly investigated.

In primary dysmenorrhea, there is usually no ultrasonographic demonstrable pelvic mass at the condition's inception. In secondary dysmenorrhea, usually there is a demonstrable pelvic disease which may or may not be detected ultrasonographically.

Changes in menstrual patterns should be carefully evaluated and differentiated from uterine bleeding unrelated to menses. Menorrhagia or hypermenorrhea involves prolonged menstrual bleeding. Metrorrhagia is irregular or actually acyclic bleeding. Menometrorrhagia is excessive or irregular uterine bleeding between as well as during menstruations. Oligomenorrhagia is a reduction of the menstrual frequency. As a result, the interval between the cycles is longer than 28 days, but usually less than 3 months. Polymenorrhea is abnormally frequent menstruation. Abnormalities of bleeding during menstruation usually have an endocrine origin.

Intermenstrual bleeding usually has ultrasonographically demonstrable benign or malignant causes. Bleeding after intercourse or douching may have malignant causes.

PAIN

The ultrasonographic importance of the history of pain is related to the fact that certain masses can produce special types of pain. For example, localized pain in the lower abdomen may arise from the uterus or vagina.

Adnexal pain is usually referable to the lower abdomen and often radiates to the medial aspect of the thigh. Sharp pain with sudden onset may be due to torsion of pedunculated fibroid.

We have a special history sheet, shown in Table 3.1, which may be completed by either the nurse, technician, examiner, or even the patient in a short period of time. The physician can thus get enough information to collate with the ultrasonographic findings for final interpretation.

PALPATION OF THE ABDOMEN BEFORE EXAMINATION

In the twelfth week of pregnancy, the uterus usually can be felt by manual abdominal examination just above the symphysis pubis. The abdominal enlargement is less pronounced in nulliparas than in multiparas.

CHANGES IN UTERINE SIZE DURING PREGNANCY

In the first few weeks of gestation, the increase in size of the uterus is in the anteroposterior direction. As time passes, the uterus becomes

TABLE 3.1 History Profile

1. BLEEDING		
Normal menstruation	yes	no
Intermenstrual bleeding	yes	no
Contact bleeding	yes	no
2. PAIN		
Is pain related to menstruation?	yes	no
Does pain radiate?	yes	no
Is pain localized?	yes	no
3. VAGINAL DISCHARGE		
Is discharge accompanied by pain?	yes	no
Is discharge heavy?	yes	no
Is discharge more than two weeks?	yes	no
Does discharge have color or odor?	yes	no
4. HISTORY OF CONTRACEPTIVE USE		
Do you have IUCD?	yes	no
Duration of use	—	—
Is this type of IUCD effective?	yes	no
Do you discharge with IUCD?	yes	no
5. HISTORY OF INTERCOURSE		
Do you have regular intercourse?	yes	no
Do you have painful intercourse?	yes	no
6. HISTORY OF MEDICAL PROBLEMS		
Do you have diabetes?	yes	no
Do you have hypertension?	yes	no
Do you have cardiac disease?	yes	no
Do you have renal disease?	yes	no
Do you have history of syphilis?	yes	no
Do you have history of TBC?	yes	no
Do you have epilepsy?	yes	no
Do you have allergies?	yes	no
Do you take any medication	yes	no
7. SURGICAL HISTORY		
Did you have any operations?	yes	no
Date of operation	—	—
Place of operation	—	—
Diagnosis	—	—
Result	—	—
8. FAMILY HISTORY		
Do you have twinning?	yes	no
Do you have hereditary disease?	yes	no
9. SOCIAL HISTORY		
Do you use tobacco?	yes	no
Do you use alcohol?	yes	no
What is your occupation?	—	—
10. BREAST HISTORY		
Do you have any breast disease?	yes	no
Do you have any discharge from nipples?	yes	no
Do you have any tenderness?	yes	no
Did you have any operations on the breasts?	yes	no

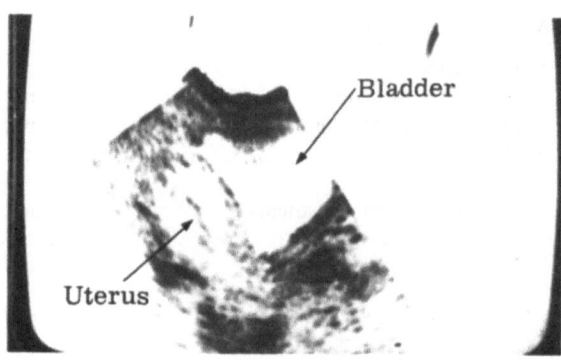

FIGURE 3.1(a)
Supine longitudinal scan. Gray scale. The distended bladder noted anteriorly. The echogenic uterus is seen posterior to the bladder. Central echoes represent uterine cavity.

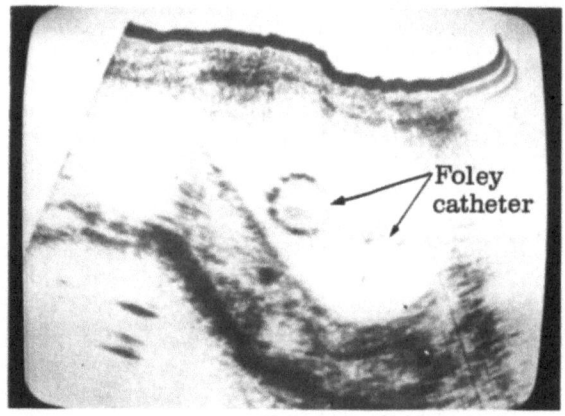

FIGURE 3.1(b)
Supine longitudinal scan. Gray scale. The rounded echoes of the Foley catheter balloon are noted in the bladder. The enlarged uterus is seen posterior to the bladder.

FIGURE 3.1(c)
Supine longitudinal scan. Gray scale. The rounded echogenic Foley catheter balloon is noted in the distended bladder.

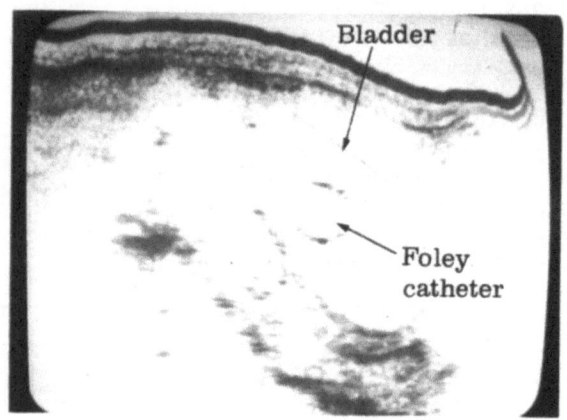

globular and by 10 to 12 weeks it measures an average diameter of 8 cm.

In pregnancy associated with inflammatory process or carcinoma of the cervix, the cervix from the early phase of gestation may remain enlarged.

SONOANATOMY

The detailed sonoanatomy of the female pelvis has been described in Chapter 2. However, a few additions deserve to be mentioned here. The skin, adipose tissue, muscular layers, and planes of the abdominal wall can be delineated by proper gain setting. The omentum and bowel have irregular, disorganized groups of echoes (3). The spine is easily identified as a posterior structure stopping sound transmission. The normal uterus is easily identified (Fig. 3.1a).

SONOLAPAROTOMY

In the nonpregnant female the symphysis pubis and small intestine shield the pelvic organs. Ultrasound consequently cannot penetrate the pelvic organs to delineate the anatomy of the uterus and adnexal structures.

Before examination, the bladder should be distended for better penetration of the ultrasonic beam. Bladder distention is accomplished by having the patient drink a large amount of fluid and instructing her not to void before examination. A filled bladder displaces the uterus posteriorly while it displaces the small intestine superiorly. Consequently, a transmitting window is created through which the beam can be more effectively angled, thus permitting better delineation of the pelvic organs. By directing the beam at various angles, the characteristic echoes of the pelvic organs can be registered with as little attenuation as possible.

In some patients it is necessary to fill the bladder with a Foley catheter in order to distend the of the menstrual frequency. As a result, the interval between the cycles is longer than 28 days, but usually less than 3 months. Polymenorrhea is abnormally frequent menstruation. Abnormalities of bleeding during menstruation usually have an endocrine origin.

Intermenstrual bleeding usually has ultrasonographically demonstrable benign or malignant causes. Bleeding after intercourse or douching may have malignant causes.

PAIN

The ultrasonographic importance of the history of pain is related to the fact that certain masses can produce special types of pain. For example, localized pain in the lower abdomen may arise from the uterus or vagina.

Adnexal pain is usually referable to the lower abdomen and often radiates to the medial aspect of the thigh. Sharp pain with sudden onset may be due to torsion of pedunculated fibroid.

We have a special history sheet, shown in Table 3.1, which may be completed by either the nurse, technician, examiner, or even the patient in a short period of time. The physician can thus get enough information to collate with the ultrasonographic findings for final interpretation.

PALPATION OF THE ABDOMEN BEFORE EXAMINATION

In the twelfth week of pregnancy, the uterus usually can be felt by manual abdominal examination just above the symphysis pubis. The abdominal enlargement is less pronounced in nulliparas than in multiparas.

CHANGES IN UTERINE SIZE DURING PREGNANCY

In the first few weeks of gestation, the increase in size of the uterus is in the anteroposterior direction. As time passes, the uterus becomes

TABLE 3.1 History Profile

1. BLEEDING		
Normal menstruation	yes	no
Intermenstrual bleeding	yes	no
Contact bleeding	yes	no
2. PAIN		
Is pain related to menstruation?	yes	no
Does pain radiate?	yes	no
Is pain localized?	yes	no
3. VAGINAL DISCHARGE		
Is discharge accompanied by pain?	yes	no
Is discharge heavy?	yes	no
Is discharge more than two weeks?	yes	no
Does discharge have color or odor?	yes	no
4. HISTORY OF CONTRACEPTIVE USE		
Do you have IUCD?	yes	no
Duration of use	—	—
Is this type of IUCD effective?	yes	no
Do you discharge with IUCD?	yes	no
5. HISTORY OF INTERCOURSE		
Do you have regular intercourse?	yes	no
Do you have painful intercourse?	yes	no
6. HISTORY OF MEDICAL PROBLEMS		
Do you have diabetes?	yes	no
Do you have hypertension?	yes	no
Do you have cardiac disease?	yes	no
Do you have renal disease?	yes	no
Do you have history of syphilis?	yes	no
Do you have history of TBC?	yes	no
Do you have epilepsy?	yes	no
Do you have allergies?	yes	no
Do you take any medication	yes	no
7. SURGICAL HISTORY		
Did you have any operations?	yes	no
Date of operation	—	—
Place of operation	—	—
Diagnosis	—	—
Result	—	—
8. FAMILY HISTORY		
Do you have twinning?	yes	no
Do you have hereditary disease?	yes	no
9. SOCIAL HISTORY		
Do you use tobacco?	yes	no
Do you use alcohol?	yes	no
What is your occupation?	—	—
10. BREAST HISTORY		
Do you have any breast disease?	yes	no
Do you have any discharge from nipples?	yes	no
Do you have any tenderness?	yes	no
Did you have any operations on the breasts?	yes	no

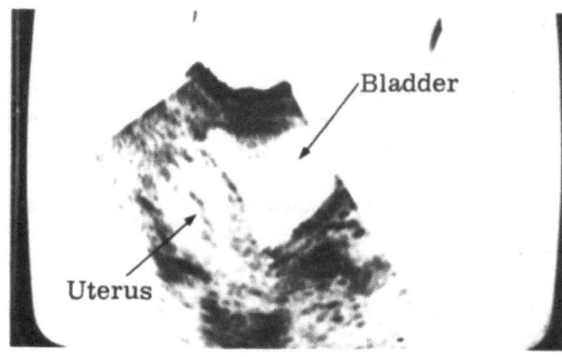

FIGURE 3.1(a)
Supine longitudinal scan. Gray scale. The distended bladder noted anteriorly. The echogenic uterus is seen posterior to the bladder. Central echoes represent uterine cavity.

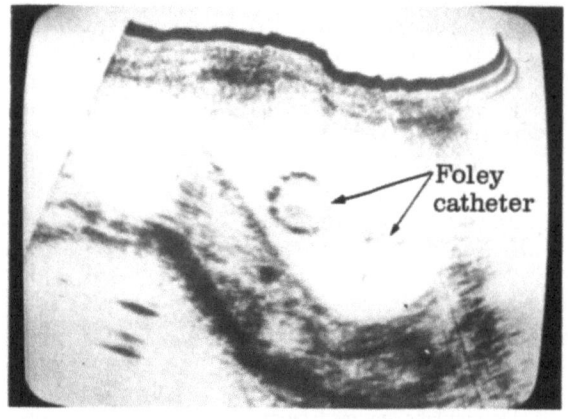

FIGURE 3.1(b)
Supine longitudinal scan. Gray scale. The rounded echoes of the Foley catheter balloon are noted in the bladder. The enlarged uterus is seen posterior to the bladder.

FIGURE 3.1(c)
Supine longitudinal scan. Gray scale. The rounded echogenic Foley catheter balloon is noted in the distended bladder.

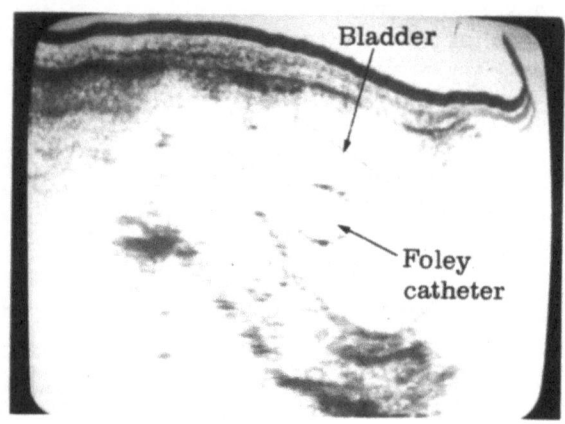

globular and by 10 to 12 weeks it measures an average diameter of 8 cm.

In pregnancy associated with inflammatory process or carcinoma of the cervix, the cervix from the early phase of gestation may remain enlarged.

SONOANATOMY

The detailed sonoanatomy of the female pelvis has been described in Chapter 2. However, a few additions deserve to be mentioned here. The skin, adipose tissue, muscular layers, and planes of the abdominal wall can be delineated by proper gain setting. The omentum and bowel have irregular, disorganized groups of echoes (3). The spine is easily identified as a posterior structure stopping sound transmission. The normal uterus is easily identified (Fig. 3.1a).

SONOLAPAROTOMY

In the nonpregnant female the symphysis pubis and small intestine shield the pelvic organs. Ultrasound consequently cannot penetrate the pelvic organs to delineate the anatomy of the uterus and adnexal structures.

Before examination, the bladder should be distended for better penetration of the ultrasonic beam. Bladder distention is accomplished by having the patient drink a large amount of fluid and instructing her not to void before examination. A filled bladder displaces the uterus posteriorly while it displaces the small intestine superiorly. Consequently, a transmitting window is created through which the beam can be more effectively angled, thus permitting better delineation of the pelvic organs. By directing the beam at various angles, the characteristic echoes of the pelvic organs can be registered with as little attenuation as possible.

In some patients it is necessary to fill the bladder with a Foley catheter in order to distend the bladder in various stages for proper evaluation of the uterus and pelvic region. The bladder may need to be filled and then emptied by degrees and then refilled for optimal diagnosis. The use of a catheter is necessary for quantitative filling of the bladder and for the patient who arrives for an ultrasonographic procedure with an incompletely filled bladder (Fig. 3.1b and c).

The distended bladder is echo free. This cystic-type structure is located below the symphysis pubis. In nonpregnant women the uterus also appears echo poor behind the bladder at low sensitivity. The size of the normal uterus varies with age, menstrual function, and parity. Clear delineation of the normal ovaries and other adnexal structures is extremely difficult. These organs may be mistaken for one another. Pathologic changes of these organs may make the recognition of individual structures easier.

Our application of the anterior transcrestal plane (ATC) and longitudinal xiphoid pubis (LXP) systems of identification over a period of four years has proven to be of great practical value. This appears, in our opinion, to be the most useful method of marking the skin in relation to the bony structures for amniocentesis and other procedures where the patient may need to be removed from the ultrasound department and have a subsequent procedure performed by other physicians.

In early pregnancy or in the case of small pelvic lesions, the interval between sections is approximately 1 cm. In later pregnancy or with large pelvic masses, sections at 2- to 4-cm intervals may be used. However, the type of sectioning and the intervals used are up to the examiner. Permanent records can be obtained through the use of a Polaroid or 90-mm filming from the oscilloscope. Gray-scale images are usually obtained from the screen of a scan converter. A series of pictures is then taken to complete the study. These include the transverse sections, ATC series, and the longitudinal sections, LXP series, which are attached in order so they may be displayed for final interpretation. The transverse pictures are arranged in an ascending manner and the longitudinal pictures (from left to right) are attached in sequence.

The screen of the oscilloscope is divided into centimeter equivalents. Therefore, the centimeter is used as a reference for measurement of the sonogram. The oscilloscope screen may be calibrated into 1-, 2-, or 3-cm divisions. Using needle-point calipers, the biparietal diameter of the head or the anterioposterior diameter of the fetal chest can be measured. Direct digital read-out systems are commercially available with electronic calipers.

SONOFLUOROSCOPY OF THE PREGNANT UTERUS

The uterus is initially examined by rapid scanning to familiarize the ultrasonographer with the location of the fetus, its lie and presentation, and site of the placenta. This screening may be performed with either the real-time scanner (Fig. 3.2), bistable unit (Fig. 3.3), or gray-scale machine (Fig. 3.4). The presence of a variable persistence oscilloscope with a rapidly fading scan image as the transducer is quickly traversing the uterus is of added value. Maximum information is obtained in the longitudinal scanning planes. Further data are acquired in the transverse plane.

The position of the fetus is first identified. The location of the head in either the breech (Fig. 3.5a) or vertex (Fig. 3.5b) presentation is studied. The cranial vault is echogenic and appears as a circle of high-amplitude echoes. The circle of echoes produced by the body is of lower echo amplitude. The fetal thorax is found and the relationship of the fetal head to the fetal body and thorax is noted (Fig. 3.6a). This is important in abnormal fetal lie where intrauterine rotational maneuvers are considered. The fetal respiratory excursions are monitored either with A-mode, M-mode, or the real-time scanner. The fetal aorta is followed from the heart as it descends into the fetal abdomen (Fig. 3.6b). The relation of the aorta to the spine is noted with the real-time scanner. The echogenic liver and spleen in

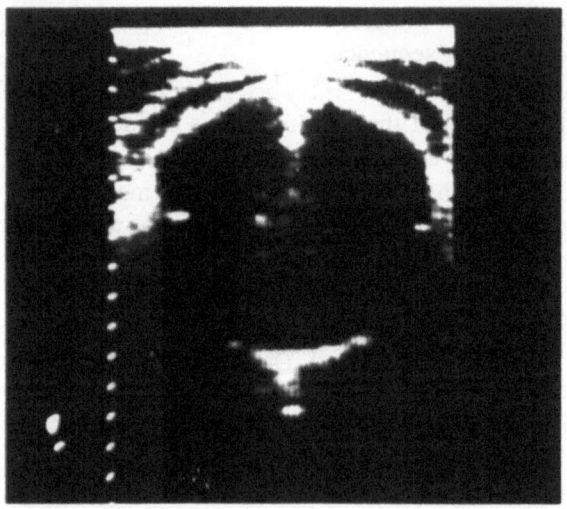

FIGURE 3.2
Supine transverse scan. Real-time scanner. The fetal head is scanned in the vertex position. The typical ovoid shape and midline echo complex are obtained by manipulation of the scanning head.

FIGURE 3.3
Supine transverse scan. B-mode. To obtain the optimal biparietal diameter, A-mode and B-mode are used. The sensitivity is decreased so that only the calvarial echoes and midline echoes are imaged. Care must be taken to position the falx echoes exactly in the middle of the cranial cavity.

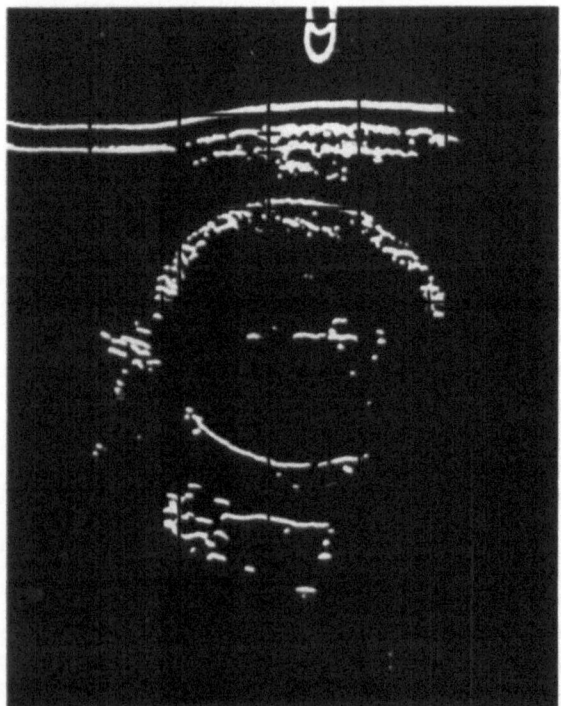

the abdomen are found as are the echo-free stomach, gallbladder, and umbilical vein. The kidneys (Fig. 3.7) are studied for possible hydronephrosis from obstructive uropathy or other renal anomaly. The bladder is identified in the pelvis (Fig. 3.8a). The fetal genitalia are searched for at the region of the perineum. The fetal scrotum and penis may be evaluated if they are not obscured by overlying fetal structures (Fig. 3.8b). The number and motion of the extremities are observed for possible fetal anomaly or nervous system disorder.

The umbilical cord is followed from the placenta (Fig. 3.9) to the insertion into the fetal umbilicus (Fig. 3.10). The position of the placenta is located (Fig. 3.11). The presence of physiologic placental degeneration is studied and pathologic placental echo patterns may be demonstrated. Shadowing of fetal parts by the posterior placenta is commonly encountered (Fig. 3.8a). The relationship of the placenta to the internal cervical os is identified.

In obese or large-for-date patients, the ultrasonographer looks for multiple gestation (Fig. 3.12), polyhydramnios, and other disorders. We find that the fetal head is best studied for twin gestation with the real-time scanner. Rapid scanning with the gray-scale unit

FIGURE 3.4
Supine transverse scan. Demonstration of fetal head with gray scale. Note midline echo pattern and anterior reverberation artifacts. Measurement of biparietal diameter is performed from the darkest anterior to the darkest distal echoes of the bony calvarium.

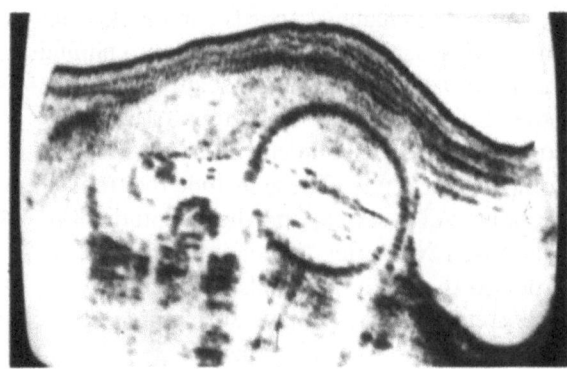

FIGURE 3.5(a)
Supine longitudinal scan. Gray scale. The fetus is in the breech presentation. The middle portion of the posterior placenta is indented by the fetal head and body.

FIGURE 3.5(b)
Supine longitudinal scan. Gray scale. The fetus is in the vertex presentation. The middle portion of the anterior placenta is indented by the flexed fetal knee which extends from the fetal hip and returns from the placenta as the fetal leg which tapers appropriately.

FIGURE 3.6(a)
Supine longitudinal scan. Gray scale. The fetal aorta appears as a parallel series of lines passing from the thorax into the abdomen. The pulsatile nature of this structure is best shown with M-mode or real-time scanning.

FIGURE 3.6(b)
Supine transverse scan. The fetal aorta appears as a parallel series of lines passing from the thorax into the abdomen.

FIGURE 3.7
Supine cross-sectional scan. Gray scale. On either side of the echogenic fetal spine are the kidney outlines. One kidney is echo-free since the cut is above the level of the calyceal system. The central echo pattern is clearly visible in the other kidney.

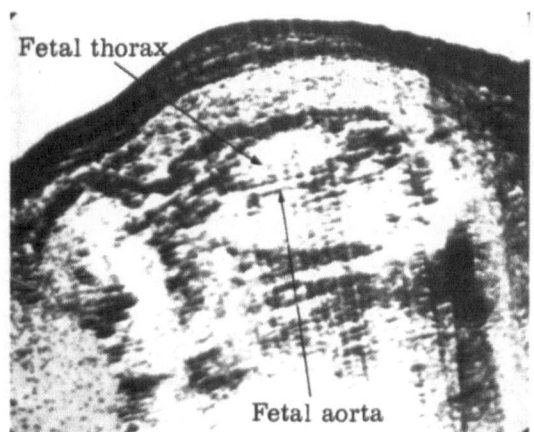

FIGURE 3-6(a)

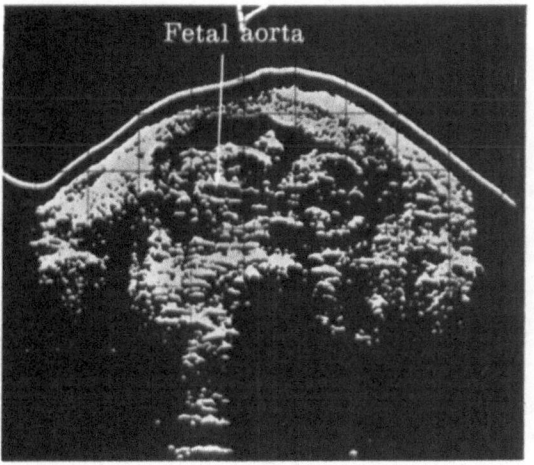

FIGURE 3-6(b)

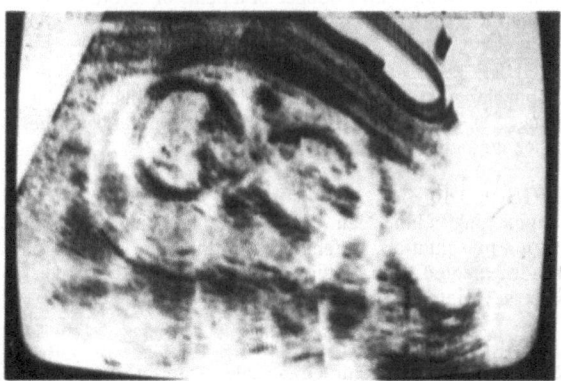

FIGURE 3-5(a)

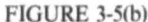
FIGURE 3-5(b)

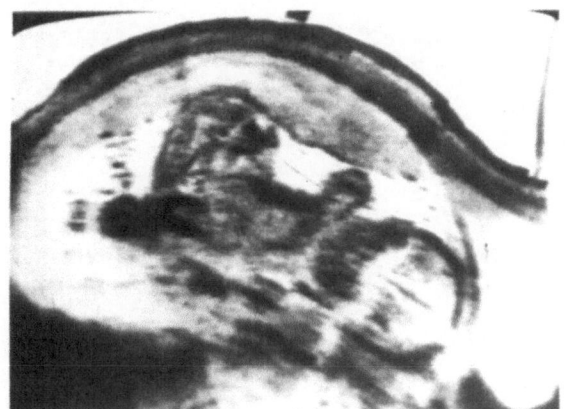

FIGURE 3-7

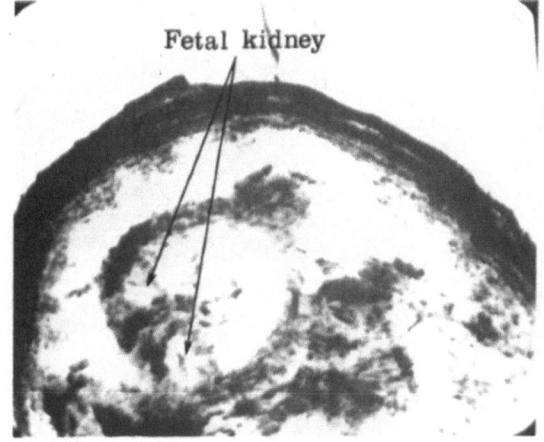

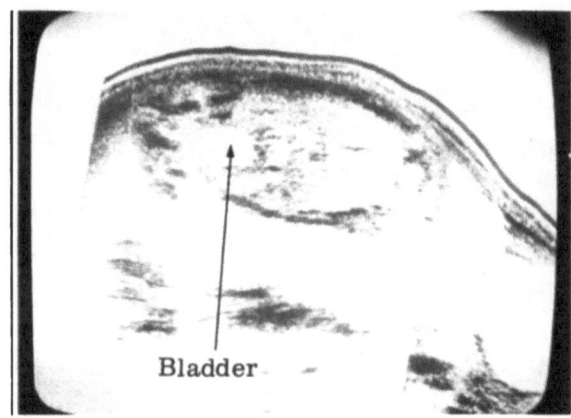

FIGURE 3-8 (a)

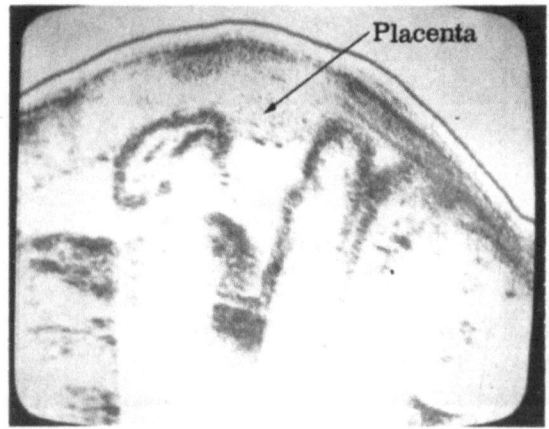

FIGURE 3-10

FIGURE 3.8(a)
Supine longitudinal scan. Gray scale. The fetal body is seen in longitudinal scan and the echo-free region in the fetal pelvis represents the fetal bladder. Note posterior placenta.

FIGURE 3.8(b)
Supine longitudinal scan. Gray scale. The fetus is in the vertex presentation. The fetal buttocks are noted facing ventrally. There is no evidence of a penis or scrotum. A female was delivered.

FIGURE 3.9
Supine longitudinal scan. Gray scale. The umbilical cord is imaged as a stepladder-type of echo passing between the placenta and the umbilicus.

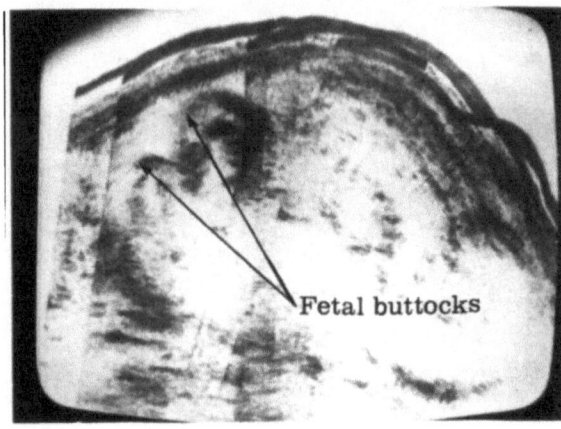

FIGURE 3-8 (b)

FIGURE 3.10
Supine longitudinal scan. Gray scale. The fetus lies in the vertex presentation. Extending from the anterior placenta is the fragmented echo pattern of the umbilical cord which enters the fetal abdomen.

FIGURE 3.11
Supine longitudinal scan. Gray scale. Anterior placenta. The fetal parts are scanned in a perpendicular manner and produce a sonic shadow so that distal structures may not be adequately imaged.

FIGURE 3-9

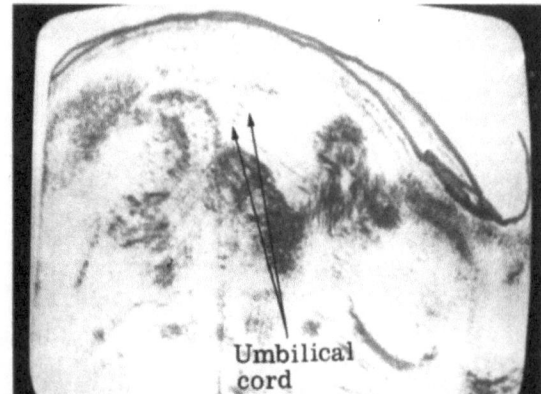

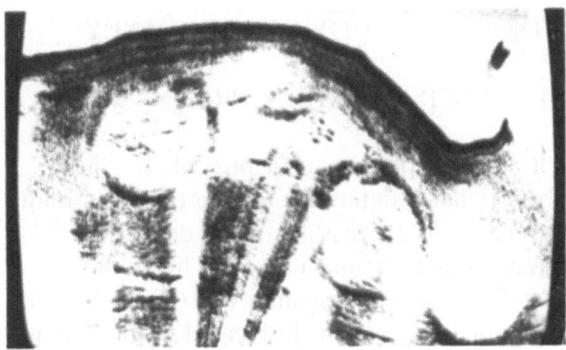

FIGURE 3.12
Supine longitudinal scan. Gray scale. Rounded high-amplitude structures appear at both poles of the uterus and represent fetal heads. Twin gestation is identified when two fetal heads and two placentas are noted. The fetal head is distinguished from the fetal thorax by the absence of fetal heart motion.

will also provide satisfactory information. If there is difficulty in observing the head, the presence of two placentas is proof of twin gestation. Care must be taken not to mistake a right or left lateral placenta with its anterior and posterior extensions as a double placenta (Figs. 3.13–3.15). The presence of two umbilical cords and two fetal heartbeats with M-mode are confirmatory findings. Three fetal heads may be observed but are difficult to image together in one plane. The appearance of more than three heads is ultrasonographically confusing at times and accurate counting may not be possible.

The small-for-date patient is studied for possible fetal anomaly, such as anencephaly or microcephaly, and the relationship of the size of the fetal head to the body is noted. The transmission of aortic pulsation can be detected by the real-time scanner or gray scale (Fig. 3.16). When sonofluoroscopy is completed, special attention may be given to each fetal structure with appropriate measurements.

FIGURE 3.13
Supine transverse scan. Gray scale. In multiple sections, a fundal placenta with anterior, posterior, and both lateral extensions is seen.

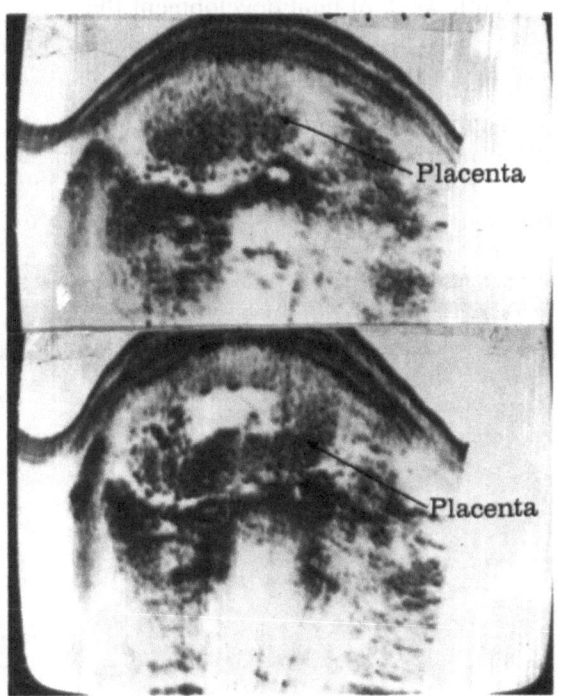

FIGURE 3.14
Supine transverse scan. Gray scale. In multiple sections a fundal placenta with anterior and posterior extensions is seen.

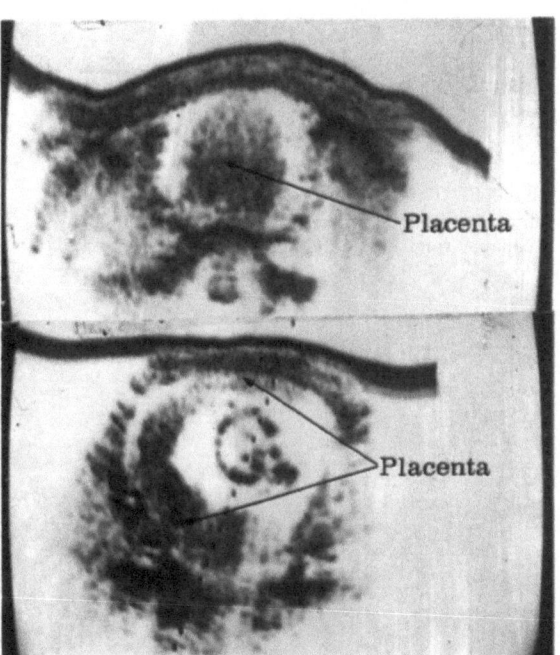

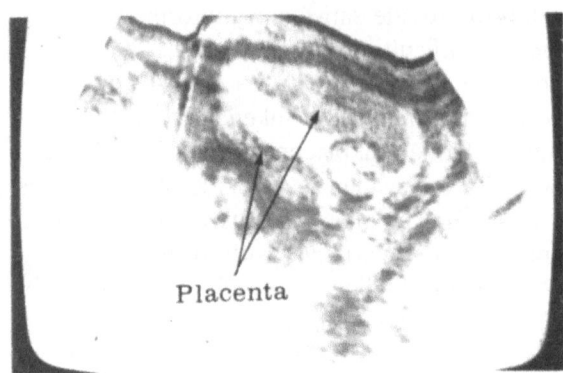

FIGURE 3.15
Supine longitudinal scan. Gray scale. Care must be taken not to mistake a right or left lateral placenta with its anterior and posterior extensions as a double placenta.

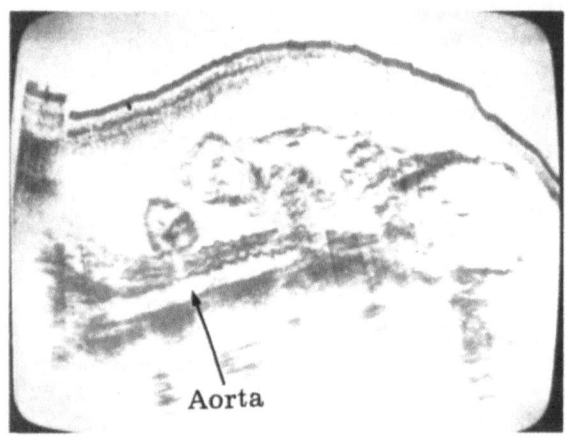

FIGURE 3.16
Supine transverse scan. Gray scale. The transmission of aortic pulsation can be detected by real-time scanner or gray scale.

FIGURE 3.17
Supine longitudinal scan. Gray scale. The gestational sac or pregnancy ring seen in the fundus of the uterus.

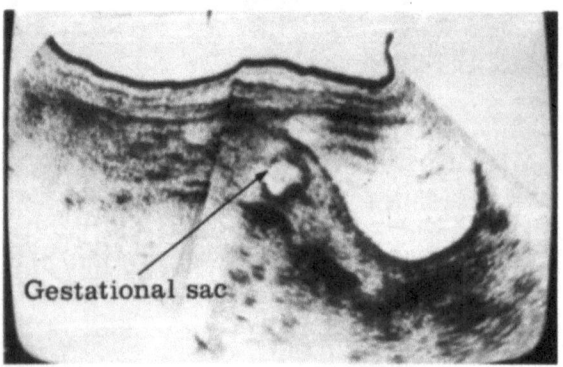

SONOPHYSIOLOGY OF PREGNANCY

DIAGNOSIS OF EARLY PREGNANCY

Ultrasonography makes it possible for the obstetrician to determine early pregnancy. In the uterine cavity there is a group of dense echoes arranged in a circular pattern. This is the gestational sac or pregnancy ring (Fig. 3.17). The gestational sac is usually located in the upper half of the uterus (Fig. 3.18). A low-lying gestational sac may signify an impending spontaneous abortion (4). Our experience has shown that the gestational sac may be found in any portion of the uterine cavity and still follow its normal course of development. The gestational sac should not be mistaken with a small cystic lesion of the endometrium (Fig. 3.19). Before examination the bladder should be distended. An overdistended bladder or the presence of a pelvic mass may flatten the gestational sac (Figs. 3.20 and 3.21). Optimally, the pregnancy ring or gestational sac can be recognized at 5 weeks gestation, which corresponds to 7 weeks from the last normal menstrual period. The identifying echoes should be regular in shape and centrally located within the uterine cavity (Fig. 3.22). From the sixth to the tenth week of fetal development the gestational sac enlarges until its edges fuse with the wall of the uterus.

As mentioned, pregnancy can be diagnosed ultrasonographically from the fifth week of

FIGURE 3.18
Supine longitudinal scan. Gray scale. The usual location of the gestational sac is in the upper half of the uterus.

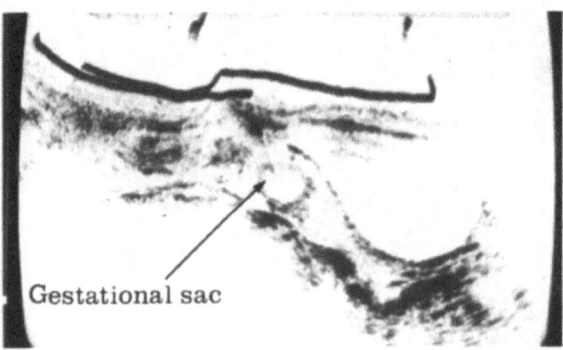

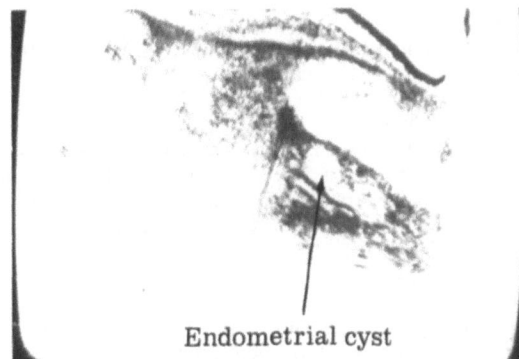

Endometrial cyst

FIGURE 3-19

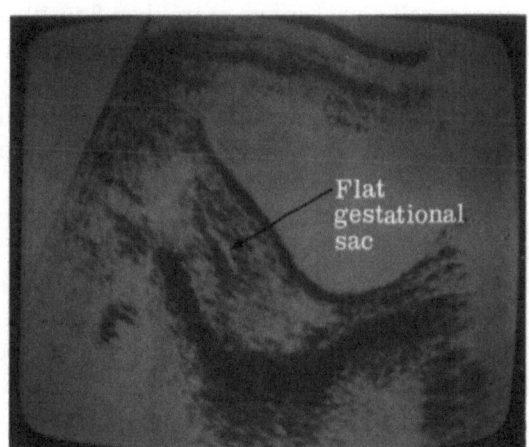

Flat gestational sac

FIGURE 3-20

FIGURE 3-21

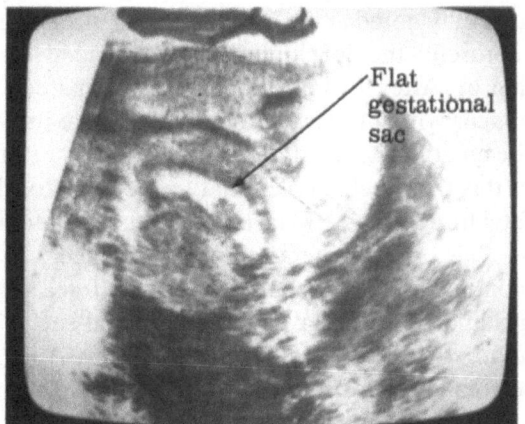

Flat gestational sac

gestation. Considering the 15 percent incidence of false positive and false negative results with immunologic pregnancy tests, ultrasonography not only adds information but is a confirmatory test.

The gestational sac is usually noted as a circular configuration of echoes within the enlarged uterus. It is extremely important to obtain echoes from the entire margin of the gestational sac to evaluate the architecture of the pregnancy ring as a three-dimensional structure and to determine whether it is intact or broken and where such interruption in the wall may occur. The initial examination is performed in the sagittal plane with sections taken in the LXP system along the plane between the pubis and umbilicus. The sectioning interval must be small

FIGURE 3.19
Supine longitudinal scan. Gray scale. The gestational sac–like structure is seen within the uterine fundus and in the midline. No echogenic boundary is noted. This differentiates this cystic structure from the gestational sac. Diagnosis, endometrial cyst.

FIGURE 3.20
Supine longitudinal scan. Gray scale. Gestational sac of early pregnancy. Flat echogenic outline may be a normal variant of the usually rounded gestational sac, and may be due to an overdistended bladder.

FIGURE 3.21
Supine longitudinal scan. Gray scale. Note flattening of the gestational sac by a posteriorly located fibroid uterus with echogenic internal echo pattern.

FIGURE 3.22
Supine longitudinal scan. Gray scale. Echo pattern of a centrally located ring is noted in the uterine fundus. This is the ideal location for the gestational sac.

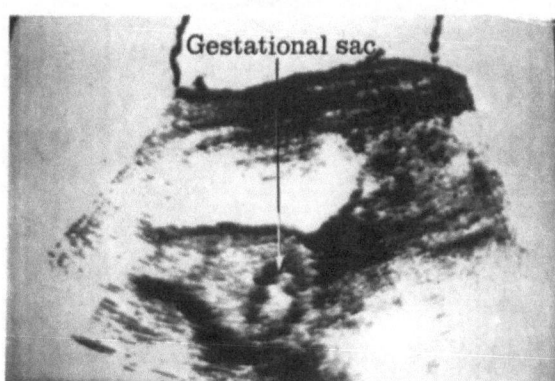

Gestational sac

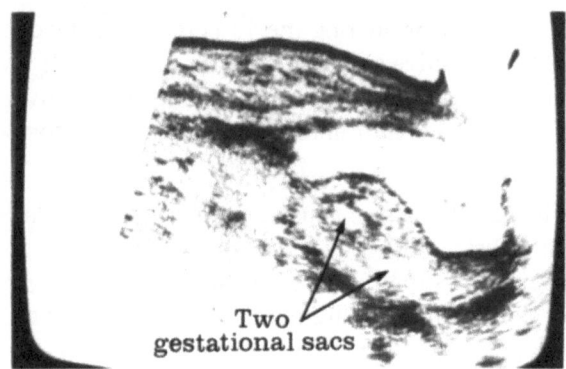

FIGURE 3-23

FIGURE 3.23
Supine longitudinal scan. Gray scale. Two gestational sacs noted inside the uterine cavity.

FIGURE 3.24(a)
Supine longitudinal scan. Gray scale. The thin echogenic rim of the gestational sac is noted with increased thickness of echoes along the periphery of the sac denoting the early placenta. Within the gestational sac scattered echoes identify the developing fetus.

FIGURE 3.24(b)
Supine transverse scan. Gray scale. Thickening of the gestational sac denotes formation of the early placenta. Fetal echoes are not yet noted.

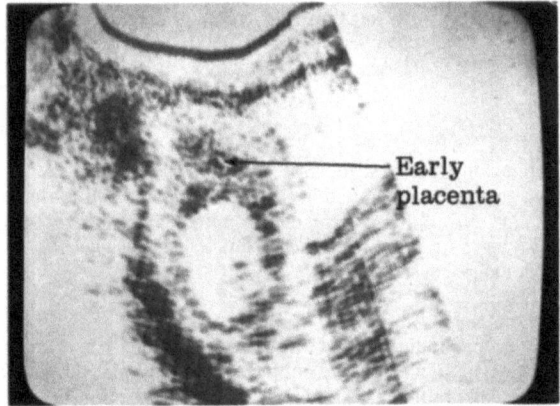

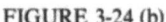

FIGURE 3-24 (a)

FIGURE 3-24 (b)

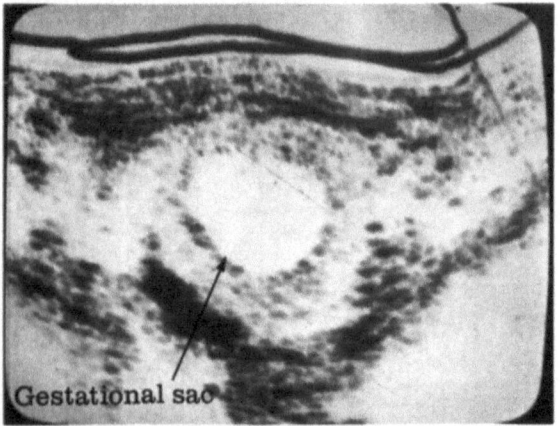

since the uterus and the contained pregnancy ring generally measure no more than 8 to 10 cm. We have found slices taken at 0.5-cm intervals satisfactory for the purpose of completely demonstrating the gestational sac. Occasionally, variations in the angulation of the transducer are needed to avoid any misinterpretation of gestational sac pathology. This is especially true if detection of more than one gestational sac is to be confirmed. The relationship of the gestational sac to the uterus is studied next in the sagittal plane to detect the shape, position, and number (Fig. 3.23). The study is then continued in the transverse plane or ATC system and the geometry of the gestational sac and uterus are corroborated to complete the three-dimensional sonolaparotomy of the uterus and the developing pregnancy. Serial examinations are added as necessary to follow the growth of the gestational sac.

A thickening of a portion of the pregnancy ring is generally noted at the eighth to ninth week which represents the developing placenta (Fig. 3.24a and b). After 9 weeks, localized internal echoes appear within the gestational sac and are due to the enlarging fetal outline (Fig. 3.25), and usually at this time the Doppler study is positive for the fetal heartbeat. At 10 to 13 weeks the gestational sac has been obliterated and is no longer identifiable by ultrasound. At about 10 weeks of gestation the border of the gestational sac approximates the wall of the uterus. As the pregnancy ring disappears gradually the placenta and fetal head will appear (Fig. 3.26).

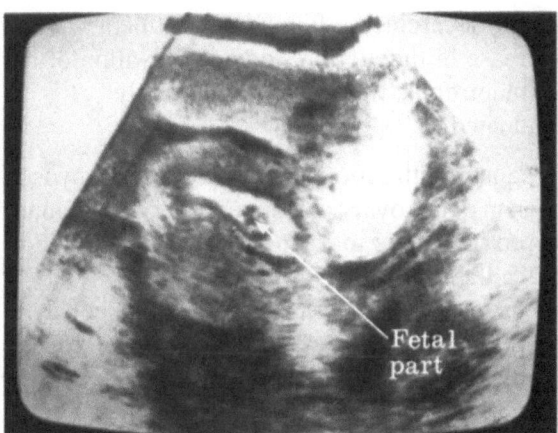

FIGURE 3-25

FIGURE 3.25
Supine longitudinal scan. Gray scale. Within the gestational sac is the amorphous echo pattern of the developing fetus. Motion is demonstrable with the real-time scanner. Nine weeks gestation.

FIGURE 3.26
Supine longitudinal scan. Gray scale. Thirteen weeks' gestation shows a placenta occupying 60 percent of the uterus. Within the echo-free amniotic fluid the early outline of the fetal head and body is demonstrable.

FIGURE 3.27
Supine transverse scan. Gray scale. The uterine outline is minimally enlarged. Scattered internal echoes are noted. Patient was in the fourth month of gestation. Incomplete abortion.

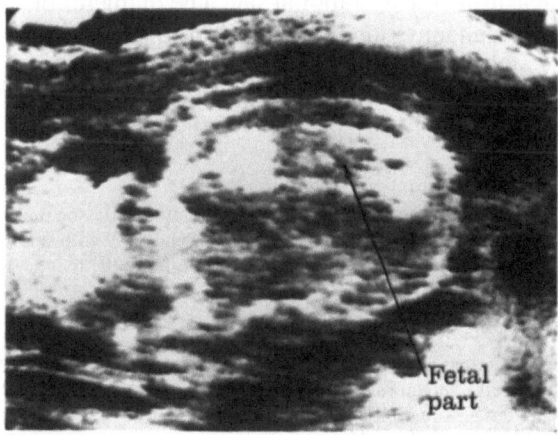

FIGURE 3-26

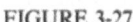

FIGURE 3-27

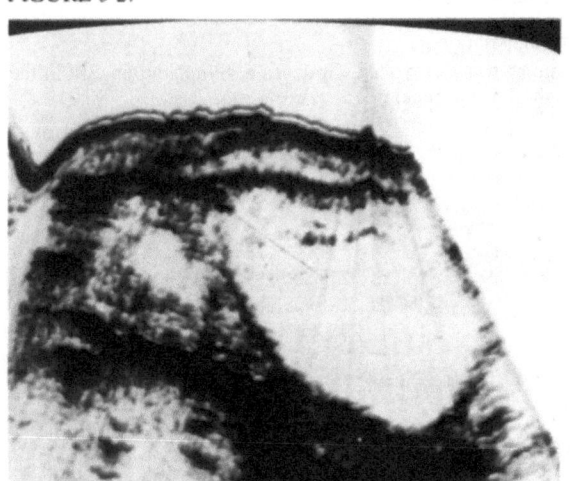

Abnormality of the gestational sac and a dilated cervix are indicative of an impending abortion. If the fetal structures do not appear within 9 to 10 weeks, a blighted ovum is suspected. When the borders of the gestational sac are ill-defined and irregular, pregnancy loss should be considered (Fig. 3.27).

As previously mentioned, the period of gestation from the tenth to the thirteenth week is the "gray zone" of ultrasonic diagnosis, since neither the gestational sac nor the fetal head can be imaged. Ultrasonography usually shows scattered formless internal echoes within the fluid-filled center of the uterus. If the initial examination is performed at this time, there may be diagnostic difficulty in distinguishing between normal pregnancy, hydatidiform mole, missed abortion, or fibroid uterus with cystic transformation (6). This problem may be ameliorated with the application of Doppler ultrasound, since the fetal heart is often detected at 12 weeks' gestation. The real-time scanner may also be used to detect intrauterine fetal motion which verifies a normal early pregnancy. The use of either Doppler ultrasound or real-time scanning during the "gray zone" of pregnancy may provide relief both to the worried patient and the ultrasonographer. Serial demonstration of fetal echoes differentiates the normal pregnancy from all conditions which cause dirty uterus when coupled with a pregnancy test when the uterus is enlarged. Development of choriocarcinoma after evacuation of hydatidiform mole, or recurrence

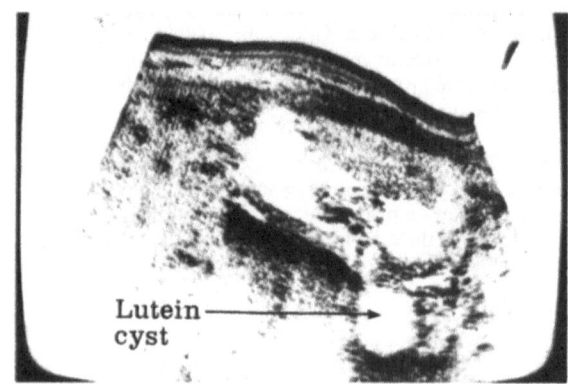

FFIGURE 3-28 (a)

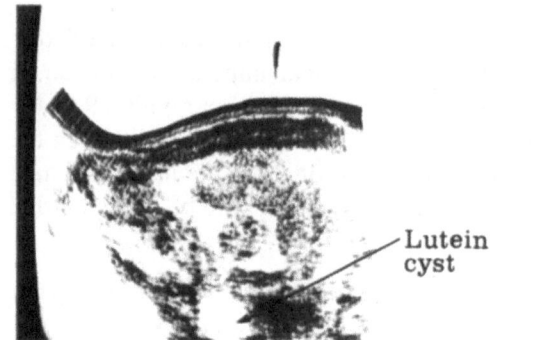

FFIGURE 3-28 (b)

FFIGURE 3-28 (c)

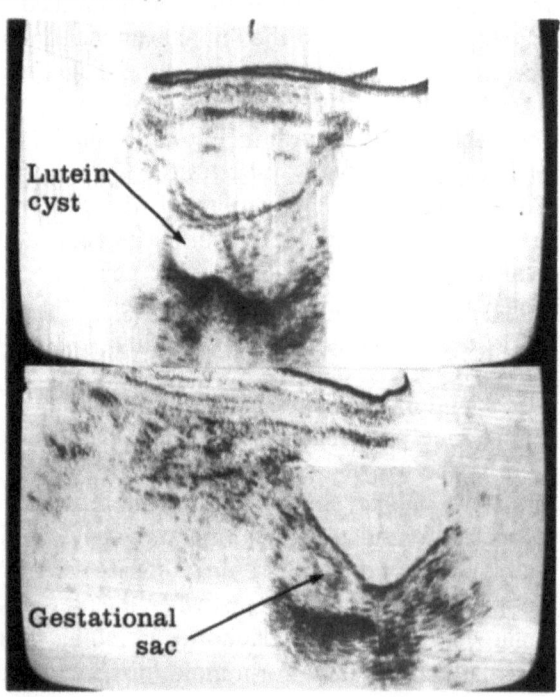

of choriocarcinoma following treatment with an increase in the uterine size and elevation of gonadotrophic titer, can be accurately evaluated.

Frequently, the corpus luteum of pregnancy is seen in either ovary and appears as a cystic mass approximately 2 to 4 cm in diameter (Fig. 3.28a,b,c, and d). With progression of pregnancy, the luteal cyst will spontaneously regress. Occasionally a luteal cyst may be large (simple or septate), and in rare instances may be hemorrhagic and cause complications of pregnancy, such as an abortion (Fig. 3.29a and b).

Evaluation of gestational age is accomplished by measuring the gestational sac. The diameter of the pregnancy ring is applied to a standard graph to obtain the gestational age. As the gestational

FIGURE 3.28(a)
Supine longitudinal scan. Gray scale. Cystic cul-de-sac mass measures 4 cm. This cyst regressed spontaneously with serial scans until complete disappearance. Asymptomatic theca lutein cyst.

FIGURE 3.28(b)
Supine transverse scan. Gray scale. Cystic mass lesion seen in the left adnexal region. This cyst regressed spontaneously with serial scans until complete disappearance. Asymptomatic theca lutein cyst.

FIGURE 3.28(c)
Supine transverse and longitudinal scan. Gray scale. The bladder is optimally distended. Gestational sac is well seen in the uterine cavity. A 3 × 3 cm lutein cyst in the left adnexal region is noted.

FIGURE 3.28(d)
Supine transverse scan. Gray scale. Simple lutein cyst in the right adnexal region.

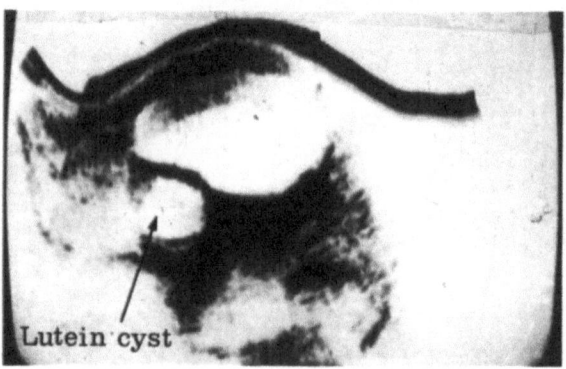

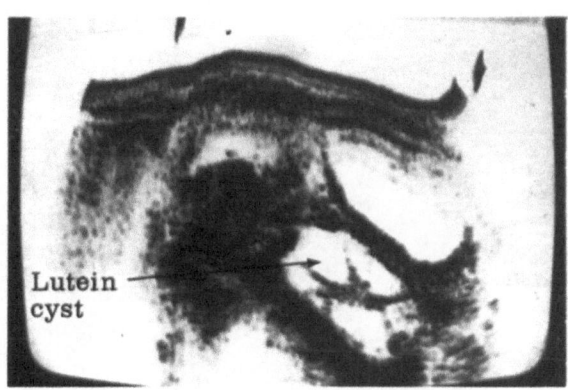

FIGURE 3.29(a)
Supine longitudinal scan. Gray scale. Large multiseptate cystic lesion in the cul de sac is noted. Patient admitted to the hospital with a diagnosis of threatened abortion. Patient underwent surgery because of enlarging cystic lesion. At operation, hemorrhagic lutein cyst was found.

FIGURE 3.29(b)
Supine transverse scan. Gray scale. Same case as in Fig. 3.29a. Multiseptate hemorrhagic lutein cyst again is noted.

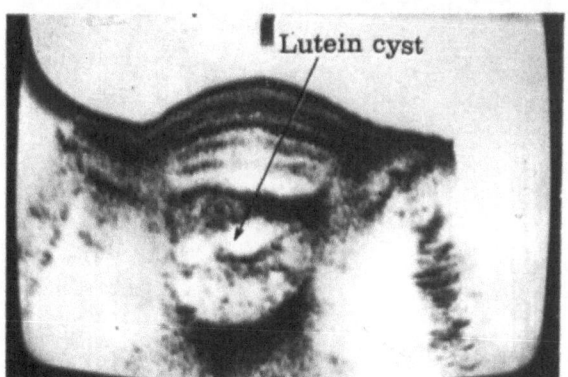

sac disappears, the head of the fetus becomes manifest. By the thirteenth week of pregnancy, the fetal skull is visible in about 75 percent of cases. In subsequent weeks, the correlation reaches 95 percent (Fig. 3.30a and b). Gestational age is most accurately determined by measuring the biparietal diameter of the fetal head and comparing the results with the standard charts.

In early pregnancy the fetal head outline is rounded and circular in shape. This is contrasted with the configuration of the head in later months when an elliptic appearance is the rule.

The fetal thorax is seen at about 15 to 17 weeks' gestation. Better estimation of fetal age and weight may be obtained by the combined use of the biparietal diameter with the fetal thoracic measurement.

In scanning the fetal head, care should be taken to identify the central linear echo pattern of the midline structures for accurate measurement of the biparietal diameter. The source of the midline echoes is considered to be from the falx cerebri or interhemispheric fissure.

By using the biparietal diameter and anteroposterior diameter of the fetal thorax with a reliable nomogram, the estimated fetal weight may be ascertained. The biparietal diameter alone may be used to estimate fetal weight, but it is not accurate. However, the biparietal diameter is highly accurate for fetal age determination (Fig. 3.31).

The fetal head is first visible at 12 to 13 weeks' gestation. This figure is important since many elective abortions by the suction technique must be carried out before 14 weeks' gestation if they are going to be performed in the first trimester. Second trimester abortions have a higher morbidity and mortality. The absence of a fetal head during scanning implies that a suction curettage is safe at this time.

To evaluate the gestational age optimally, it is best to wait until approximately the seventeeth week of gestation (Fig. 3.32a and b). If a patient is unsure of her dates, serial measurements at 3-week intervals will show the rate of growth on

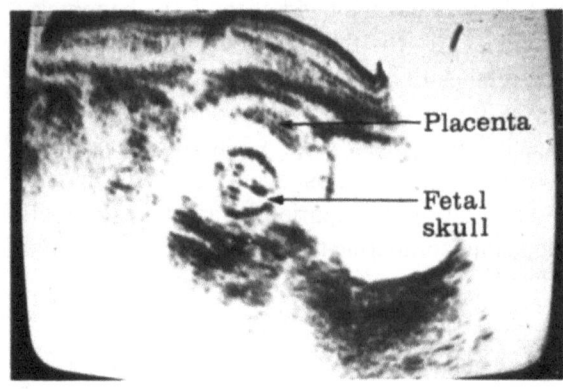

FIGURE 3.30(a)
Supine longitudinal scan. Gray scale. The crescent-shaped echoes of the placenta are best visualized when the fetal head is separated from the placenta by some distance, so that the amniotic fluid provides a good interface with the placenta.

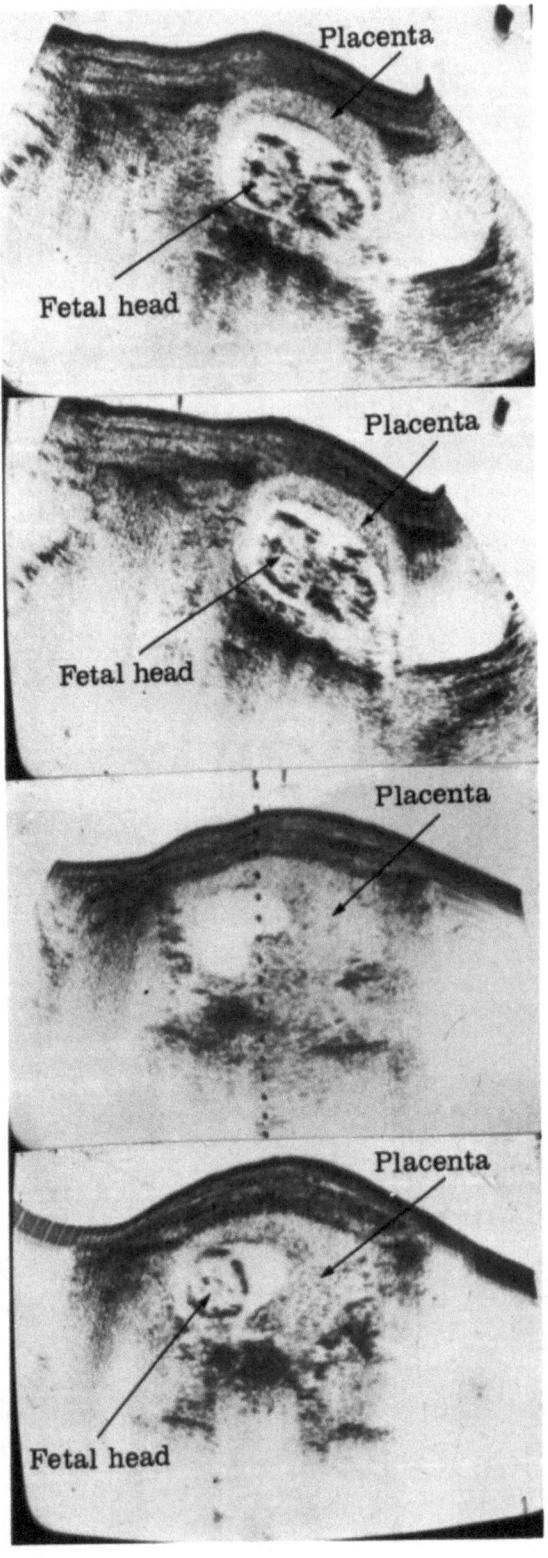

FIGURE 3.30(b)
Supine longitudinal and transverse scan. Gray scale. Demonstration of the fetal head, fetal body, and placenta in the early second trimester.

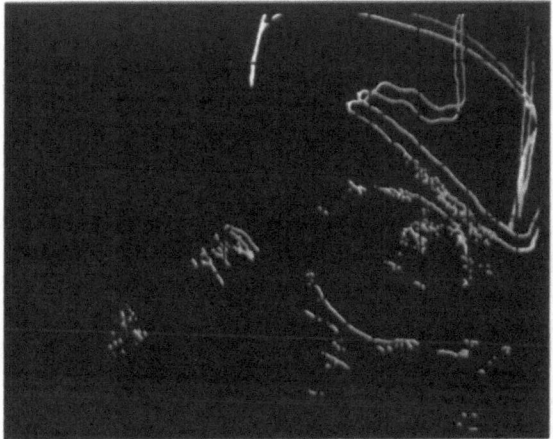

FIGURE 3-31

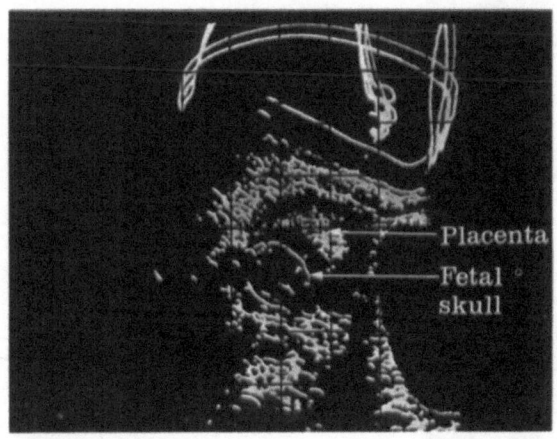

FIGURE 3-32 (a)

FIGURE 3-32 (b)

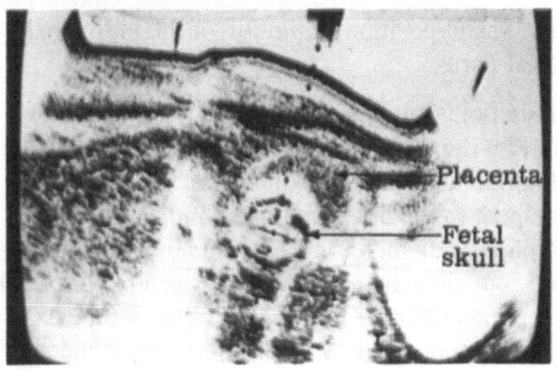

FIGURE 3.31
Supine longitudinal scan. B-mode. The biparietal diameter is highly accurate for fetal age determination. The midline echoes are demonstrated for accurate location and measurement.

FIGURE 3.32(a)
Supine longitudinal scan. B-mode. For accurate evaluation of gestational age it is best to wait approximately 17 weeks of gestation.

FIGURE 3.32(b)
Supine longitudinal scan. Gray scale. The fine echo pattern of the placenta is noted between the echo-poor space of the uterine wall and the echo-free zone of the amniotic fluid. At 17 weeks' gestation the fetal head may be clearly imaged.

the standard tables. It has been noted that fetal head sizes may be placed into one of three percentile ranks. Large is denoted as being greater than the 75th percentile, average as between the 25th and 75th, and small as less than the 25th. Under normal conditions fetuses falling within one group will remain at the same cephalic level during growth until birth. One group studying fetal development for intrauterine growth retardation found it optimal to take a first measurement at 22 weeks' gestation and again at 32 weeks' gestation (7). We make multiple serial measurements between 20 and 36 weeks for the most accurate assessment of fetal growth and development. It must be noted that, late in pregnancy, the diabetic fetus will have a larger biparietal diameter due to the macrosomic condition. Fetal well-being may not be established by measuring the biparietal diameter in this group. A mature fetus with weight greater than 2500 g may be diagnosed when the biparietal measurement is at least 8.7 cm.

MEASUREMENT OF THE BIPARIETAL DIAMETER

Prior to the evolution of the ultrasonic method, the physician had to rely on roentgenographic studies to measure the size of the fetus and biparietal diameter. X-ray studies allow a reliable and accurate measurement of the fetal skull in relation to the bony pelvis (Fig. 3.33), if the head is located in the pelvis and lies in

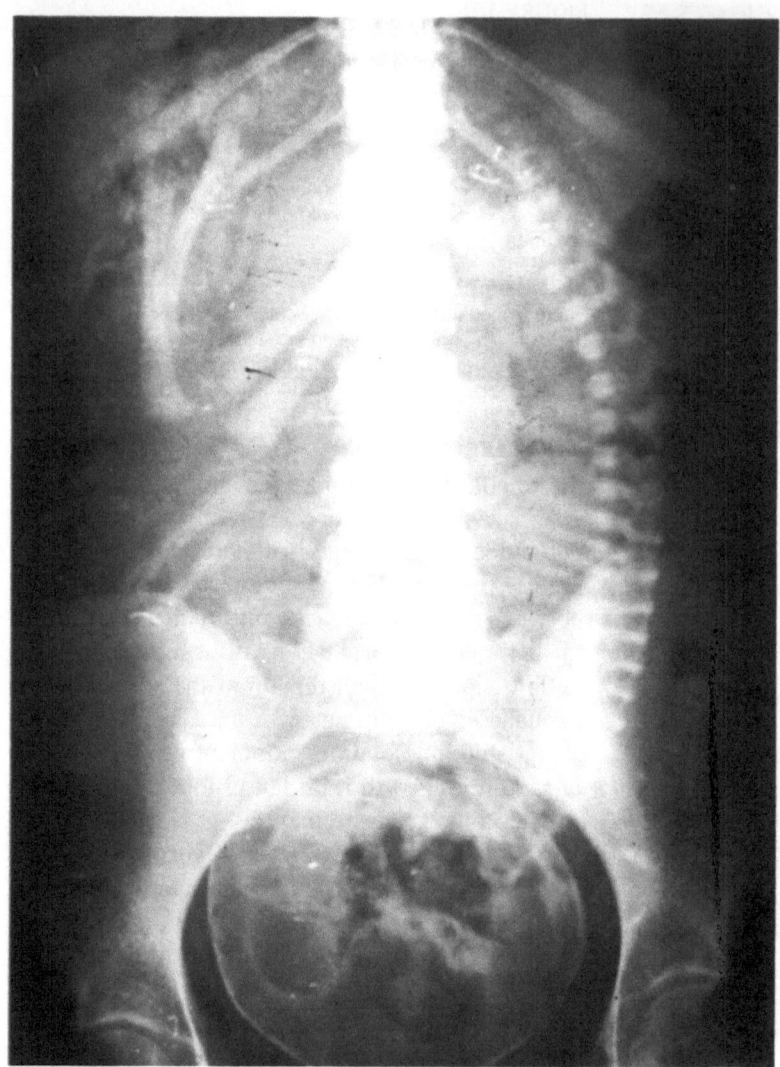

FIGURE 3.33
Flat plate of the abdomen. Single fetus in the vertex presentation. The small fetal parts are on the left. Ribs and spine are noted. The bony structures are well visualized by X-ray. The soft tissues are optimally imaged by ultrasound. Relationship of calvarium to the bony pelvis for cephalopelvic disproportion determination can be optimally evaluated by using X-ray pelvimetry.

certain particular planes, eg, the lateral or anteroposterior planes. If conditions do not meet the optimal pelvimetry criteria and the amount of magnification cannot be estimated precisely, the reliable dimensions of the fetal head cannot be ascertained. Using ultrasound, the most accurate measurements may be obtained disregarding the fetal position and lie.

The majority of fetuses are in the cephalic presentation. The discernment of another orientation is extremely important in obstetric management. Information regarding fetal presentation is best obtained with longitudinal

sections to localize the fetal head and fetal thorax. The real-time scanner permits the ultrasonographer to detect immediate changes in fetal head position or motion of the individual fetal parts.

Exact measurement of the biparietal diameter (BPD) depends upon precise localization of the fetal lie and the angle of the fetal head with respect to the investigating sound waves. The biparietal diameter is defined as the maximum reproducible distance between the fetal temporal or parietal bones. The midline echo of the falx must be centered between the strong echoes of

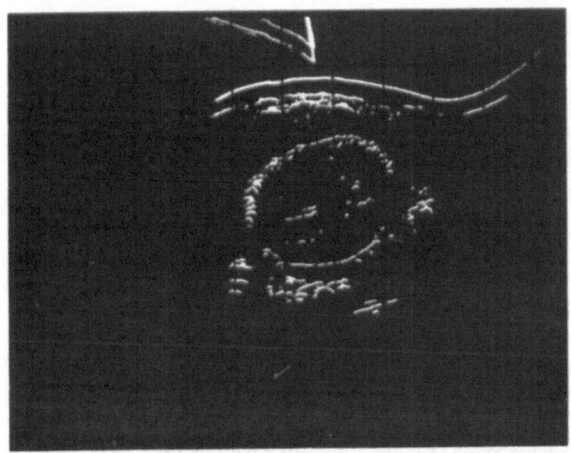

FIGURE 3.34
Supine transverse scan. B-mode. The maximum biparietal diameter is best obtained when the sensitivity is lowered to most clearly delineate the cranial outlines. Note the exquisitely sharp skull contour.

the cranium. A-mode and B-mode measurements are made directly from the screen (Fig. 3.34).

Gray-scale scanners produce a thicker skull outline and the output must be reduced to depict the calvarium as a single line (Fig. 3.35a). Electronic calipers may be used to measure the biparietal diameter. Digital read-out or a permanent record on a Polaroid print will provide the measuring landmarks, or simultaneous comparisons can be made between bistable and gray scale (Fig. 3.35b). Using black and white, or leading edge for BPD, simultaneous A-mode and B-mode display can be superimposed in some units (Fig. 3.36a).

In scanning the vertex presentation, with the head on the side, a longitudinal scan will determine the plane of the dorsal flexure of the head within the maternal pelvis. This angle of flexure is corrected by proper angulation of the transducer in the transverse scanning plane.

FIGURE 3.35(b)
Supine longitudinal scan. Simultaneous comparison between bistable and gray scale for the measurement of the biparietal diameter.

FIGURE 3.35(a)
Supine transverse scan. Gray scale. Gray-scale scanners produce a thicker skull outline and the output must be reduced to depict the calvarium as a single line.

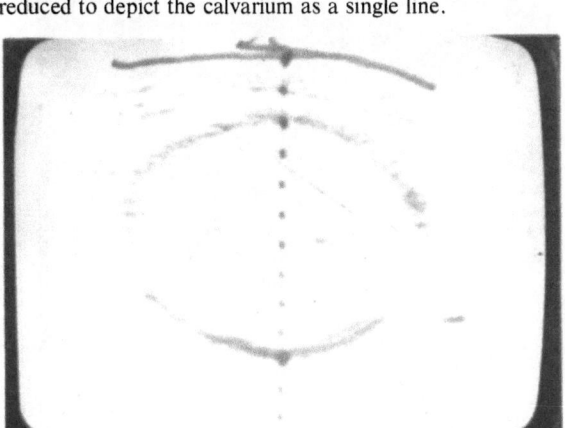

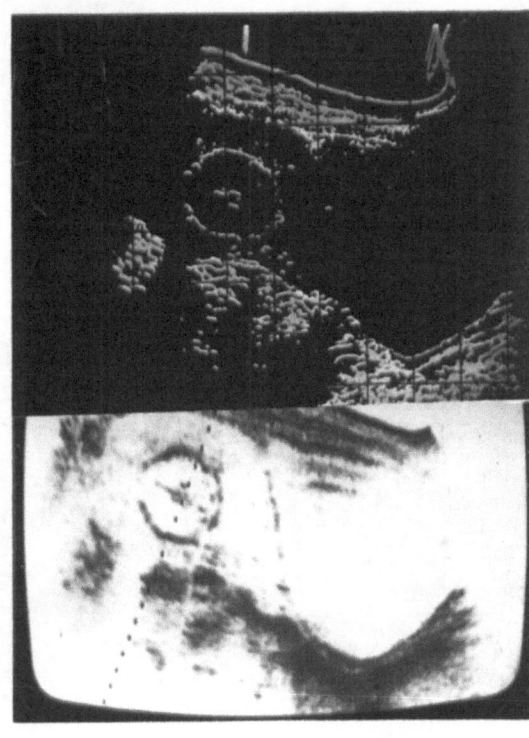

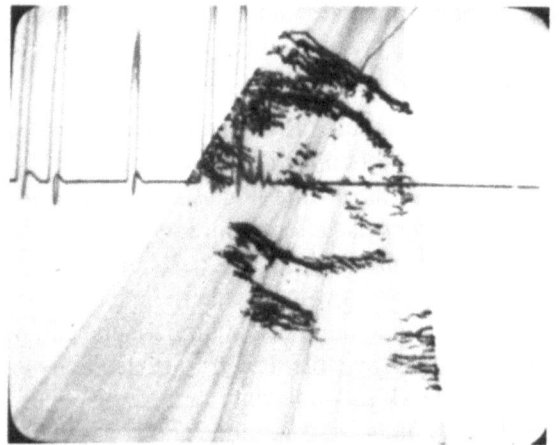

FIGURE 3-36 (a)

Appropriate transverse scans are made until the maximum intracranial distance is located. This is most easily accomplished with the real-time scanner since any change in the fetal skull position due to inherent fetal movements may be immediately noted and corrected by the ultrasonographer.

FIGURE 3.36(a)
Supine transverse scan. Gray scale. Measurement of the BPD. After detection of the calvarium and midline echo with leading edge, A-mode translation may be performed and superimposed over the scan.

FIGURE 3.36(b)
Supine transverse scan. Gray scale. Nonperpendicular studies produce false echo pattern which is not valid for the measurement of the biparietal diameter.

FIGURE 3.36(c)
Supine transverse scan. Gray scale. Another diameter that presents perpendicular surfaces is that of the occipitofrontal plane. The occipitofrontal diameter is much larger than the biparietal diameter. This also is not a valid measurement.

FIGURE 3.36(d)
Supine transverse scan. Occasionally, midline echoes appear as a curve. This is still a valid reading.

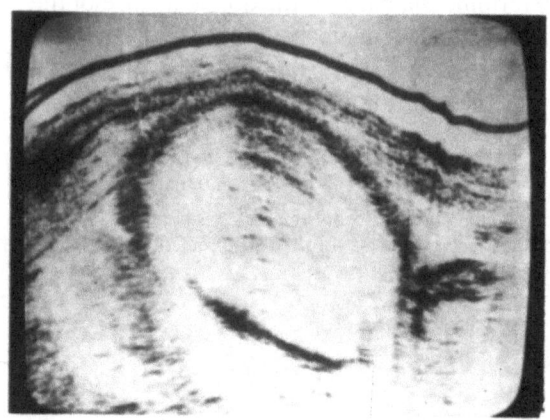

FIGURE 3-36 (b)

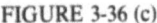

FIGURE 3-36 (c)

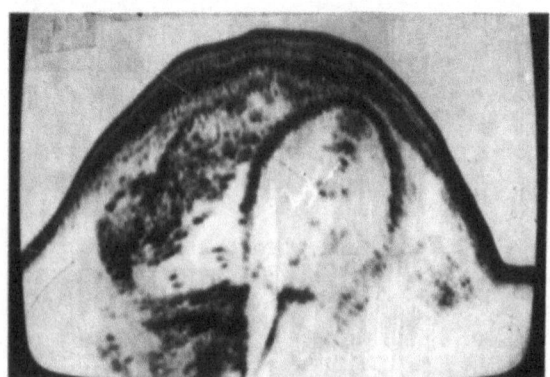

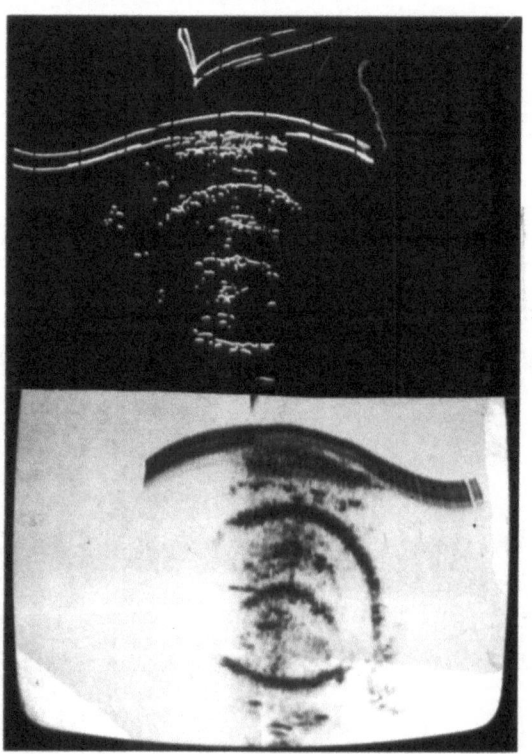

The examiner should move the transducer over the abdomen until strong and equal-amplitude echoes are received from the near and far sides of the skull with A-mode. Since the abdomen of the pregnant subject is round in late gestation, the transducer can move in various angulations up to 90° from the vertical plane. This maneuver facilitates accurate measurement of the BPD.

Studying the patient with A-mode and B-mode in combination with gray scale yields the maximum information. In A-mode study, the echoes from the fetal skull usually are equal when both sides of the skull are perpendicular to the sonic beam. In the vast majority of cases, the distance between the equal-amplitude echoes signifies the BPD. It should also be kept in mind that the only other diameter that occasionally presents perpendicularly is that of the occipitofrontal plane. Using the knowledge that the occipitofrontal diameter is much larger than the BPD (Fig. 3.36b and c), these two diameters may be differentiated. Also, if two nonperpendicular surfaces are measured, the vertical deflections are not equal in height. Again, it should be emphasized that the absence of midline echoes invalidates the reading.

As described above, the widest diameter of the fetal skull that is perpendicular to the midline echoes is considered to be the maximum biparietal diameter. Occasionally, midline echoes appear as a curved line; this still implies a valid reading (Fig. 3.36d). There are a number of charts and tables available for fetal age evaluation from the biparietal diameter. Unfortunately, large variations in gestational age determination exist between these tables (8–10). Most of these differences may be explained on the basis of geographic locality, socioeconomic status, or racial differences.

We use the placental appearance and the data listed in Table 3.2 for our determinations. These data are comparable with those in the literature. If the BPD is calculated to be more than 105 mm, the study should be repeated and, if the reading is constant, hydrocephalus should be considered. To avoid any confusion, accurate measurements should be obtained.

TABLE 3.2 Approximation of Gestational Age From Biparietal Diameter (BPD)

BPD (cm)	GESTATIONAL AGE
2.5	14.0
2.6	14.0
2.7	14.5
2.8	14.5
2.9	15.0
3.0	15.5
3.1	16.0
3.2	16.5
3.3	16.5
3.4	17.0
3.5	17.5
3.6	17.5
3.7	18.0
3.8	18.5
3.9	18.5
4.0	19.0
4.1	19.5
4.2	19.5
4.3	20.0
4.4	20.5
4.5	20.5
4.6	21.0
4.7	21.5
4.8	21.5
4.9	22.0
5.0	22.5
5.1	22.5
5.2	23.0
5.3	23.5
5.4	23.5
5.5	24.0
5.6	24.5
5.7	24.5
5.8	25.0
5.9	25.0
6.0	25.5
6.1	26.0
6.2	26.0
6.3	26.5
6.4	27.0
6.5	27.5
6.6	27.5
6.7	28.0
6.8	28.5
6.9	28.5
7.0	29.0
7.1	29.5
7.2	29.5
7.3	30.0
7.4	30.0
7.5	30.5
7.6	30.6
7.7	31.0

TABLE 3.2 (*Continued*)

BPD (cm)	GESTATIONAL AGE
7.8	31.5
7.9	31.9
8.0	32.6
8.1	33.0
8.2	33.5
8.3	34.1
8.4	34.7
8.5	35.0
8.6	35.4
8.7	36.0
8.8	36.4
8.9	37.0
9.0	37.1
9.1	38.0
9.2	38.5
9.3	39.0
9.4	39.2
9.5	39.8
9.6	40.0
9.7	40.5
9.8	41.0
9.9	41.8
10.0	41.9

For the measurement of BPD, our experience shows that usage of the A-mode or simple bistable mode is still superior. If the single spike is seen for the measurement in the trace, the two points of the takeoff from the baseline become the actual measurement. The confusing factor is the presence of multiple spikes. To overcome this obstacle, the simplest method is to decrease the gain setting and slightly change the angulation of the transducer until three clear spikes are seen. In some commercially available units, the study can be done simultaneously with the leading edge or black-and-white pattern on the television screen and with special maneuvers the two studies can be superimposed. This is important because the errors can be minimized to less than 2 mm.

In measuring the biparietal diameter, the ultrasonographer must be aware of the tilting of the fetal skull as it enters the pelvic inlet. In this situation, the biparietal diameter may be obtained in an oblique plane relative to the true transverse plane. In these cases, the midline echoes will not lie in the exact midline or may be completely absent. The optimal study is obtained when the degree of asynclitism of the fetal head is determined from the sagittal scan and the ultrasonographer adjusts the transverse scan plane angle in an appropriate manner to register the biparietal diameter in the plane perpendicular to the midline structures.

MATERNAL PELVIS

Although pelvimetry may be performed with ultrasound, X-ray pelvimetry is still considered the best method for examination of the bony pelvis. Indications for X-ray pelvimetry include the following.

1. If the diagonal conjugate is less than 11.5 cm

2. Presence of diseases which already affect the bony pelvis

3. Very prominent ischial spines with flattened sacrum

4. Failure of progression of labor

5. Breech, face, and other abnormal presentations

6. Narrowed intertuberous diameter accompanied by narrow subpelvic angle

HEAD

The calvarium produces a strong echo to the interrogating ultrasound and appears as a regular, circular, or elliptic outline on the bistable oscilloscope. The increased sensitivity of gray-scale equipment reveals not only the bony structures but also the pericranial soft tissues such as fat, muscle, and hair. These are displayed as a region of low-amplitude echoes adjacent to the high-amplitude calvarial echoes. The exact shape of the fetal head is best delineated without the peripheral echoes (which increase the thickness of the bony outline for measurement purposes) by decreasing the gain of the unit. The optimal outline of the head can be obtained through bistable study (Fig. 3.37a).

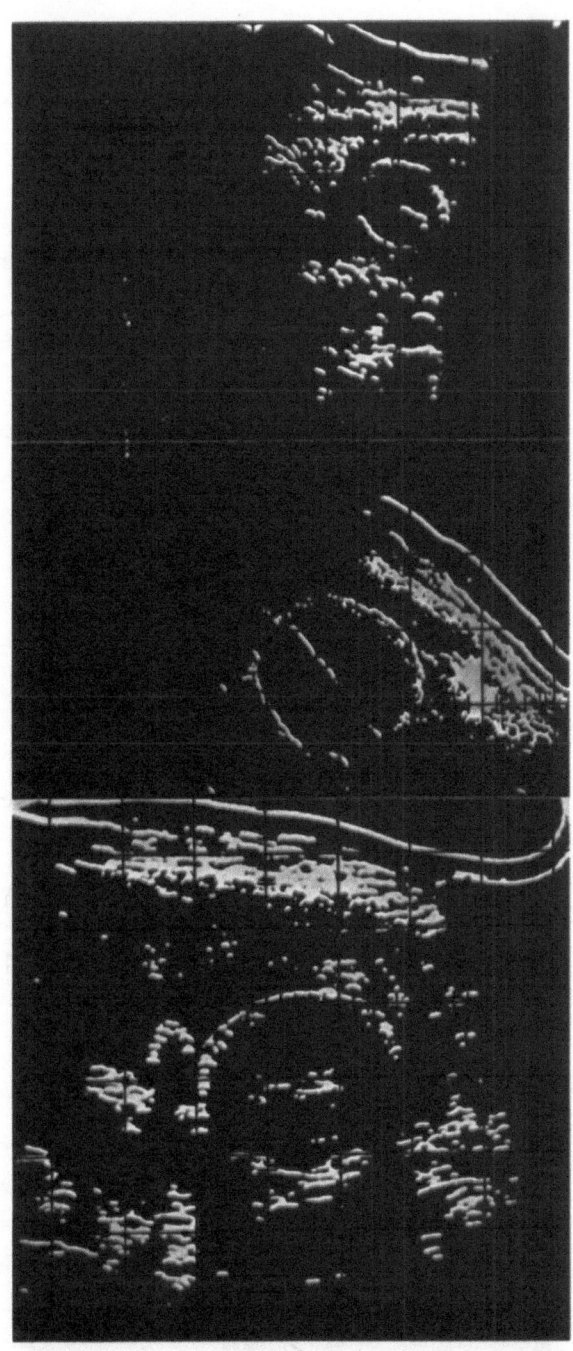

FIGURE 3.37(a)
Supine transverse scan. B-mode. The optimal outline of the head can be obtained through bistable study.

The linear midline structure of moderate echogenicity that parallels the posteroanterior axis of the calvarium is thought to represent the interhemispheric region, including the intracranial falx cerebri and the third ventricle. There is a consistent set of symmetric echoes lateral to the anterior portion of the falx, most likely representing the lateral portion of the anterior horn of the lateral ventricle (11). Another pair of anteriorly located C-shaped structures appear at the junction of the frontal bone with the facial bones and represent the bony orbits. When the correct plane of fetal skull orientation is demonstrated, a band of reverberation artifacts is often seen which originates from the near table and should not be mistaken with any other structures. Occasionally, motion of the fetus may produce some difficulties in measuring BPD (Fig. 3.37b).

SPINE

Distal to the head, a pair of strongly echogenic lines connect the thorax with the head. This is the ultrasonic appearance of the cervical spine in sagittal section (Fig. 3.38a). This structure continues with a dorsal curvature into the rest of the spine, ending at the strong echo complex of

FIGURE 3.37(b)
Supine transverse scan. Occasionally, motion of the fetus may produce some difficulty in measuring BPD.

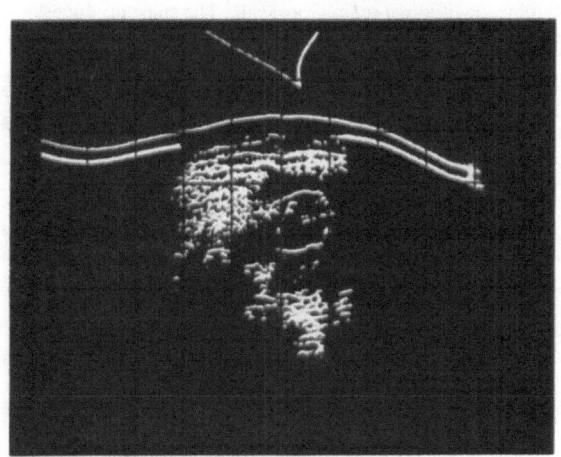

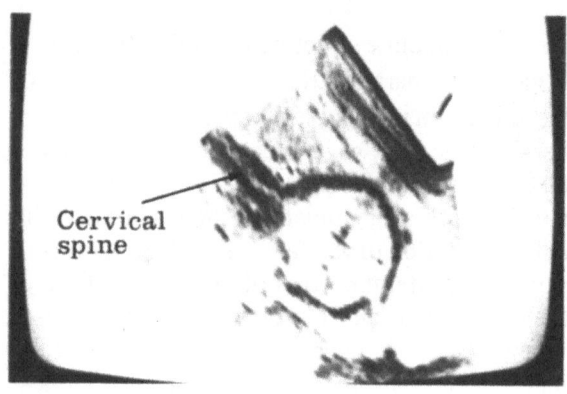

FIGURE 3.38(a)
Supine longitudinal scan. Gray scale. Distal to the head, a pair of strongly echogenic lines connect the thorax with the head. This is the ultrasonic appearance of the cervical spine in sagittal section.

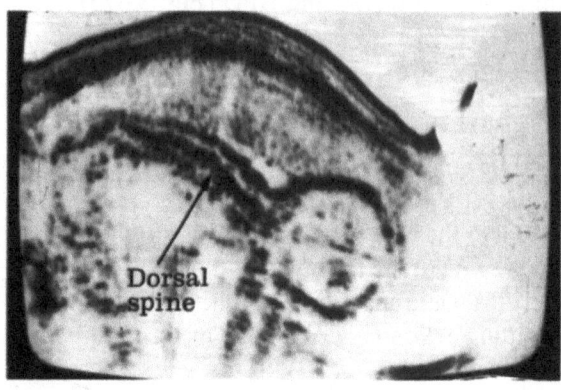

FIGURE 3.38(b)
Supine longitudinal scan. Gray scale. The cervical spine continues with a dorsal curvature into the rest of the spine, ending at the strong echo complex of the pelvis.

FIGURE 3.38(c)
Supine longitudinal scan. Gray scale. The spine produces a sonic shadow in later weeks of pregnancy.

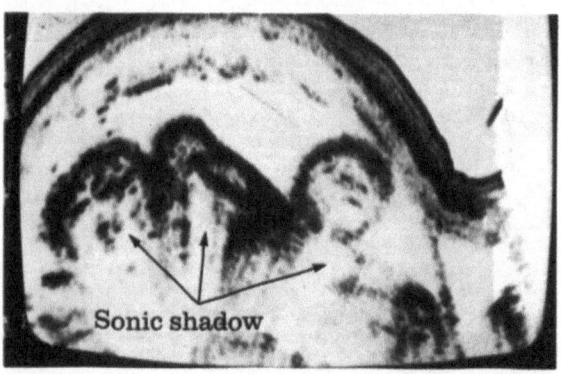

the pelvis (Fig. 3.38b). The spine produces a sonic shadow in later weeks of pregnancy (Fig. 3.38c). Ribs appear as parallel lines projecting from the spine (Fig. 3.38d). Along the spine— and of a similar configuration—lies the aorta. This may be differentiated from the spine by the sharper appearance of the parallel lines and the lack of sonic shadowing which may be often demonstrated when the spine lies ventrally adjacent to the transducer. The aorta is best distinguished from the vertebral column by the typical, synchronous pulsations shown with the fine real-time scanner.

FETAL HEART

The fetal heart becomes a functional pumping organ at 35 to 45 days' amenorrhea. One investigator, using A-mode echography, was able to detect fetal heart motion as early as 45 days' amenorrhea (12). It is possible to observe fetal heart motion with A-mode or M-mode at 7 to 10 weeks' gestation (13). The application of M-mode or real-time scanning makes evaluation of fetal death a straightforward process when coupled with Doppler studies. The unequivocal signs of fetal death by radiologic imaging occur long after fetal demise. The ultrasonic signs by bistable or gray scale are indirect signs.

FIGURE 3.38(d)
Supine longitudinal scan. Gray scale. The fetus is in the vertex presentation. Linear parallel echoes extend from the dorsal spine representing the posterior rib cage. A sonic shadow is produced by the dorsal spine.

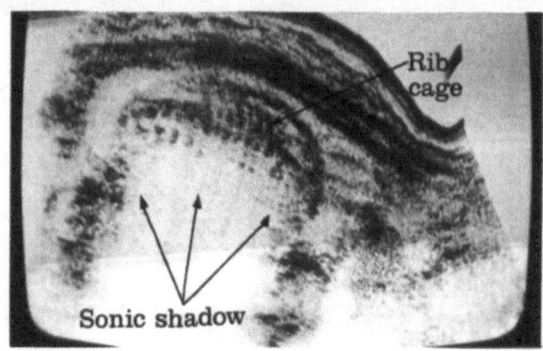

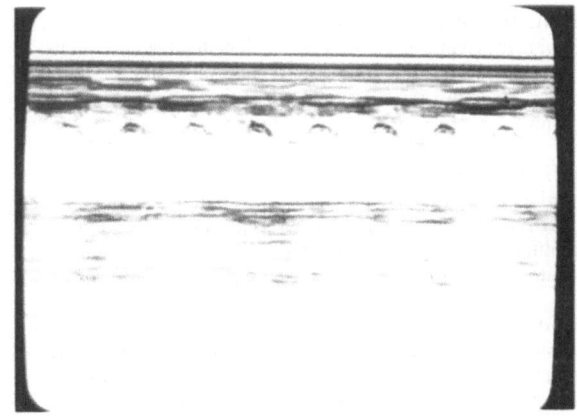

FIGURE 3.39(a)
M-mode scan over the maternal abdomen and fetal thorax. The fetal heart appears as an echo-free area with a clearly demonstrated rapid and cyclic echo of the contracting ventricle. The beating heart identifies the fetal thorax.

FIGURE 3.39(b)
M-mode scan over the maternal abdomen and fetal thorax. Demonstration of fetal heart and fetal respiratory motion.

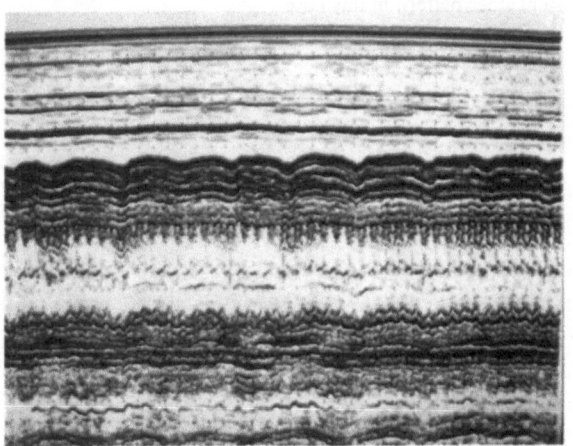

However, when motion studies are available, the beating fetal heart is rather easy to image (Fig. 3.39a and b). The absence of a fetal heartbeat when expected is the most definite sign of nonviability of the fetus.

MONITORING THE FETAL HEART RATE

The fetal heart motion can be easily detected by the real-time scanner. However, at present, in our experience, irregularity of the fetal heart cannot be adequately judged by the real-time scanner. For precise evaluation the fetal heart signal should be registered through a chart recorder. Doppler ultrasound can be used for continous monitoring of the fetal heart rate. The normal fetal heart rate is 120 to 140 beats per minute. A unit with a multiple transducer array permits continuous tracking of the fetal heart, even if the fetus moves. Tracking with this instrument, the fetal heart signals will be transmitted to a counting circuit and chart recorder. The other channel of the unit records a simultaneous tracing showing uterine contractions. Any irregularity of the fetal heart rate can easily be registered during the course of labor and followed throughout delivery. The unit can be adjusted so that any decrease or alteration in the fetal heart motion can be detected and the physician can thus be alerted to possible fetal distress.

FETAL THORAX

Cross section of the chest reveals the rounded outline of the vertebral column due to the vertebral body and the elements of the neural arch. The fetal heart has already been discussed; however, the identification of this structure most accurately locates the fetal thorax (Fig. 3.40a and b). Rib detail may often be imaged as a series of closely parallel echogenic linear structures (Fig. 3.38d). In late pregnancy, the fetal thorax produces a sonic shadow over the placenta (Fig. 3.41). The motion of thorax can be demonstrated by M-mode (Fig. 3.39b).

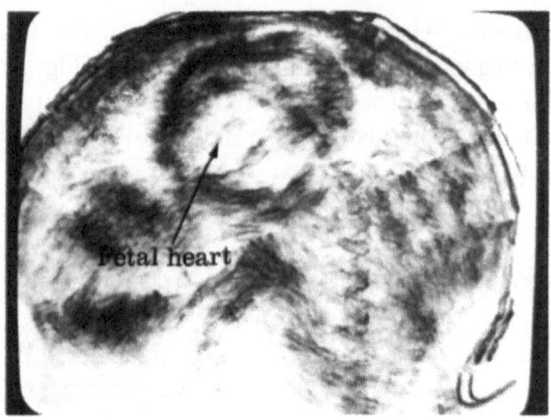

FIGURE 3-40 (a)

FIGURE 3.40(a)
Supine transverse scan. Gray scale. The fetal heart with its internal septum may be localized by gray scale. Verification of this structure is made with M-mode or the real-time scanner.

FIGURE 3.40(b)
Supine longitudinal scan. Gray scale. The fetal body is seen in cross section and an echo-free region with a dividing septum is noted to represent cardiac chambers. Note sonic shadowing by fetal parts.

FIGURE 3.41
Supine longitudinal scan. Gray scale. The fetal thorax may occasionally produce a sonic shadow sign as a normal variation. Echo-free area represents fetal heart.

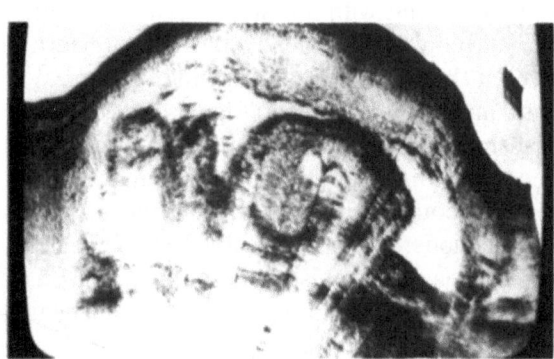

FIGURE 3-40 (b)

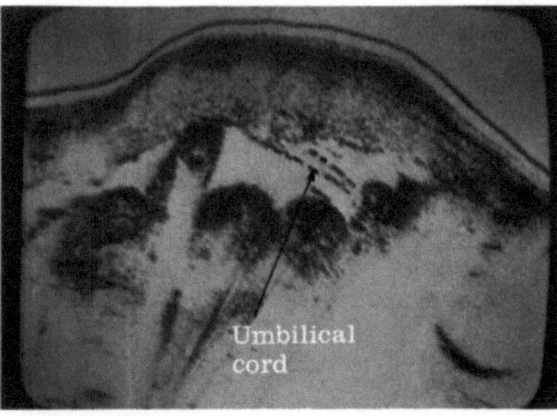

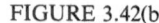

FIGURE 3.42(a)
Supine longitudinal scan. Gray scale. The flat chorionic plate of the anterior placenta protrudes into the amniotic cavity and extrudes the umbilical cord. The cord generally appears as an interrupted linear array of parallel echoes due to its tortuous course and motion.

FIGURE 3.42(b)
Supine longitudinal scan. Gray scale. The cord appears as a stepladder pattern in this case.

FIGURE 3-41

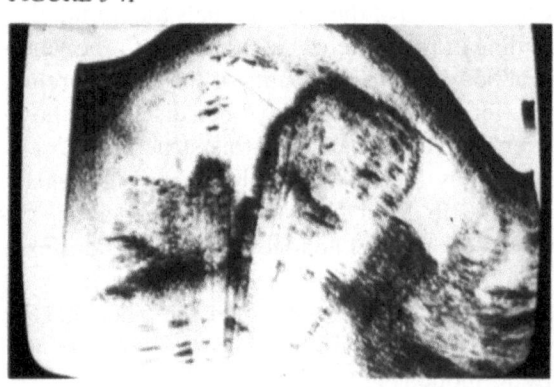

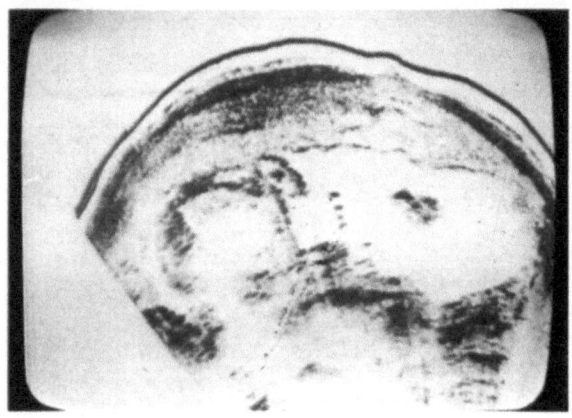

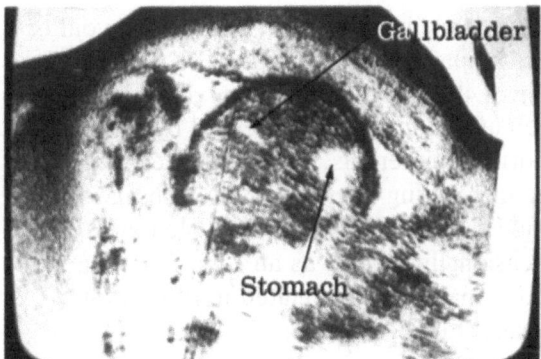

FIGURE 3-43

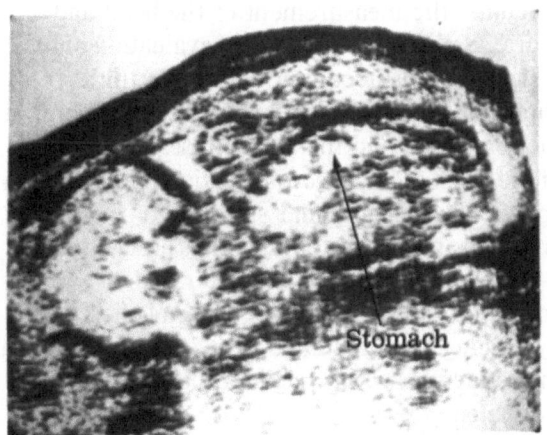

FIGURE 3-44

FIGURE 3-45

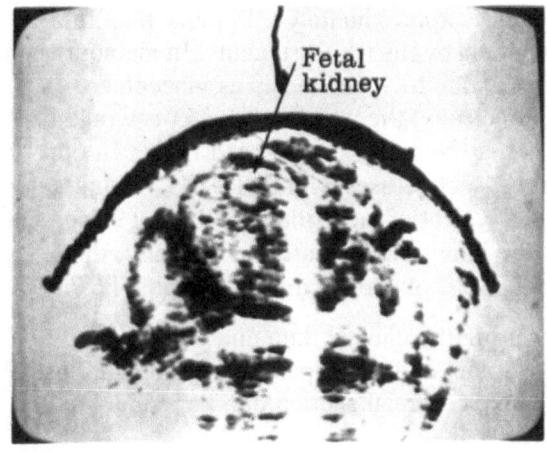

FIGURE 3.43
Supine longitudinal scan. Gray scale. Cross section through the fetal upper abdomen demonstrating the fetal gallbladder in the right upper quadrant as a pearshaped echo-free structure surrounded by echoes of the liver. In the left upper quadrant is the fluid-filled fetal stomach. The fluid is due to fetal swallowing.

FIGURE 3.44
Supine longitudinal scan. Gray scale. The fetal heart is noted as an echo-free zone within the thoracic cavity divided by a linear echo representing the interventricular septum. Immediately cranial and to the left of the cardiac chambers is noted a rounded echo-free structure in the fetal left upper quadrant characteristic of the fetal stomach.

FIGURE 3.45
Supine transverse scan. Gray scale. Cross section through the fetal abdomen. The placenta is posterior. The fetal back is ventral to the maternal abdominal wall and the spine casts a sonic shadow. On either side of the spine are the ovoid renal outlines.

FETAL ABDOMEN

The fetal abdomen is a rounded image in cross section and is most easily separated from the fetal thorax by a lack of cardiac pulsations. The attachment of the umbilical cord at the fetal umbilicus (Fig. 3.42a) may be noted as an interrupted series of linear parallel echoes (Fig. 3.42b) with gray scale, or as a pulsatile structure with the real-time scanner. The fetal liver is echogenic. In the right upper quadrant are noted two anechoic structures representing the gallbladder and stomach (Fig. 3.43).

The gallbladder may appear ovoid or linear in shape and is shorter than the umbilical vein. The umbilical vein has an anteroposterior course from the umbilicus to the region of the venous union near the dorsal spine. These two structures are best separated by the pulsations of the vein with the real-time scanner. In the left upper quadrant, the fluid-filled fetal stomach is seen as an echo-free space of variable appearance (Fig. 3.44).

The fetal kidneys are miniature versions of the adult organs. They have an echo-free periphery and an echogenic interior and are lateral to the dorsal spine (Figs. 3.45 and 3.46). Intrauterine hydronephrosis may be identified by cystic transformation of the renal outlines (Fig. 3.47).

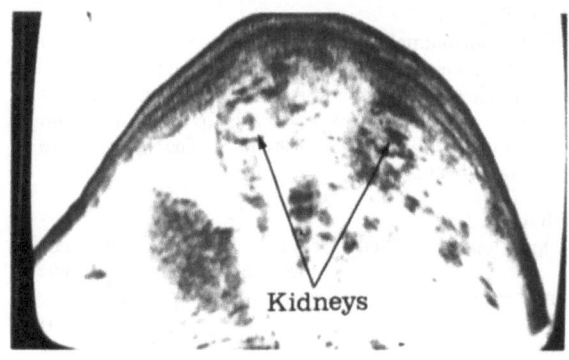

FIGURE 3.46
Supine transverse scan. Gray scale. Cross section through the fetal abdomen. The thorax produces a sonic shadow sign. The fetal back is ventral to the maternal abdominal wall and the spine casts a sonic shadow. On either side of the spine are the ovoid renal outlines.

FIGURE 3.47
Supine transverse scan. Gray scale. Section through the fetal kidneys shows multiple disorganized echo-free areas instead of the expected renal outline. Fetus born with massive bilateral hydronephrosis which after autopsy was proven to be due to posterior urethral valves.

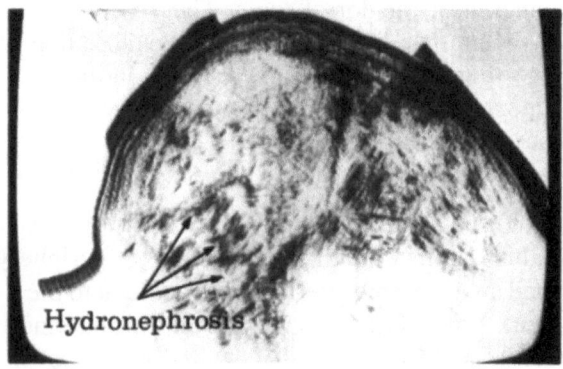

The urinary bladder is imaged as an ovoid or rectangular echo-free area in the fetal pelvis. (Fig. 3.48a and b). This organ varies in size and fetal urination may be observed by gray scale at short time intervals, or with the real-time scanner during micturition after observing bladder distension. The fetal colon may be occasionally imaged as an echo-free area in the abdominal cavity unrelated to other cystic organs (Fig. 3.49).

FETAL WEIGHT

With optimal calibration of the ultrasonograph machine, the measurement of the head and thorax is obtained and used in evaluation of fetal weight. This is accomplished in the third trimester by measuring the biparietal diameter of the fetal head and the anteroposterior diameter of the chest (14). The cross section of the chest is shown when the circular structure of the thorax is visible and the vertebral bodies are delineated. By using the biparietal diameter and anteroposterior diameter of the fetal chest and by placing a straightedge across the nomogram, the estimated age or weight of the fetus can be evaluated (15).

In 80 percent of our cases, the estimated weight by using both BPD and anteroposterior diameter of the chest is within 0.5 pounds (lb) of the actual birth weight. In the remaining 20 percent, there are a number of reasons to explain these differences. For instance, in diabetes, the fetal weight is approximately 1 lb more than that predicted by the measurements. In malnourished fetuses due to such causes as placental insufficiency, the weight of the fetus would be less than that of the estimated range. In our series, such fetuses with BPDs of 9 cm or greater had a weight of more than 5.5 lb, and 98 percent of the infants were mature. Normally, the fetus with a BPD of over 9 cm has a weight of 6.7 lb.

By using the clinical data and combined ultrasonic studies proper decisions regarding elective cesarean section can be made.

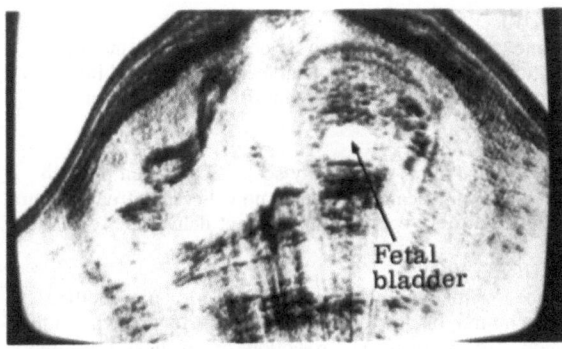

FIGURE 3.48(a)
Supine transverse scan. Gray scale. Rectangular outline of the echo-free fetal bladder. Note echogenic area of the fetal spine with distal sonic shadowing.

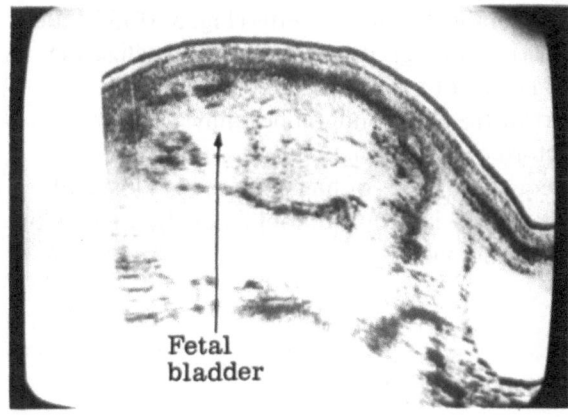

FIGURE 3.48(b)
Supine longitudinal scan. Gray scale. Round echo-free bladder in the fetal pelvis is seen. Note posterior placenta.

FIGURE 3.49
Supine transverse scan. Gray scale. A small echo-free area is noted near the echo-free bladder. Multiple scans showed this to have the typical configuration of the fetal colon.

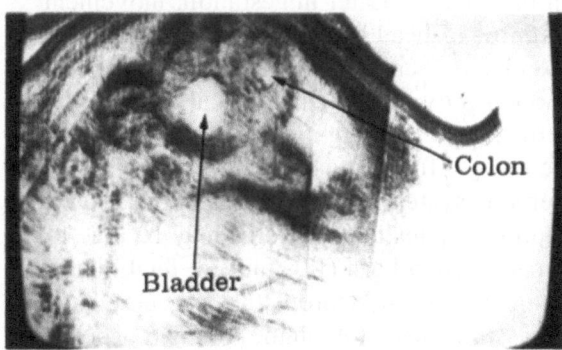

SEX DETERMINATION

The higher resolution of gray-scale systems now permits detailed imaging of the fetal perineum. The fetal orientation is noted and then the perineum is localized by finding the landmarks of the fetal bladder and fetal pelvis. Sections are made parallel to the long axis of the fetus to detect the fetal penis or scrotum connected to the fetal perineum. This physical attachment must be demonstrated to rule out the possibility of fetal limbs simulating the rounded appearance of the scrotum. The penis appears as a short linear echo pattern and the scrotum as an echo-free compartment with a central median septum (Fig. 3.50a,b,c,d,e, and f). The low-level echoes of the testes appear as symmetric low-amplitude echoes within the fetal scrotal compartments. The female sex is ascertained by exclusion of the presence of the penis and scrotum by ultrasonic imaging. The best time for scanning is at 30 to 32 weeks' gestation. The determination of fetal sex is useful for genetic counseling of parents who may be suspected of having children with sex-linked disorders, such as hemophilia (16).

FETAL EXTREMITIES

The upper and lower limbs of the fetus are best studied with a combination of high-resolution gray-scale scanning and real-time scanning. The real-time scanner is most suitable for observing the motion of the arms and legs. The presence of appropriate fetal movements assures that gross neurologic function is intact. Sonofluoroscopy of the uterus shows the coordinated motion of the upper and lower limbs with respect to the fetal trunk. Mental integration of the movement allows the ultrasonographer to decide which extremity is part of the upper trunk and which limb is associated with the lower portion of the fetus. After real-time scanning has located and identified the fetal limbs with accuracy, the gray-scale unit may study these regions with either a 2.25 or a 3.5-MHz transducer to image the bony structures of the arms and legs as well as the

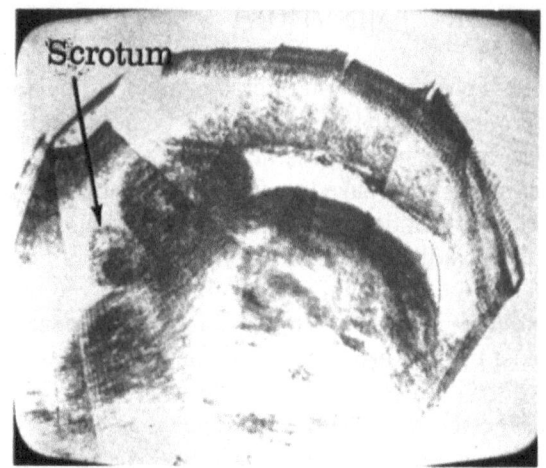

FIGURE 3-50 (a)

FIGURE 3.50(a)
Supine transverse scan. Gray scale. The echogenic fetal scrotum appears at the perineum between the fetal buttocks. Courtesy of D. J. Flanigan, Santa Barbara, California.

FIGURE 3.50(b)
Supine longitudinal scan. Gray scale. Scan taken through fetal perineum. Search produced no echoes protruding from the fetal buttock region. Female infant delivered.

FIGURE 3.50(c)
Supine longitudinal scan. Gray scale. Vertex presentation. The echo-free bladder clearly outlines the fetal pelvis. In the region of the perineum no projections of a penis or scrotum are noted. Female infant delivered.

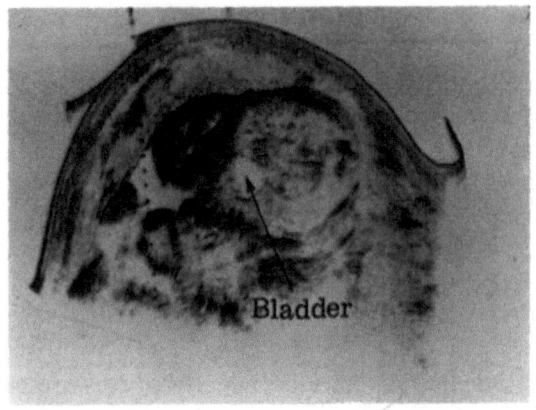

FIGURE 3-50 (b)

FIGURE 3-50 (c)

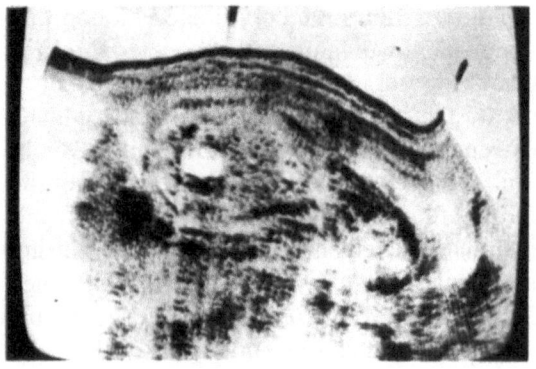

digits of the developing fetus (Fig. 3.51a,b,c,d,e, and f). Although it is difficult to visualize the phalanges of the hands and feet, effort on the part of the ultrasonographer may produce a picture clearly depicting the presence of an adequate number of fingers or toes. This is of great value in suspected fetal genetic defects or other anomalies.

FETAL MOTION

Early fetal motion may be detected between 8 and 10 weeks' gestation with a real-time scanning system and consists of changes of position of the fetus within the uterine cavity and limb motion without alteration of the fetal position in the gestational sac (17). In our experience with the real-time scanner, fetal heart motion can be detected at 14 weeks of gestation in most cases. Later in gestation, movement patterns of head bobbing and chest wall excursion become discernable. Each type of motion provides specific clinical data about the fetus. Head bobbing implies a certain degree of neurologic function is present in the fetal nervous system. The presence of chest wall motion implies that the fetus may be able to breathe when born (17). Indeed, fetal motion sometimes is so vigorous that one may have great difficulty in obtaining true and accurate

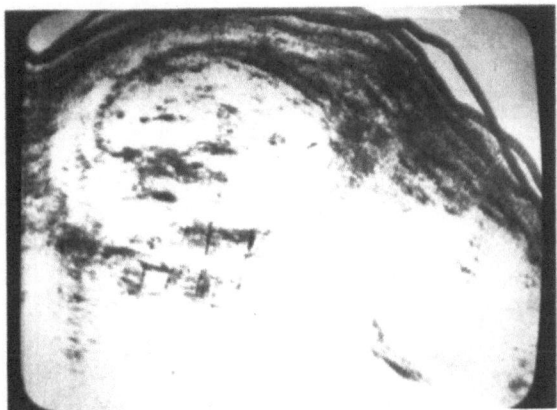

FIGURE 3-50 (d)

FIGURE 3.50(d)
Supine longitudinal scan. Gray scale. The fetal buttocks are anterior and in the superior part of the uterus. Ultrasonographic searching could not demonstrate a penis nor a scrotum. Female infant delivered.

FIGURE 3.50(e)
Supine oblique scan. Gray scale. The fetal penis sppears as a linear echo extending from the fetal perineum. On either side are noted shorter and rounder echogenic structures representing the fetal scrotum with its testicles. Courtesy of D. J. Flanigan, Santa Barbara, California.

FIGURE 3.50(f)
Supine longitudinal scan. Gray scale. The fetal penis extending from the fetal perineum. Note both fetal knees.

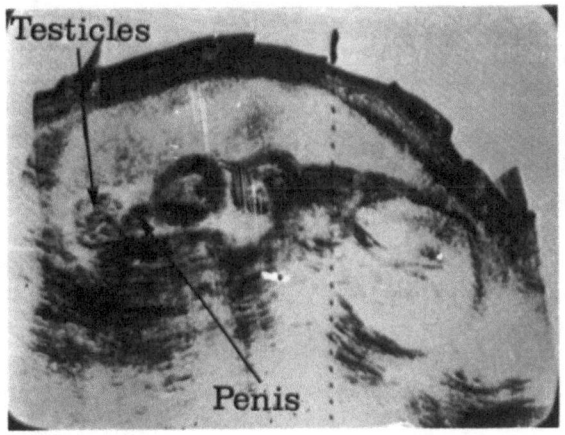

FIGURE 3-50 (e)

FIGURE 3-50 (f)

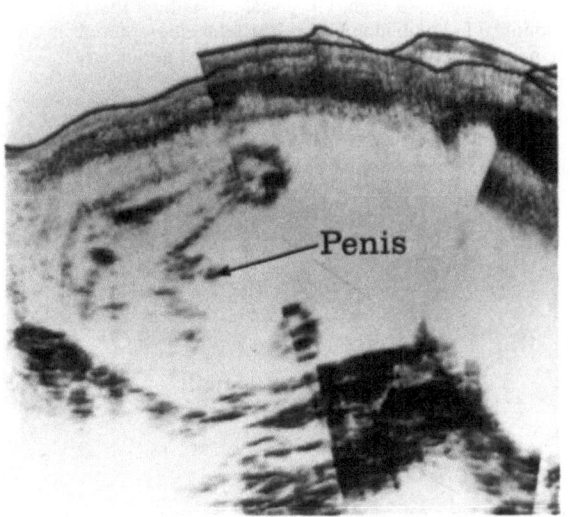

fetal measurements, such as thorax size and biparietal diameter (Fig. 3.52). Movement may be so rapid that two fetal heads may be observed if the scanning speed is slow enough to record a single fetal head in two different positions. Real-time scanning affords the best imaging of various fetal movements.

FETAL GROWTH

For determination of fetal growth, ultrasonic cephalometry is one of the most valuable tools when combined with clinical correlation. At the beginning of gestation, fetal growth can be followed by measuring the size of the gestational sac. As growth progresses, the fetal heart may be detected by the real-time scanner. As time passes, the BPD can be monitored sequentially. The average increase in the BPD is approximately 1 to 2 mm per week. Sudden changes in the growth rate of the fetal head suggest certain pathologic conditions; eg, a sudden decrease in fetal head size may indicate either placental insufficiency or fetal death. In cases of twin gestation, the BPD of both fetuses should be followed. On occasion during examination, the identification as to which twin is which may be difficult. In abnormal pregnancy, such as is associated with anencephaly or hydrocephalus, the BPD

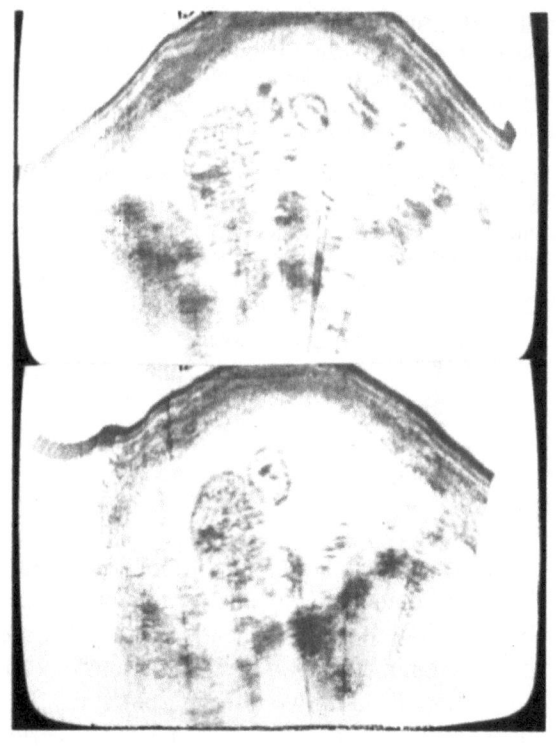

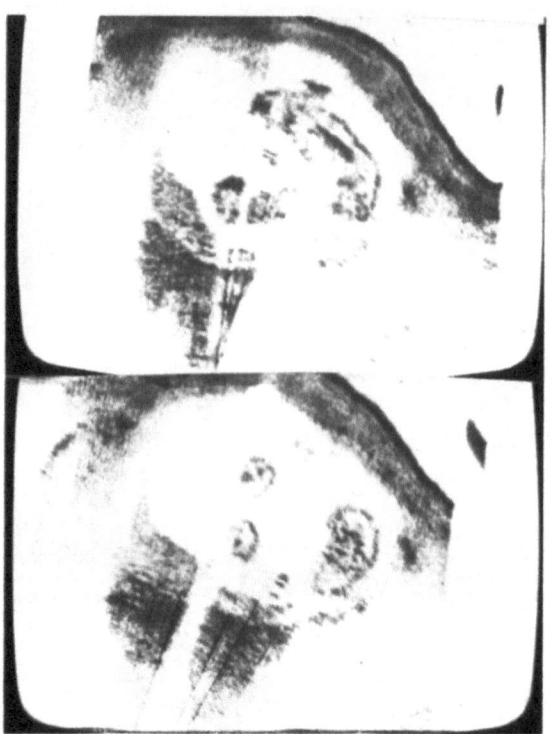

FIGURE 3.51(a)
Supine longitudinal scan. Gray scale. The fetal lower limbs are seen in cross section. Fetal extremities are seen as discrete echogenic areas. Sonic shadow is present.

FIGURE 3.51(c)
Supine transverse scan. Gray scale. The fetal thorax is identified in an oblique plane. The fetal elbow, forearm, and hand with distinct echoes from the digits are clearly displayed.

FIGURE 3.51(b)
Supine transverse scan. Gray scale. Anterior placenta. Fetal extremities are noted.

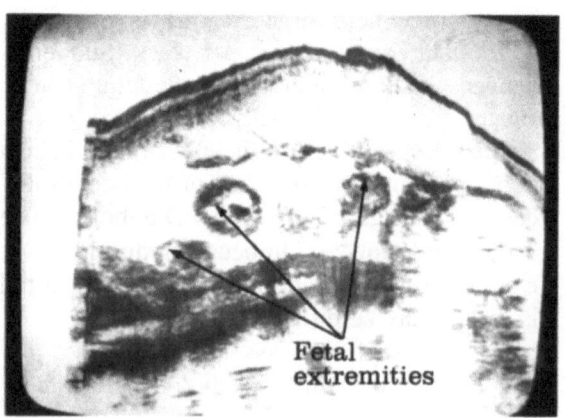

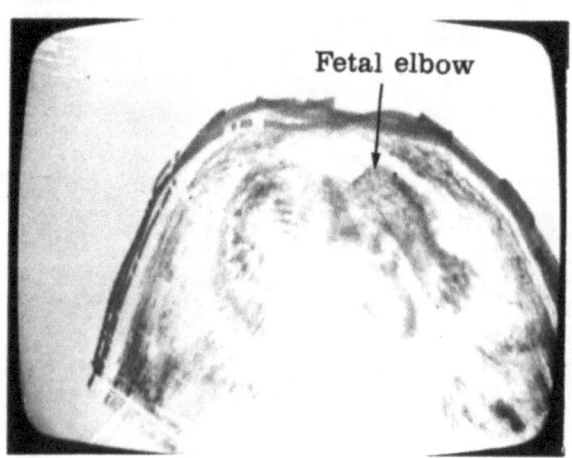

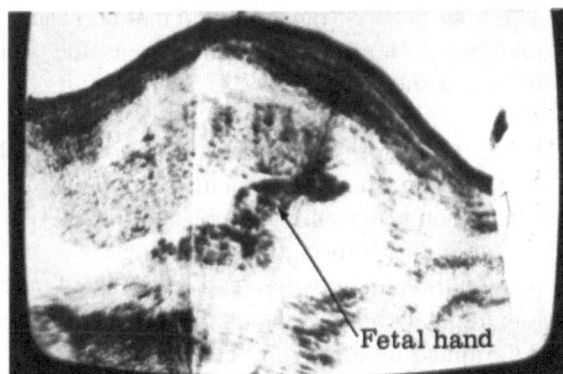

FIGURE 3-51 (d)

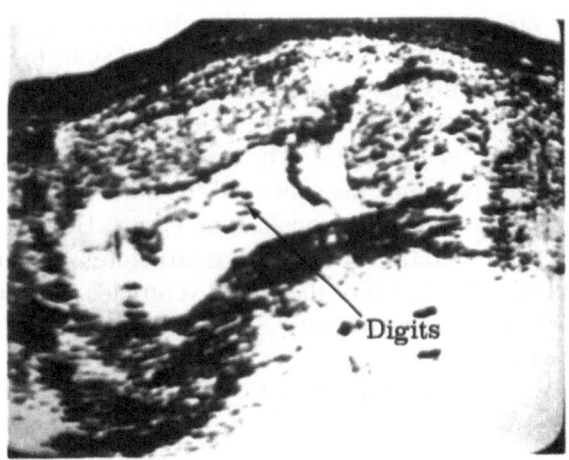

FIGURE 3-51 (e)

FIGURE 3-51 (f)

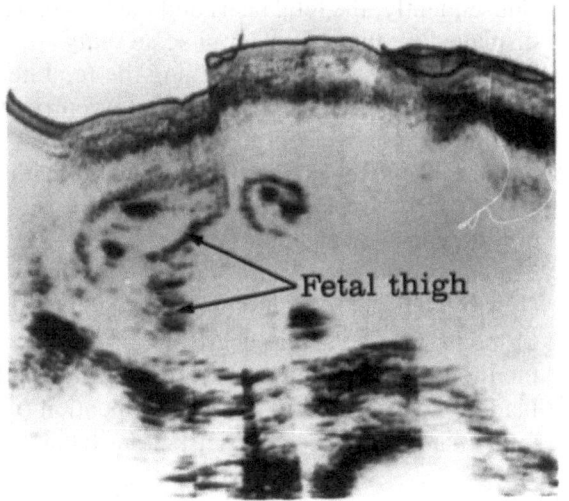

measurement and follow-up is extremely helpful for final termination of the pregnancy.

PRESENTATION AND POSITION

Ultrasonography is an excellent method for evaluation of presentation and position. Ultrasonography is especially valuable when there is difficulty in palpation. Obesity, muscular resistance of the abdominal wall, or a very thick anterior placenta are among the commonest obstacles to palpation of the fetus. With ultrasonic study, the muscles of the anterior abdominal wall and their fascial attachments can be seen in detail. If the patient is heavy and obese, Scarpa's fascia is occasionally outlined (18).

FIGURE 3.51(d)
Supine transverse scan. Gray scale. The fetal elbow, forearm, and hand are clearly displayed.

FIGURE 3.51(e)
Supine transverse scan. Gray scale. Anterior placenta with a prominent umbilical cord is visualized. The fetal hand with distinct digits is imaged clearly with high-resolution gray scale.

FIGURE 3.51(f)
Supine transverse scan. Gray scale. Clearly displayed fetal perineum.

FIGURE 3.52
Supine longitudinal scan. Gray scale. Vertex presentation. There is a double outline due to the fetal skull. Also noted is a double outline to the distal bladder wall. Real-time scanner revealed vigorous fetal movement against the bladder.

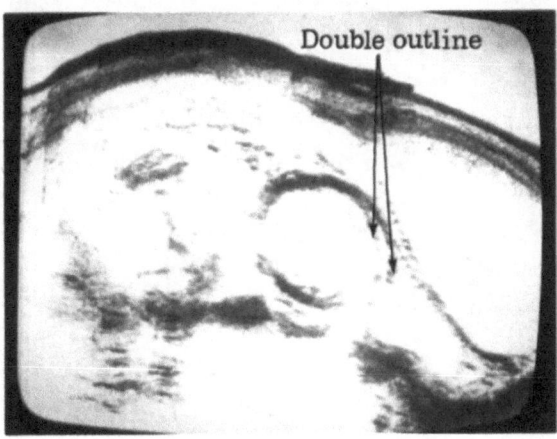

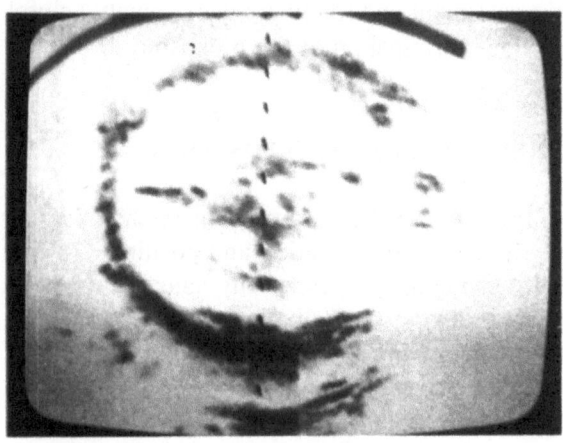

FIGURE 3.53
Supine scan. Demonstration of midline echoes emanating from such structures as falx cerebri, third ventricle, and lateral ventricle.

FIGURE 3.54
Supine longitudinal scan. Gray scale. In the cephalic presentation the fetal head can be localized in the lower part of the uterus.

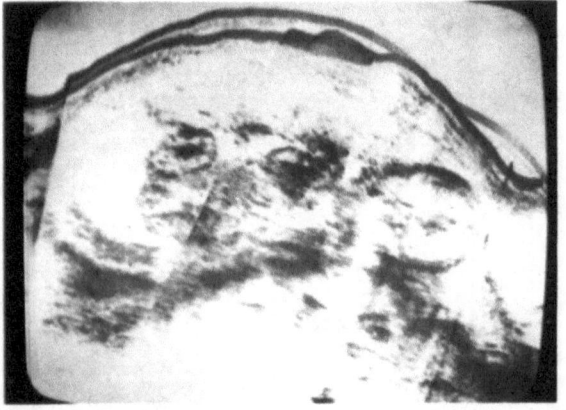

The fetal head is transonic and can be easily identified as a round structure on one side of the uterus or the other.

Since the majority of fetuses are in the cephalic presentation, the discernment of another orientation is extremely important in obstetric management. Information regarding presentation and position can be obtained in the longitudinal section. The fetal attitude is easily determined by localizing fetal parts in both longitudinal and horizontal ultrasonic studies.

The longitudinal scan is taken for identification of the fetus and its lie. Then horizontal sections are performed at selected levels for verification of presumptive diagnostic findings. Taking the total fetus into consideration, stronger echoes will be returned from the skull than from any other fetal part (18). The reflecting bony calvarium, including the echoes of the inner and outer tables, makes the localization easier. However, demonstration of the midline structures, such as the falx cerebri or the lateral ventricles, is absolutely diagnostic (Fig. 3.53). Difficulties arise when the head is engaged and penetration through the pubic bone is not possible.

The fetal trunk can first be identified by the detection of the fetal spine and fetal heart with the real-time scanner. For further evaluation, different sections at different levels, including oblique projections, are necessary. Subsequently, the fetal heart and kidneys can be displayed by bistable or gray-scale units. Difficulties arise in distinguishing the fetal heart from the fetal bladder when the interventricular septum cannot be identified. By slicing at various levels, the position of the bladder with respect to the rest of the trunk can be ascertained. Cardiac contractility can be evaluated and the pulsations of the fetal heart (120 to 140 beats per minute) can be captured by M-mode. Grossly, fetal heart motion can be monitored by the real-time scanner, whereas the bladder echo has no motion. Identification of fetal anatomy has been described in detail.

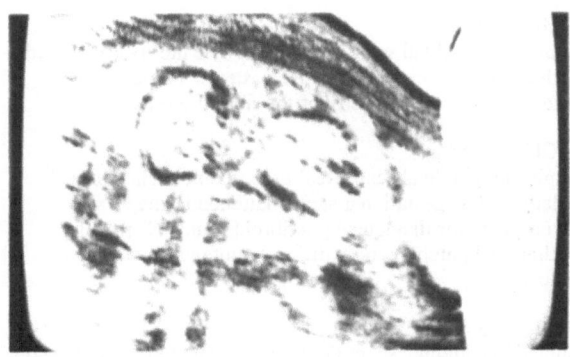

FIGURE 3.55
Supine longitudinal scan. Gray scale. In the breech presentation the fetal head can be localized in the upper part of the uterus.

CEPHALIC PRESENTATION

The fetal head can be localized in the lower part of the uterus (Fig. 3.54). Detection of the head and its display echo does not present any difficulty. The only problem, as previously described, arises when the head is engaged and thus difficult to image.

The shape of the returned echo is extremely important for assessing fetal head position. When the head is well flexed, the plane of section goes through both the parietal and suboccipitobregmatic diameters. Consequently, the displayed echo appears perfectly circular in shape. With further extension of the head, other diameters can be identified and the head loses its circular shape.

BREECH PRESENTATION

In breech presentation, the head can be localized in the upper part of the uterus (Fig. 3.55). In contrast to the cephalic presentation, detection of the head and its display echoes may present some difficulties, especially when there is excessive movement of the fetus. The problem arises in distinguishing the fetal head from the fetal trunk; but the best landmarks for differentiation of these two structures are the fetal spine and fetal heart. Longitudinal sections are of great value for detection of the breech (18).

FIGURE 3.56
Supine scan. Gray scale. In the transverse lie the fetal head and trunk are located in the transverse position.

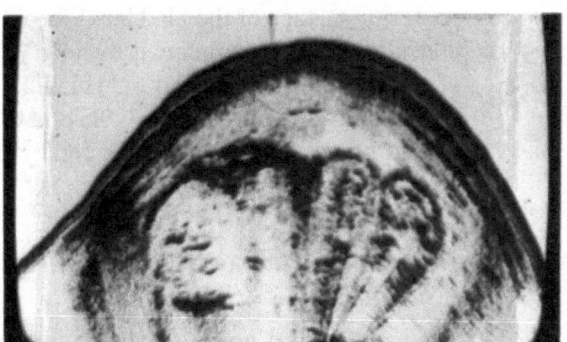

TRANSVERSE LIE

In transverse lie, the head and trunk are ususally located at the same level and fetal parts (eg, hands, feet) are generally located above or below the trunk (Fig. 3.56). The main difficulty in detecting transverse lie is that its appearance must be differentiated from that of twins. The only way to achieve absolute certainty is to obtain multiple sections at different times. The cause of the malpresentation must be further

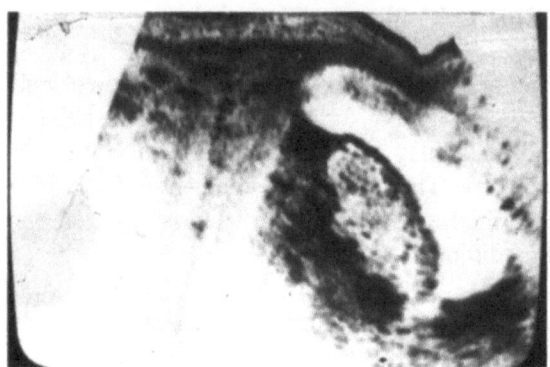

FIGURE 3-57

FIGURE 3.57
Supine longitudinal scan. Gray scale. The uterus is enlarged with extrinsic pressure over the posterior border of the bladder. Note echogenicity of the fibroid uterus.

FIGURE 3.58(a)
Supine longitudinal scan. Real-time scanner. The uterus is enlarged. The gestational sac is flattened in the anteroposterior diameter by a fibroid tumor of irregular outline and patchy echo pattern. Spontaneous abortion followed.

FIGURE 3.58(b)
Supine longitudinal scan. Gray scale. The uterus is enlarged. Infarcted fibroid nodule with internal echoes is seen in the uterine fundus. Clear, well-defined gestational sac is located in lower portion of the uterus.

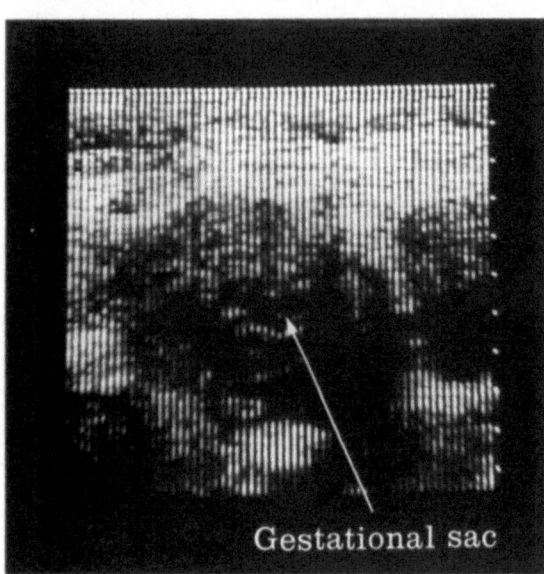

Gestational sac

FIGURE 3-58 (a)

FIGURE 3-58 (b)

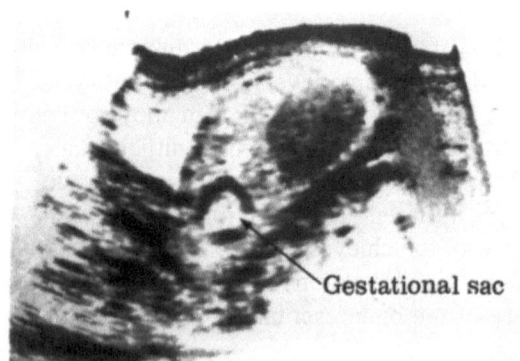

Gestational sac

investigated (19). If the real-time scanner is available, the diagnostic workup is made more simple.

DIFFERENTIAL DIAGNOSIS

Any pelvic mass of sufficient size or any enlarged uterus should be investigated for possible pregnancy. The following conditions require full investigation.

1. In a simple, uncomplicated fibroid, the uterus demonstrates as an echo-free space (20), but in pregnancy, fetal parts have their own echo patterns. On the other hand, in myomatous degeneration (21), the fibroid usually has some internal echoes (Fig. 3.57). Another valuable criterion is the fact that the fibroid is much firmer than the pregnant uterus, and, as a result, this usually produces an indentation on the posterior surface of the bladder. Fibroid uterus may be accompanied by pregnancy (Fig. 3.58a and b). Headlike calcified fibroid uterus (Fig. 3.59a and b) should not be mistaken for the fetal head and will be discussed in detail.

2. The distinction of a bladder diverticulum from a pregnant uterus is easily made.

3. Recognition of a nonpregnant uterus in an abnormal position relative to other

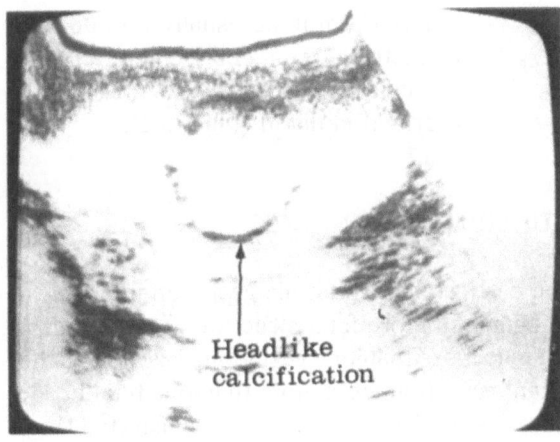

FIGURE 3-59 (a)

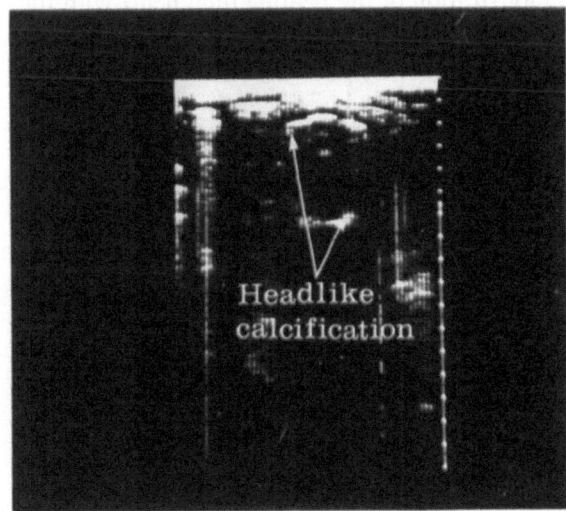

FIGURE 3-59 (b)

FIGURE 3-60

organs automatically excludes pregnancy (22).

4. Ovarian cysts usually are echo free (Fig. 3.60) unless the cysts are loculated.

5. Carcinoma of the ovary does not have a specific echographic pattern and only the mass can be outlined (23).

6. Ectopic pregnancy may be suggested by confirmation of the pregnancy ring outside of the uterus, fetal parts seen outside the uterus, or enlargement of the uterus with diffuse amorphous internal echoes and no fetal parts. (Fig. 3.61) The clinical correlation is of extreme help.

FIGURE 3.59(a)
Supine transverse scan. Gray scale. Rounded incomplete ring of echoes is noted within a large fibroid uterus. Distal to the posterior wall of the calcific mass is an artifactual reverberation echo simulating the distal boundary of the fibroid. This may be confused with a fetal head. Ring-shaped calcified fibroid.

FIGURE 3.59(b)
Supine transverse scan. Real-time scanner demonstrates calcified fibroid simulating a fetal head. Note the sonic shadowing distal to the calcific interface. Sonic shadowing is generally better appreciated with the real-time scanner due to its linear beam path.

FIGURE 3.60
Supine transverse scan. Gray scale. Ovarian cyst in the right side is seen. Ovarian cysts are usually echo-free unless the cyst is loculated.

FIGURE 3.61
Supine transverse scan. Gray scale. Rounded adnexal mass with scattered internal echoes represents ectopic gestational sac.

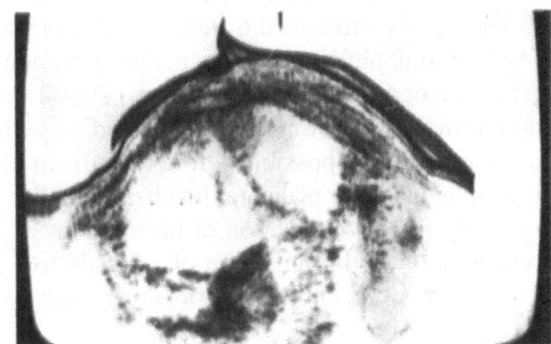

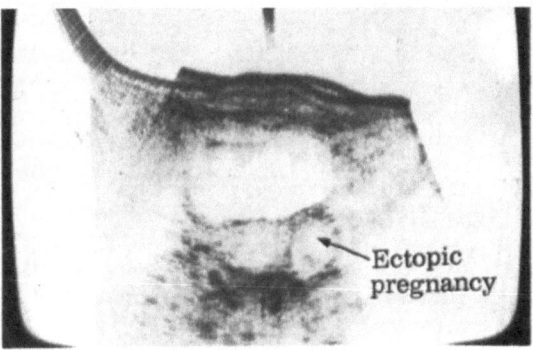

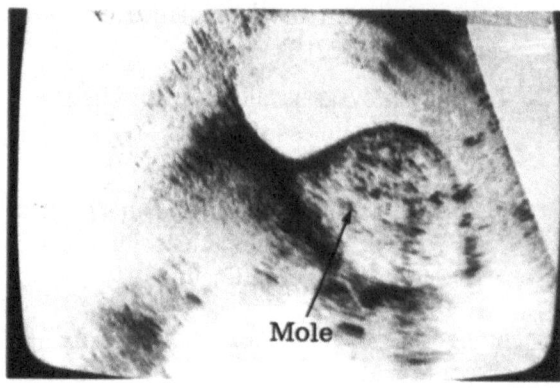

FIGURE 3.62
Supine longitudinal scan. Gray scale. The uterus is diffusely enlarged and indents the bladder. Through transmission is high. Fine echoes fill the uterine cavity. Hydatidiform mole.

FIGURE 3.63(a)
Supine longitudinal scan. B-mode. Two fetal heads are noted at opposite ends of the uterus in the vertex and breech presentations. This is the usual appearance of twin gestation. A posterior placenta is noted.

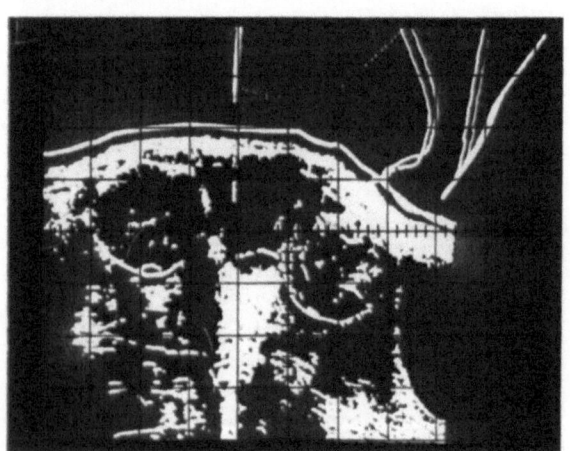

7. Hydatidiform mole usually produces symmetric uterine enlargement and has a specific echo pattern which is described in detail (Fig. 3.62).

MULTIPLE PREGNANCY

The early state of multiple gestation may be recognized before fetal structure is observed. There is more than one gestational sac and as the pregnancy progresses more than one fetal head, thorax, and placenta may be demonstrated (Fig. 3.63a,b, and c). Separate gestational sacs may be identified at as early as 6 weeks' gestation (Fig. 3.63d). The problem of the round fetal body simulating a second head is easily resolved with demonstration of the beating fetal heart with the real-time scanner.

SPURIOUS PREGNANCY OR PSEUDOCYESIS

Pseudocyesis usually occurs near menopause or in women with an intense desire for a child. These patients may have increased abdominal size with usually normal menstruation. Morning sickness may exist. Ultrasonography is one of the best tests for these patients since it can automatically exclude pregnancy. The patient will usually be convinced of the actual situation.

THE PLACENTA

Determination of the placental position in the uterus with respect to the cervix has been a major achievement of ultrasound. The normal placenta may be followed from its earliest phase to the various physiologic degenerative changes that occur near term. Abnormalities of position and internal structure may now be studied with an accuracy never possible before the advent of ultrasound. Precise placental localization is necessary for the evaluation of bleeding in pregnancy or for the insertion of a needle for atraumatic amniocentesis. Ultrasonographic

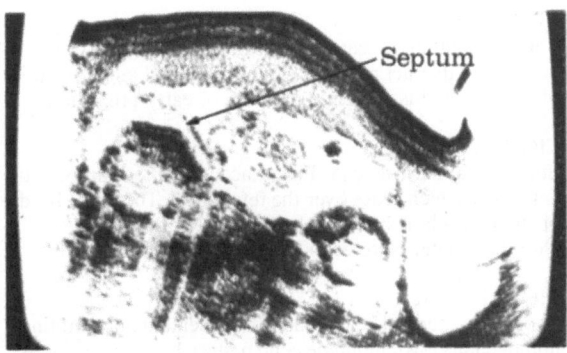

FIGURE 3.63(b)
Supine longitudinal scan. Gray scale. Anterior and posterior placentas are noted. Fetal heads appear at both poles of the uterine cavity. A linear echogenic septum marks the separation of the twin pregnancy.

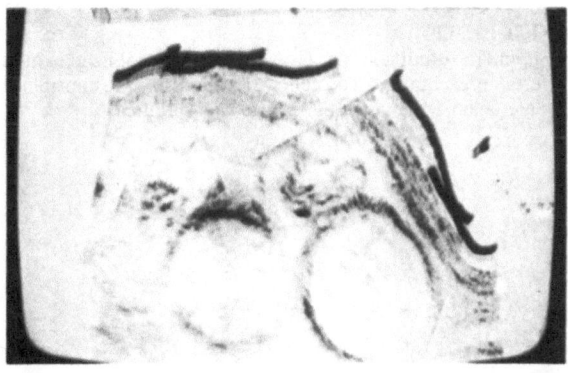

FIGURE 3.63(c)
Supine oblique scan. Gray scale. Two rounded fetal heads are adjacent to each other. Optimal documentation of twins is provided when both heads are shown in the same plane; oblique sections may be necessary. The real-time scanner will show twins easily with sonofluoroscopy.

FIGURE 3.63(d)
Supine longitudinal scan. Gray scale. Two gestational sacs may be identified as early as 6 weeks' gestation. Note two gestational sacs inside the enlarged uterus.

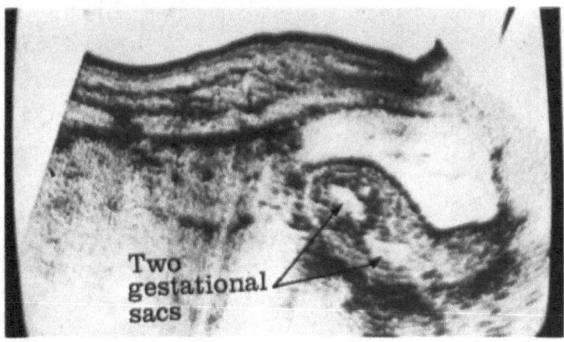

placental localization has completely replaced the procedure of radioisotopic scanning, which was the preferred method of localization before the development of B-scan ultrasound (24–30).

NORMAL PLACENTA

The placenta is first seen at about 10 weeks' gestation and at this time it may occupy between one-half and three-fourths of the uterine cavity. The placental tissue at this time is moderately echogenic. Several weeks later it assumes the low-amplitude homogeneous echo pattern that will characterize this organ for the majority of the pregnancy (Fig. 3.64a) (31).

Routine study with B-mode or gray scale demonstrates the placenta as a thick speckled band of echoes in the echo-free background of the amniotic fluid (Fig. 3.64b and c). This homogeneous band is surrounded by a thin echogenic boundary facing the intrauterine cavity and represents the chorionic plate of the placenta (Fig. 3.65a and b). At low sensitivity the placenta is echo free, while at high gain settings it completely fills in with echoes. The margins of the placenta may be determined with great accuracy and correlated with external physical landmarks.

Echoes inside the placenta arise from the internal texture of the placenta, the chorionic villi, and are easily recorded with high amplification (Fig. 3.66). Between the echoes of the chorionic villi, which are a diffuse reflector of ultrasound, and the fetus is an echo-free zone corresponding to the amniotic fluid.

If the position of the placenta is difficult to determine, the transverse scan is very helpful in establishing the primary site of this structure. This is particularly important in amniocentesis where, for instance, an anterior placenta may not entirely cover the anterior wall, and the ultrasonographer may be able to localize an area for puncture of the uterus through the anterior abdominal wall under which no placental tissue is present.

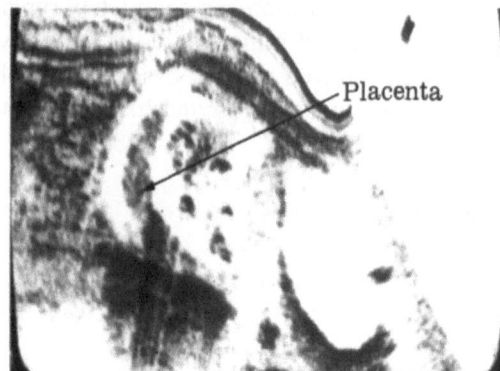

FIGURE 3-64 (a)

FIGURE 3.64(a)
Supine longitudinal scan. Gray scale. After 12 to 13 weeks of gestation a distinct placenta can be identified in the majority of cases. Fundus posterior placenta of early pregnancy.

FIGURE 3.64(b)
Supine longitudinal scan. Fine placental echoes are noted anteriorly which cross over the fetal body. The distal border of the placenta is bounded by the dark echoes of the chorionic plate. Note echo-free area of amniotic fluid.

FIGURE 3.64(c)
Supine longitudinal scan. Anterior placenta demonstrating homogenous low-amplitude echo pattern bounded by high-amplitude echoes of the chorionic plate.

FIGURE 3.65(a)
Supine longitudinal scan. Gray scale. The fetal head is in the vertex presentation. The anterior placenta shows the echogenic margin of the chorionic plate. Sonic shadow is cast by fetal parts in a normal fetus.

FIGURE 3.65(b)
Supine longitudinal scan. Gray scale. The fetal head is in the vertex presentation. The echogenic margin of the chorionic plate against the amniotic fluid is well outlined.

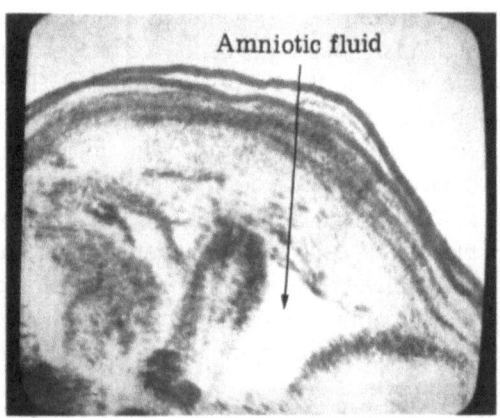

FIGURE 3-64 (b)

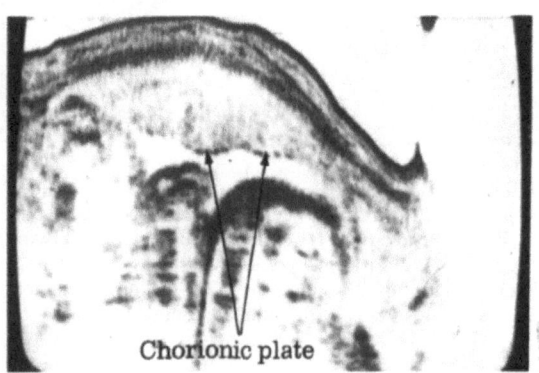

FIGURE 3-65 (a)

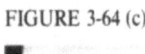

FIGURE 3-64 (c)

FIGURE 3-65 (b)

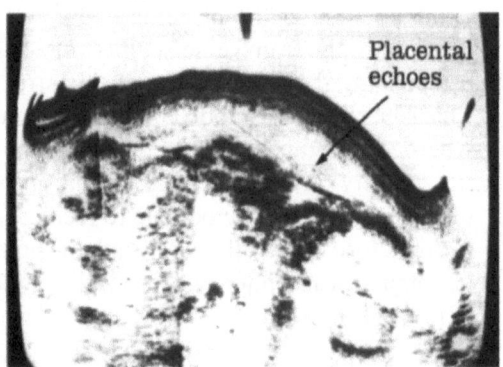

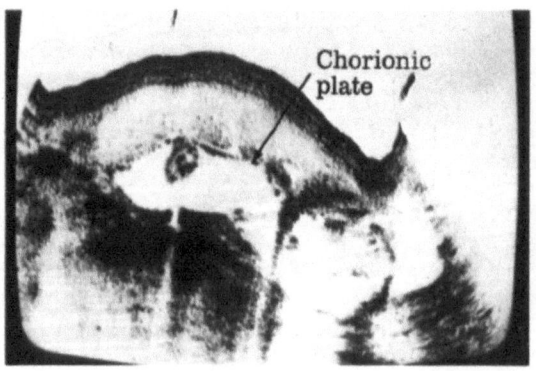

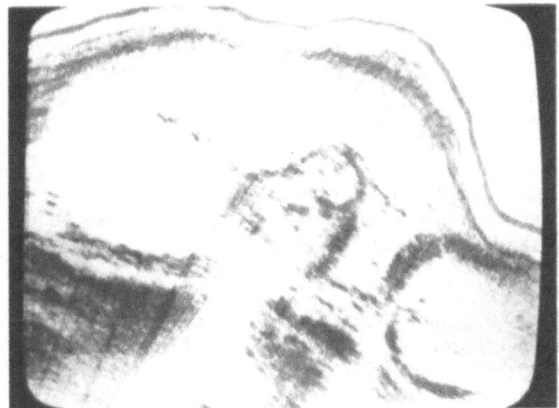

FIGURE 3-66

Gray-scale imaging reveals new dimensions in placental growth and pathology. Between 13 and 28 weeks, the internal echoes of the placenta lie within the chorionic plate and the uterine wall echoes are low amplitude in intensity (Fig. 3.67). Since the placenta is a diffuse reflector, compound scanning techniques generally produce the best imaging of this structure. Difficulties arise in the diagnosis of the posterior placenta. The overlying fetus generally attenuates much of the sound beam so that the weak echoes of the posterior placenta may not be of sufficient intensity to register on the oscilloscope (Fig. 3.68a and b). This sonic

FIGURE 3.66
Supine longitudinal scan. Gray scale. Echoes inside the placenta arise from the internal texture of the placenta, the chorionic villi, and are easily recorded with high amplification. The placenta is anterior. There is an indentation in the midportion of the placenta due to pressure by a fetal extremity.

FIGURE 3.67
Supine longitudinal scan. Gray scale. Between 13 and 28 weeks, the internal echoes of the placenta lie within the chorionic plate and the echoes of the uterine walls are low amplitude in intensity.

FIGURE 3.68(a)
Supine longitudinal scan. Gray scale. The posterior placenta is echo free and poorly imaged. Posterior placenta should always be suspected when the fetal body and head are anterior and separated from the posterior uterine wall by any significant distance.

FIGURE 3.68(b)
Supine longitudinal scan. Gray scale. The overlying fetus generally attenuates much of the sound beam, so that the weak echoes of the posterior placenta may not be of sufficient intensity to register on the oscilloscope.

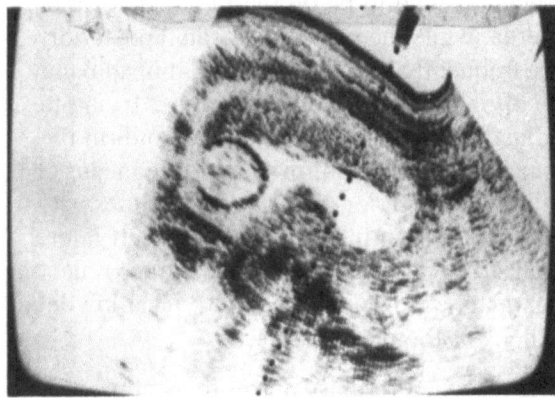

FIGURE 3-67

FIGURE 3-68 (a)

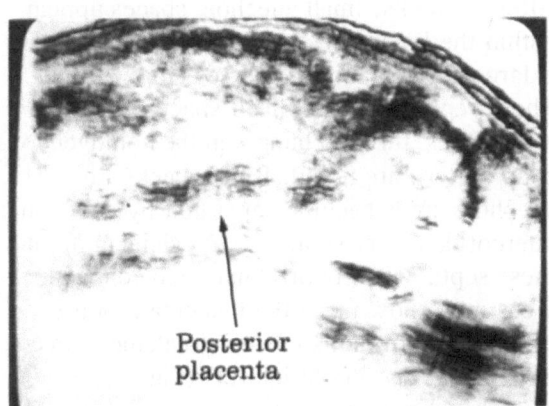

Posterior placenta

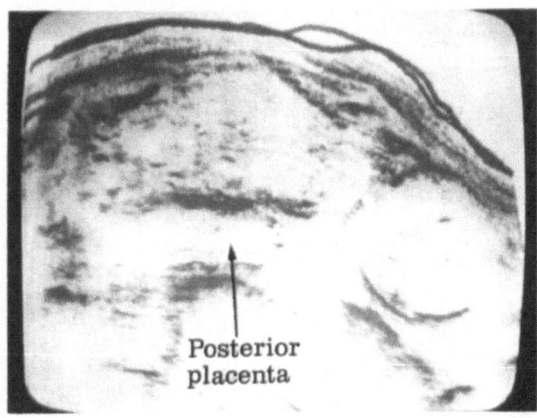

Posterior placenta

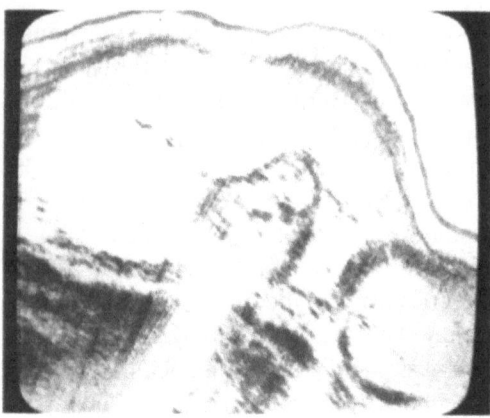

FIGURE 3-69 (a)

FIGURE 3.69(a)
Supine longitudinal scan. Gray scale. The fetal head is in the vertex presentation. The anterior placenta shows the interrupted echogenic margin of the chorionic plate. Sonic shadow is cast by fetal parts in a normal fetus.

FIGURE 3.69(b)
Supine transverse scan. Gray scale. The placenta may enlarge markedly in the presence of edema. This is seen in erythroblastosis fetalis. Posterior placenta.

FIGURE 3.70
Supine longitudinal scan. Gray scale. The uterus is markedly distended with a large echo-free area due to polyhydramnios. Note the thin rim of placental tissue from rapid uterine expansion.

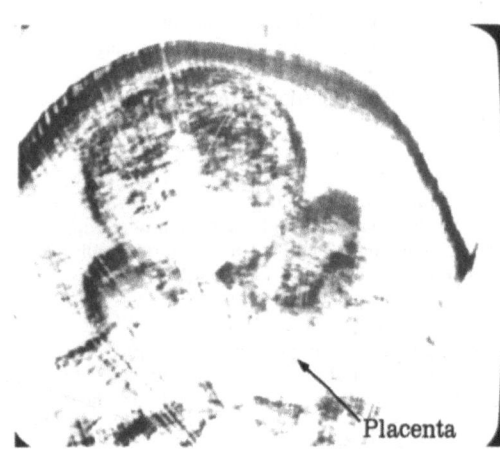

Placenta

FIGURE 3-69 (b)

FIGURE 3-70

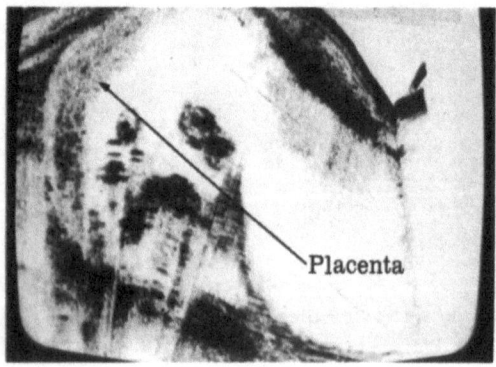

Placenta

shadowing effect is common and its very presence is one of the diagnostic criteria of a posterior placenta. The majority of anterior placentas tend to be on the right side of the uterus, while the placentas located posteriorly are frequently left sided. This relationship may be of value to the ultrasonographer trying to adjust the scanning technique to confirm the location of a posterior placenta. One means of filling the posterior placenta with echoes is to compound scan from the right and left lateral walls to the abdomen, using the diffuse reflecting characteristics to produce the typical low-level echoes of the placental tissue.

The placental form is subject to local pressure changes (Fig. 3.69a). It may enlarge markedly in the presence of edema. This is seen in erythroblastosis fetalis (Fig. 3.69b). The placenta may be thinned and depressed when adjacent to some fetal structure or in the distended uterus of polyhydramnios (Fig. 3.70) (32).

After 28 weeks, small anechoic spaces appear within the homogeneous echo pattern and enlarge as gestation progresses (Fig. 3.71). These represent blood-filled spaces. As term approaches, further changes in the homogeneous echo pattern are noted. By 36 weeks, the anechoic areas become separated by echogenic intercotyledonary septa due to calcification of these septa. Also, poorly margined echogenic areas may show up in the placenta and are irregular, amorphous placental calcifications most likely due to old infarcts (Fig. 3.72a,b,c,d,e, and f).

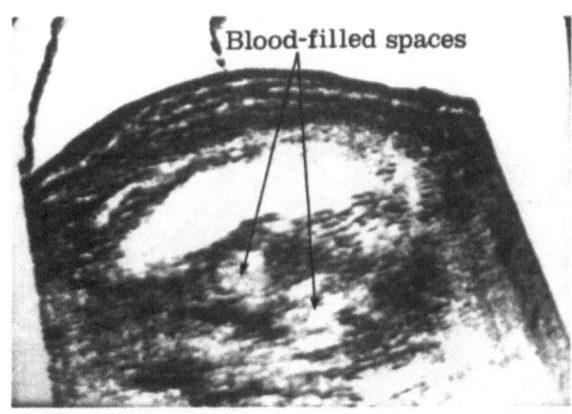

Blood-filled spaces

FIGURE 3.71
Supine longitudinal scan. Gray scale. Areas of degenerative changes within the placenta may appear as echo-poor regions with a random distribution.

TYPES OF PLACENTA

The anterior placenta is located along the anterior wall of the uterus. The fundal placenta lies in the uterine fundus.

A corporeal placenta is adjacent to the body of the uterus. Thus, an anterior fundocorporeal placenta extends the entire length of the uterus in an anterior position. Posterior placentas are against the posterior uterine wall and the above classification applies in a similar manner. Lateral placentas occur on either the right or left lateral wall. This type is unusual and may extend anteriorly or posteriorly. The tendency for posterior placentas to be left sided and anterior placentas to be found on the right side may be due to the rotation of the uterus as it grows out of the pelvic cavity (33).

The posterior placenta presents unique problems since it is often shielded from the incident ultrasound beam by the fetal parts, and the speckled echoes of the chorionic villi and the continuous band of the chorionic plate may not be well visualized. We may be able to appreciate part of the placenta or observe a separation between the fetus and the posterior wall of the uterus that is made from failure to localize any placental structure inside the uterus (Fig. 2.41B).

PLACENTA PREVIA

The diagnosis of placenta previa is made when placental tissue overlies the internal cervical os (Fig. 3.73a,b,c,d,e,f,g,h, and i). A full bladder is most important to provide a sonic window to detect low-intensity placental echoes in the region of the internal os. This is especially true in the case of posterior placenta previa where the filled bladder may displace the overlying fetal structures away from the cervical canal, thus permitting better imaging. Early detection of placenta previa is vitally important for patient care.

The normal placenta will separate the fetal skull in the vertex presentation from the maternal sacrum by a distance of less than 1.6 cm.

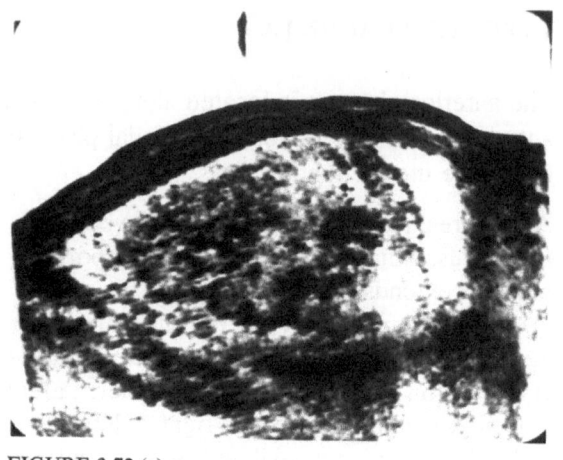

FIGURE 3-72 (a)

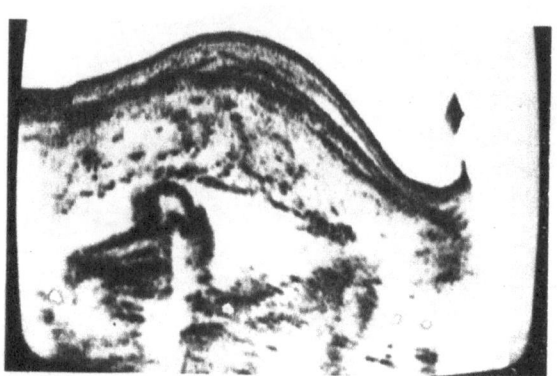

FIGURE 3-72 (d)

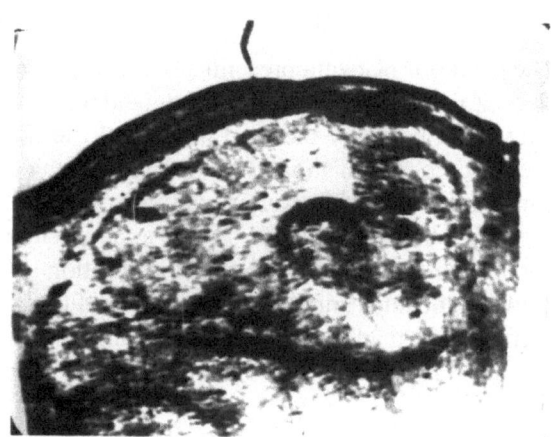

FIGURE 3-72 (b)

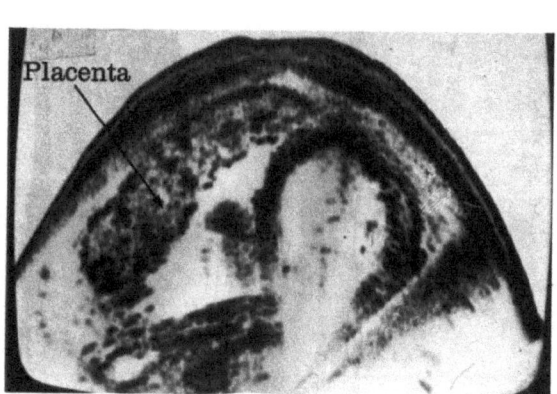

FIGURE 3-72 (e)

FIGURE 3-72 (c)

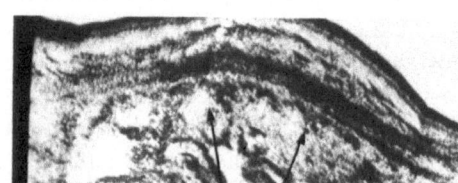

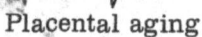

FIGURE 3-72 (f)

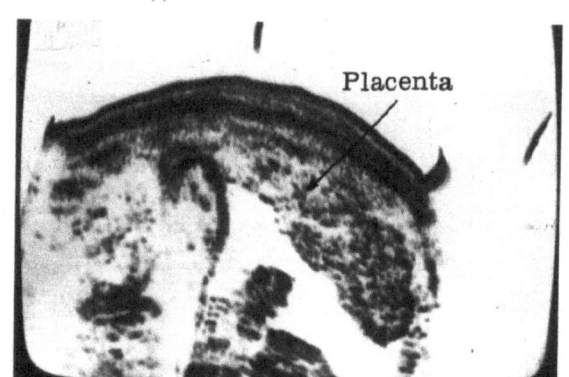

FIGURE 3.72(a)
Supine longitudinal scan. Gray scale. Scan through lateral placenta showing irregularity of the normally homogeneous placental tissue with echo-poor and strongly echogenic regions. Echo-poor areas represent degenerative changes. Echogenic zones are diffuse calcifications of the placenta. Normal fetus delivered.

FIGURE 3.72(b)
Supine longitudinal scan. Gray scale. Scan over this posterior placenta shows multiple echogenic interfaces with sonic shadowing, indicative of heavy areas of calcification in regions of previous placental degenerative changes.

FIGURE 3.72(c)
Supine longitudinal scan. Gray scale. The anterior placenta has an irregular echo pattern with scattered high-amplitude regions. Placental degeneration changes at 37 weeks' gestation.

FIGURE 3.72(d)
Supine transverse scan. Gray scale. Same case as in Fig. 3.72c. Anterior placenta has an irregular echo pattern with scattered high-amplitude regions. Placental degenerative changes at 37 weeks' gestation.

FIGURE 3.72(e)
Supine transverse scan. Gray scale. The anterior placenta multiple areas of high- and low-amplitude echoes which represent calcifications and infarctions.

FIGURE 3.72(f)
Supine longitudinal scan. Gray scale. Same case as in Fig. 3.72e. Anterior placenta with multiple areas of high- and low-amplitude echoes which represent infarctions and calcifications.

Therefore, any separation less than this makes a placenta previa unlikely (34). This measurement may only be applied when the fetal head lies in the pelvis. To achieve this position, the mother may stand for a time or gentle manual maneuvers may be tried if the fetus is in another position. To differentiate a floating head from a placenta previa producing separation of the fetal skull from the sacrum, manual compression of the head in an anteroposterior plane will push the freely floating head against the sacrum. If the placenta is between the skull and sacrum, no decrease in distance will be noted. If the amniotic fluid is between the fetal head and the bony pelvis, there will be a notable narrowing of the distance on the precompression and the postcompression scans.

In the transverse lie or breech presentation, detection of placenta previa is difficult. Placenta previa may be marginal, partial, or total, which completely covers the cervical os. To be certain, the fornix should be identified. If the longitudinal section is performed off midline, lateral placenta may mimic placenta previa. It is thus essential that the fornix and the midline be identified for detection of placenta previa. If the lower border of the placenta extends to the internal cervical os the placenta previa is of the marginal type. The placental tissue covers the entire cervical os and is of great thickness at this site in total placenta previa. Difficulty often arises in the diagnosis of placenta previa when the placenta is posterior and the fetus is in the vertex presentation. In this case, the fetal head produces sonic shadowing of the placenta and placental echoes are not visualized. Our experience with the real-time scanner has shown that under sonofluoroscopy, the fetal head may be pushed into a more cephalic position, and the posterior placenta that had been previously covered by the fetus now returns many echoes and can be precisely localized. This maneuver may be performed manually or in the Trendelenburg position. Occasionally, nidation may be the predisposing factor in placenta previa formation. Routine ultrasonography during early pregnancy is recommended to locate the position of the pregnancy ring to prepare for possible placental abnormalities (35).

A large series of placenta previas were followed from midtrimester at 2- to 3-week intervals. Serial study showed a significant increase in the distance between the lower segment of the placenta and the cervix as compared with that found upon initial examination. As the end of pregnancy approached, the diagnosis of placenta previa was less justifiable. Of a total of 112 patients in the second trimester with ostensible placenta previa, 102 placental migrations occurred sufficiently to rule out the diagnosis of placenta previa at term (36). Our experience has shown that there is little placental migration after 32 weeks' gestation. Thus, after 32 weeks' gestation, the diagnosis of placenta previa may be firmly offered.

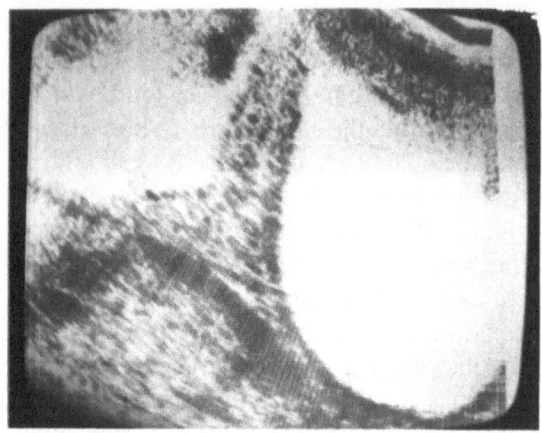

FIGURE 3-73 (a)

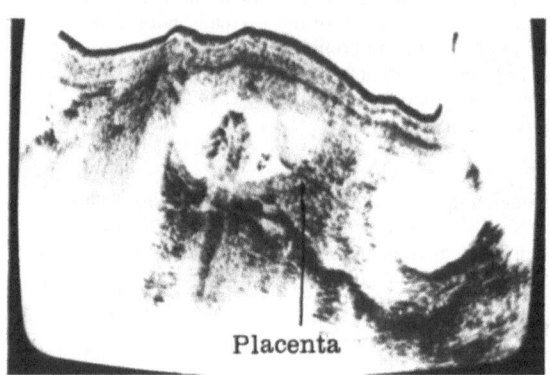

FIGURE 3-73 (d)

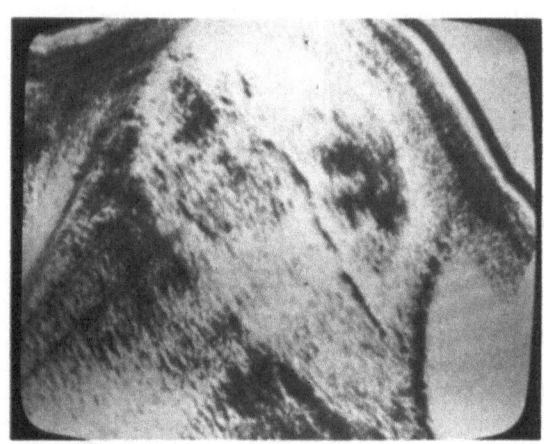

FIGURE 3-73 (b)

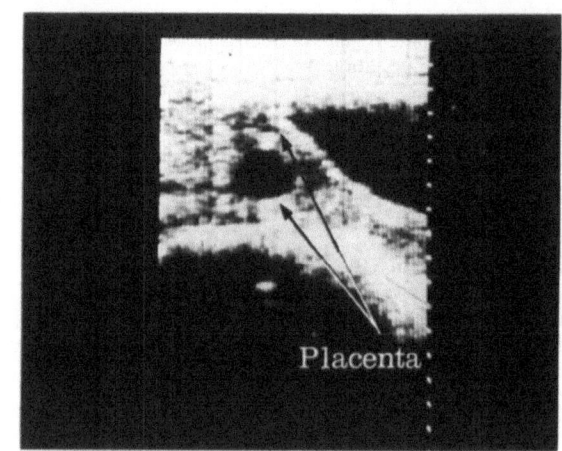

FIGURE 3-73 (e)

FIGURE 3-73 (c)

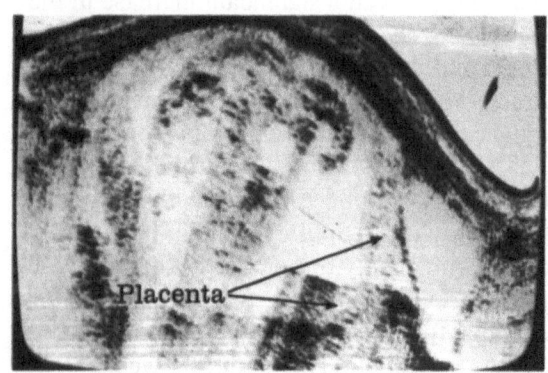

FIGURE 3-73 (f)

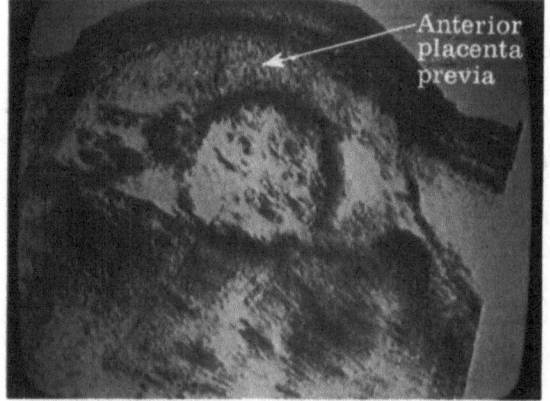

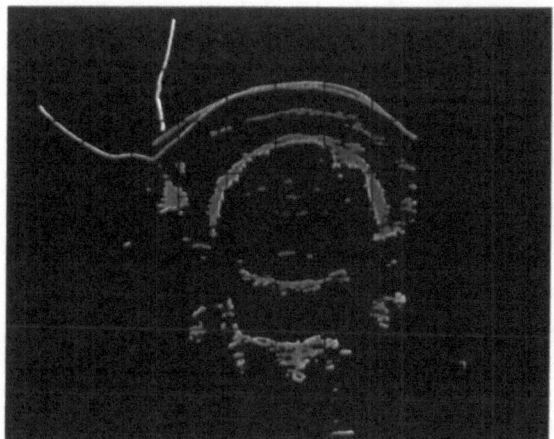

FIGURE 3-73 (g)

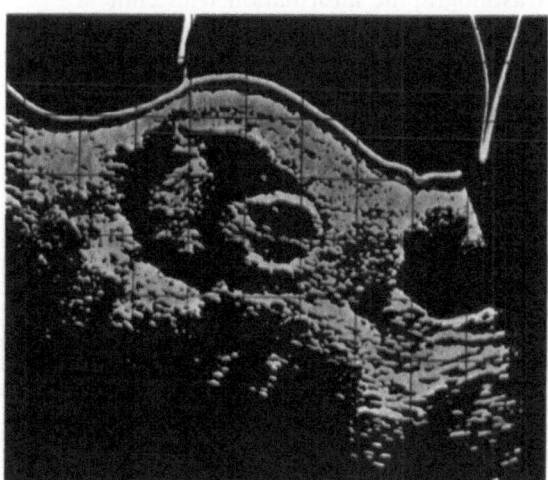

FIGURE 3-73 (h)

FIGURE 3-73 (i)

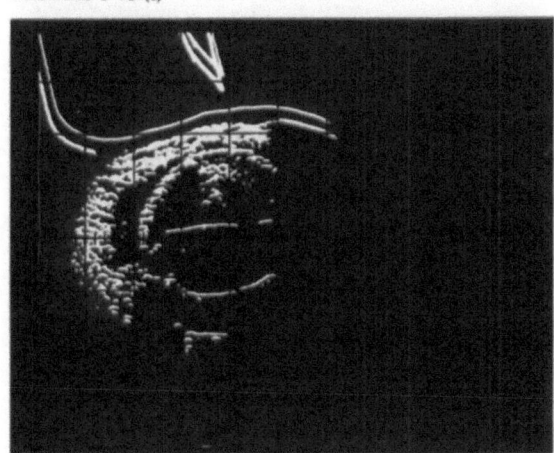

FIGURE 3.73(a)
Supine longitudinal scan. Gray scale. Magnified view of total placenta previa with medium-amplitude echoes covering the internal os of the uterus. The chorionic plate is difficult to image in this type of placental position.

FIGURE 3.73(b)
Supine longitudinal scan. Gray scale. The placenta occupies one-half of the uterus on the posterior wall. There is anterior extension of the placenta over the internal cervical os producing placenta previs. Fetal structures are noted within the amniotic fluid cavity.

FIGURE 3.73(c)
Supine longitudinal scan. Gray scale. The posterior fundal-corporeal-isthmic placenta extends completely over the internal cervical os. Note sonic shadowing of the placenta by the fetal spine.

FIGURE 3.75(d)
Supine longitudinal scan. Gray scale. Early detection of placenta previa. Sixteen weeks' gestation showing placental echoes completely covering the internal cervical os.

FIGURE 3.75(e)
Supine longitudinal scan. Real-time scanner. The echo-free bladder is fully distended. The echoes of the placenta extend from anterior and posterior directions and completely cover the internal cervical os. The echo-free amniotic fluid separates the anterior and posterior leaves of the placenta previa.

FIGURE 3.73(f)
Supine longitudinal scan. Gray scale. The speckled anterior placental echoes extend over the internal cervical os in this placenta previa.

FIGURE 3.73(g)
Supine transverse scan. Scan is taken over the engaged fetal head. The distance between the sacral wall echoes and the fetal head is 3 cm. The normal distance is less than 1.6 cm. The placenta is posterior and separates the head from the sacrum by a distance greater than normal in placenta previa. This distance did not change after pressure was applied.

FIGURE 3.73(h)
Supine longitudinal scan. Middle pregnancy with placenta previa. Note cephalic presentation of fetal head. Serial scans may show migration of placenta upward to a normal position.

FIGURE 3.73(i)
Supine transverse scan. B-mode. The fetal midline and lateral ventricular walls are demonstrated within the fetal head. The calvarium is separated from the sacrum by a distance greater than 1.6 cm due to the presence of a posterior placenta previa.

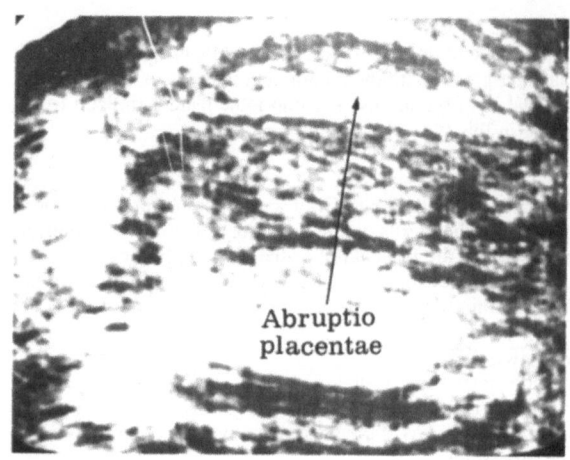

FIGURE 3.74
Supine longitudinal scan. Gray scale. The placenta is separated from the uterine wall by an echo-free space representing retroplacental hematoma. This mid-trimester bleeding patient had abruptio placentae.

ABRUPTIO PLACENTAE

Premature separation of the placenta from the uterus resulting in hemorrhage is the gross pathologic change in abruptio placentae (Fig. 3.74). The blood hemorrhaging between the placenta and the maternal uterus generally appears as an echo-free zone with a crescentic shape conforming to the anatomic location of the blood. There may be an associated outward bulge of the placental contour into the amniotic cavity. Signs of fetal distress or fetal demise should be searched for by the ultrasonographer.

Some difficulties may arise in determination of abruptio placentae; however, a combination of ultrasonographic information with clinical findings greatly facilitates diagnosis. To rule out abruptio placentae, ultrasonographic study reveals the following.

1. Exclusion of placenta previa by prior ultrasonographic study
2. Presence of numerous echoes making the placental image thicker, due to placental separation in abruptio placentae
3. Detection and/or exclusion of retroperitoneal hematoma
4. Falsely appearing abruptio placentae caused by tangential study of normal placenta; this is clarified by further sectioning.

PLACENTAL SIZE

The placenta may increase in size in various physiologic and pathologic states. The placenta enlarges with multiple gestations deriving their blood supply from one placental site, and in diabetes, syphilis, and Rh disorders. The volume of the placenta decreases in the presence of fetal demise or organizing infarct. One report stated that the development of echo-poor spaces within the near-term placenta is an indication of fetal maturity (37).

FETAL EVALUATION

DOPPLER EXAMINATION IN PREGNANCY

The Doppler principle of change in frequency with motion of a reflector of an ultrasonic signal has proven to be great use in obstetric management. Doppler studies record signals when motion is present and record no signals when the reflecting surface is motionless. Doppler ultrasound involves a type of motion sensor as contrasted with the imaging sensor of B-scan ultrasound. It has been used to detect early fetal heart motion, locate the placenta, identify vaginal or pelvic arteries, and study the fetal heart rate in late pregnancy stress tests and labor (38).

The stethoscope has been used for the evaluation of fetal heart rate patterns for many years. It has been found that this type of auscultation can only detect prolonged and severe tachycardia and bradycardia (39). Doppler ultrasound permits continuous fetal heart rate monitoring between uterine contractions as well as during contractions. Doppler technique may be audible or recorded on a strip-chart device (40). Doppler ultrasound is more sensitive than is phonocardiography since there is less interference with extraneous noise.

Abnormal fetal heart rate patterns have been classified into three main categories: (1) early deceleration due to fetal head compression; (2) late deceleration characterizing uteroplacental insufficiency; and (3) variable deceleration occurring from umbilical cord compression. The continual use of fetal heart rate monitoring has been found to improve perinatal outcome (41).

The observation of the fetal heart rate response to the stress of uterine contractions has been of use in predicting fetal jeopardy. The oxytocin challenge test (42) using external fetal heart rate monitoring to show the effect of contractions on the fetus has also been of value.

AMNIOCENTESIS

Many antenatal diagnostic studies rely on the analysis of amniotic fluid components. Chromosome analysis is used in the study of Down's syndrome in patients with increased maternal age or a previous child with a trisomy 21 or other trisomy disorder. Also, translocations of the 21 chromosome and X-linked disorders such as hemophilia may be evaluated in this manner. Amniotic fluid is used for enzyme assay in fetuses with suspected inherited biochemical disorders. Chromosomal linkage analysis is of value in certain autosomal dominant abnormalities. The intrauterine diagnosis of spina bifida or anencephalic states may be aided by the level of α-fetoprotein in the amniotic fluid.

Most sampling of amniotic fluid is performed at 16 weeks' gestation, since at this time there is adequate amniotic fluid volume and the cellularity of the fluid is increased. This early tapping allows the performance of a second trimester abortion after the biochemical and cytogenetic tests are completed after 2 to 6 weeks. Cells in the amniotic fluid settle rapidly. It is advisable for placental localization to be performed by scanning and then for the patient to be ambulatory until shortly before puncture. Although amniocentesis entails more risk when twins are present, continual visual monitoring with the real-time scanner will allow for proper guidance of the needle.

In placental localization prior to amniocentesis, it is important to place the needle through the uterus in an area devoid of placental tissue or through the thinnest portion of an anterior placenta as far away from the umbilical artery and vein as possible (Fig. 3.75). Failure to do this may result in a bloody tap which can contaminate the specimen and render it useless for analysis. The needle may transect the umbilical vessels resulting in fetal demise. Significant retroplacental bleeding may endanger the mother.

The procedure may be performed with the real-time scanner or with the puncture transducer.

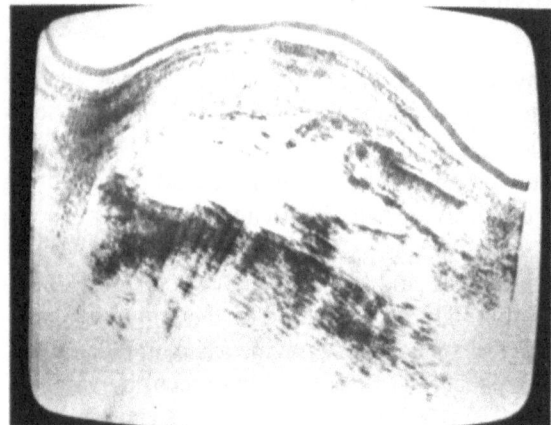
FIGURE 3-75

The placenta is scanned and the transducer is placed over the largest area of amniotic fluid. Since a smooth metallic needle will only be imaged when the beam is perpendicular to the axis of the needle, a specially grooved needle with a teflon sheath is used. It is inserted obliquely through the anesthetized skin to lie within the amniotic fluid under the transducer beam. Since the needle is small, if it is not initially detected, the transducer should be angled through a gentle arc to pick up the needle echoes. Sometimes the needle will appear within the amniotic cavity and no fluid will return. It is most likely that the membranes have been displaced by the needle and a brisk push on the needle may puncture the membranes. This is of no danger since the real-time scanner monitors the position of both the needle and the fetus. (43).

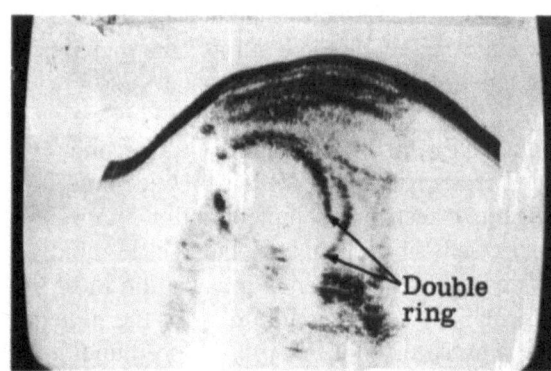
FIGURE 3-76

FIGURE 3.75
Supine longitudinal scan. Gray scale. The low-amplitude echoes of the placenta are contained within the echogenic boundary of the chorionic plate. Fetal parts are noted.

FIGURE 3.76
Supine transverse scan. Gray scale. The outline of the fetal skull is irregular with overlapping of the strong cranial echoes. Fetal demise.

FIGURE 3.77
Supine longitudinal scan. Double-ring contour to the fetal head is due to fetal motion during the scanning procedure. This problem does not occur with real-time scanning.

FIGURE 3.78
Supine transverse scan. Gray scale. Section through distal part of cranium. Note massive edema of scalp surrounding the oval outline of the fetal skull. High through transmission noted distal to edematous tissues of the pericranium. Erythroblastosis fetalis.

FIGURE 3-77
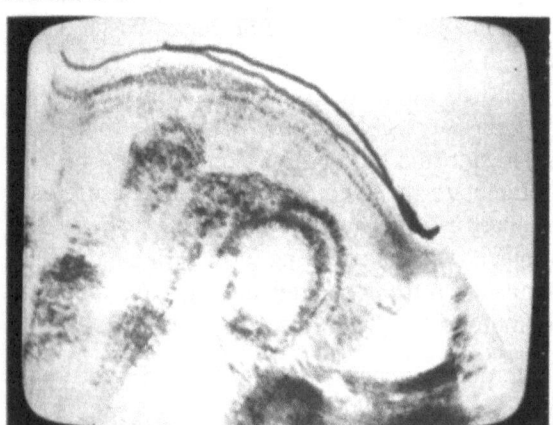

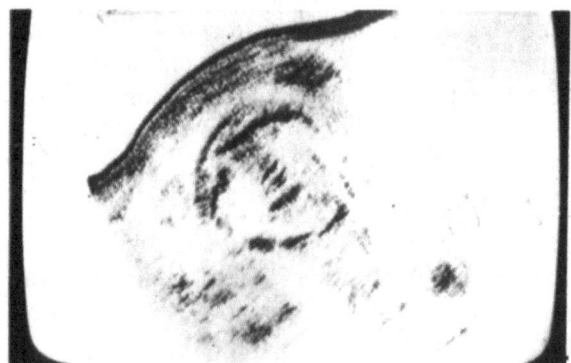

Amniocentesis may also be performed with the puncture transducer with a central bore. The direction of the probe and the needle site are marked by the electronic line on the oscilloscope which may be superimposed upon the B-scan. This visibly depicts the path of intended puncture. The distal echoes represent the fetus or fetal parts and this distance may be monitored with either the A-mode or M-mode displays. The area selected is prepared and draped. A sterilized aspiration transducer with a central lumen is then attached to the ultrasonic unit. The exact depth of the amniotic fluid within the uterus is determined from the sonogram study, by using either digital read-out or A-mode monitoring. The needle is advanced through the central lumen of the aspiration transducer into the amniotic fluid. The procedure can be continuously monitored and the echo from the tip of the needle will be registered in the same fashion as echoes from needles directed ultrasonographically into the uterine cavity for saline abortions. Ultrasonography has also been utilized in the placement of endoscopes when direct visual monitoring of the fetus and placenta is needed. The exact depth of the tip of the endoscopic needle can be evaluated easily (43).

In our experience amniocentesis using ultrasonic guidance is not necessary if a posterior placenta has been documented. Sonofluoroscopy is indicated during amniocentesis when the placenta is in the anterior position.

ANOMALIES OF PREGNANCY

FETAL DEATH

The ultrasonic determination of fetal demise depends upon the duration of the pregnancy. In early gestation the death of the fetus may be represented by fragmentation of the gestational sac, which may appear as a circular or triangular echo-free zone interrupted by scattered strong echoes within the uterus. The uterus is generally small for the expected dates. Later in pregnancy, Doppler ultrasound and M-mode recording may be used to evaluate fetal viability. After 8 weeks'

gestation, fetal motion may be detected by Doppler techniques, M-mode, or the real-time scanner. These methods are the only means to check the fetus during the "gray zone" of ultrasonic diagnosis occurring between the tenth and thirteenth week of gestation, when there is no clearly defined gestational sac or fetal head. The absence of fetal motion or fetal heart beat signifies fetal death. Doppler ultrasound may accurately record fetal heart motion at 12 weeks' gestation; in addition, the real-time scanner and M-mode can detect fetal activity at about 8 weeks' gestation. After 13 weeks' gestation, the characteristic deformities of the nonviable fetus are imaged with the gray-scale scanner. Following a given period of time, certain echographic changes are noted on the sonogram. A double ringlike contour to the normal single ring appearance of the fetal skull appears (Fig. 3.76). This ultrasonic appearance is equivalent to the radiographic "halo" sign, which is noted in a matter of days subsequent to fetal death as a radiolucency adjacent to the fetal skull, most likely representing edema of the fetal scalp or layering out of fat within the scalp tissue planes. This sign is nonspecific and may be seen in fetuses of diabetic mothers (43); in normal fetuses, either with or without fetal movement during contact B-scanning (Fig. 3.77); in erythroblastosis fetalis (Fig. 3.78); or when the fetal head deeply indents the bladder wall and may produce a double interface echo pattern that simulates a double skull contour at the point of contact of the fetal head with the bladder. This pseudo–double ring shape is localized and does not appear to completely encircle the fetal head (Fig. 3.79).

The chest wall becomes irregular in a similar manner to the fetal skull after a longer period subsequent to fetal demise. This is then followed by the appearance of a disorganized echo pattern within the fetal head and thoracic cavity (Fig. 3.80). Subsequently, it is noted that the outlines of the head and thorax become grossly distorted and that evidence of fetal growth on follow-up sonograms has ceased. Air within the fetus due to internal decomposition may produce a sonic shadow (Fig. 3.81). Often it is necessary to wait

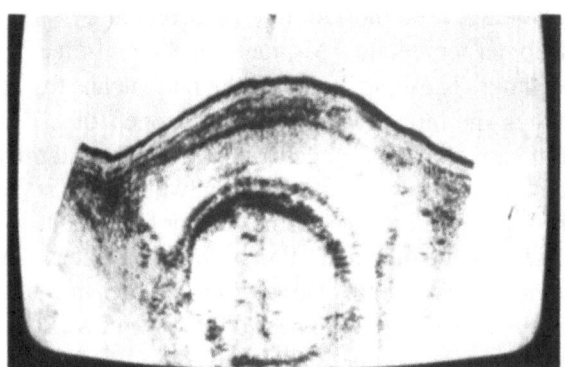

FIGURE 3-79

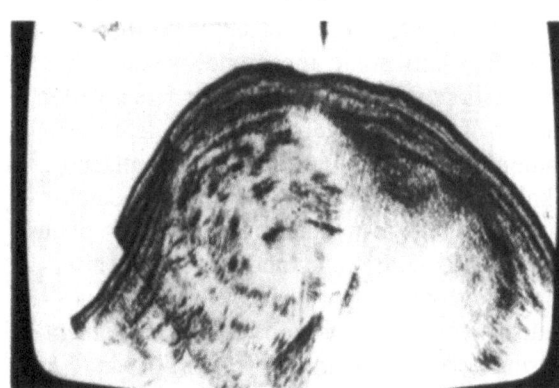

FIGURE 3-80

FIGURE 3-81

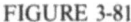

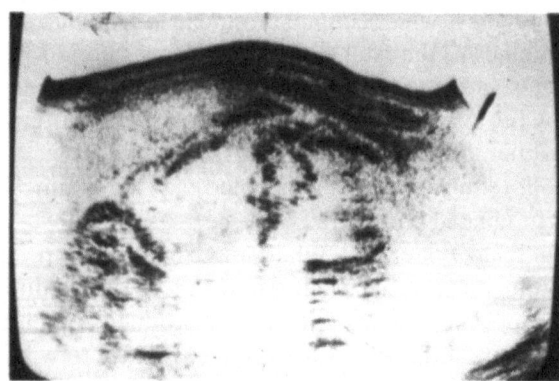

FIGURE 3.79
Supine transverse scan. Gray scale. The fetal head deeply indents the bladder. This produces a pseudo–double skull contour which should not be mistaken for fetal demise. Note the single layer of the fetal head posteriorly.

FIGURE 3.80
Supine transverse scan. Gray scale. Scan through the fetal body shows no recognizable anatomic structures. Internal disorganization is due to fetal demise of several days length.

FIGURE 3.81
Supine longitudinal scan. Gray scale. The distal border of the fetal body is not imaged due to sonic shadowing. Large amounts of gas were present intraabdominally due to tissue decomposition resulting from fetal death.

2 to 6 days to document these changes, approximately 5 to 7 days after the fetal death diagnosis can be established. Immediate and definitive proof is obtained when there is no fetal heart motion discernable with the real-time scanner. The optimal determination will be obtained by usage of the real-time scanner and Doppler technique. Alternatively, gray scale will image the cardiac chambers and M-mode may be used to record the presence or absence of cardiac contractility.

RADIOLOGIC SIGNS OF FETAL DEATH

The following radiologic signs may be observed.

1. Spalding's sign. There is gross overlapping of skull bones, due to liquefaction of the brain. This usually develops several days after fetal death.

2. Exaggerated curvature of the fetal spine. This situation needs more time to develop and depends on maceration of spinous ligaments.

3. Gas in the fetus. This is the most reliable sign.

ABORTION

DIAGNOSIS OF ABORTION

Ultrasonographic findings are extremely useful in the management of suspected spontaneous abortion. Ultrasound can determine whether the

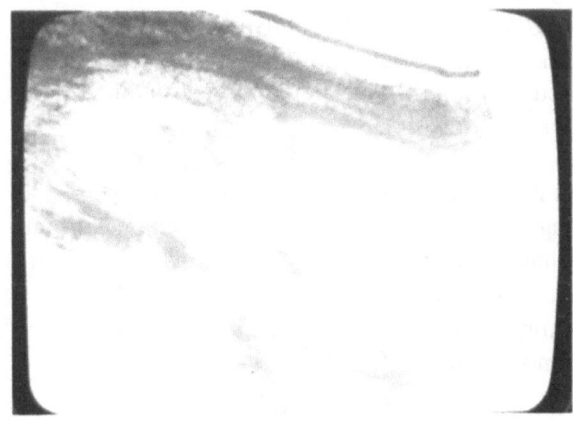

FIGURE 3.82(a)
Supine longitudinal scan. Gray scale. The uterus is of fibroid type. The pregnancy ring has an irregular shape with an area of interrupted echo pattern. This configuration when coupled with appropriate clinical data represents threatened abortion.

FIGURE 3.82(b)
Supine longitudinal scan. Gray scale. Large multiseptate cystic lesion in the cul de sac is noted. Patient admitted to the hospital with a diagnosis of threatened abortion. Patient underwent surgery because of enlarged cystic lesion. At operation, a hemorrhagic luteal cyst was found.

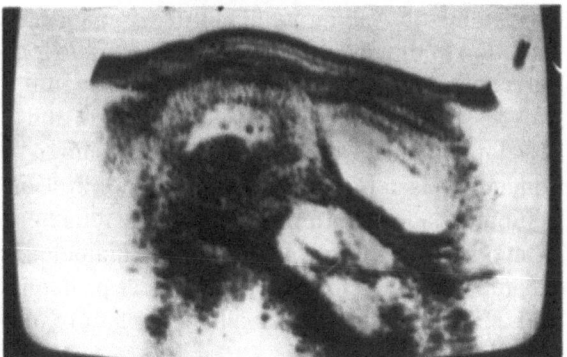

fetus or gestational sac is within the uterus or has already passed, and can also evaluate the status of the products of conception. The decision to perform surgery on the bleeding pregnant patient, treat her with bed rest, or send the patient home without a curettage is assisted by the ultrasonic findings within the uterine cavity. The actively bleeding patient with a uterus full of echoes should have surgery performed; while the patient with diminishing vaginal hemorrhage and a uterine cavity without echoes may be spared an unnecessary dilation and curettage. The early application of ultrasonography in the diagnosis of abortion will save both the patient and the clinician much valuable time and trouble.

THREATENED ABORTION

In threatened abortion the status of the gestational sac of the bleeding patient must be carefully evaluated. The pregnancy ring may be circular and intact or it may be incomplete or defective in some areas (Fig. 3.82a). We have found that small gaps in the structure of the sac in the bleeding patient follow a normal course of events. Similarly, an irregular sac may be associated with a spontaneous abortion. We suggest serial evaluation of the gestational sac as the optimal method of following threatened abortion (Fig. 3.82b). A partially open pregnancy ring may enlarge and close up to form a complete and intact sac on subsequent scans. The absence of growth of the uterus is another important factor in the analysis of abortion. The normal gestational sac should enlarge within 1 week while the aborting uterus may show a decrease in size of the pregnancy ring. The ultrasonographic diagnosis of abortion becomes extremely complex during the "gray zone" of pregnancy at 10 to 13 weeks' gestation where the pregnancy ring is no longer present. The ultrasonographer should not confuse the irregularity of the gestational sac fusing into the walls of the uterus with the broken pregnancy ring of the aborting gestational sac. The use of real-time scanning to evaluate fetal motion and provide proof of fetal viability appears to be useful in experienced hands. We have observed intrauterine echoes with motion that have still progressed to spontaneous abortion. The application of motion techniques should be coupled with the clinical data and information of the gray scale B-scans.

MISSED ABORTION

The ultrasonographic diagnosis of missed abortion is based on the lack of definite evidence of fetal life. The gestational sac, fetal parts, or definite fetal movements are not identifiable and the uterus is enlarged with only scattered amorphous echoes in its center. This ultrasonic appearance is not specific since other conditions may mimic a missed abortion (1). Hydatidiform mole, fibroid uterus, ovarian tumor, and the "gray zone" may be confused with a missed abortion. Clinical data, laboratory tests, and the use of serial sonograms for follow-up are the optimal tools for determining missed abortion (Fig. 3.83).

SUMMARY

Early bleeding in pregnancy generally occurs at 8 to 11 weeks and is usually due to a blighted ovum. The following criteria for the diagnosis of abortion have been described.

1. Loss of definition of the gestational sac or fragmentation of the pregnancy ring with a break in its contours

2. Absence of fetal echoes within the gestational sac after 10 weeks' gestation

3. A gestational sac that is small for the expected date

4. Failure of growth of the pregnancy ring with serial examinations

5. Low position of the gestational sac in the uterine cavity with or without an open cervix

Real-time scanning combined with Doppler and M-mode study yields optimum information in early pregnancy while the patient is bleeding. No sign of fetal movement after 10 weeks' gestation implies that the pregnancy is in jeopardy (13). The usual outcome of a blighted ovum is a spontaneous abortion. The application of these criteria may obviate long hospital stays since the various types of abortion may be suggested. An accuracy rate of 97.5 percent was obtained in a recent series (44).

As mentioned, threatened abortion may be diagnosed when bleeding occurs with or without definite evidence of fetal motion by M-mode or real-time scanning. In missed abortion with retained fetal tissue, scanning will usually demonstrate the following:

1. Uterus small for date

2. Failure of uterine growth on repeat serial studies

3. Abnormal and amorphous uterine contents or grossly distorted fetal outline

4. Absence of fetal motion

Incomplete abortion is suspected when there is no evidence of normal fetal structure and a series of echoes in line with the endometrial cavity is noted.

Complete abortion has occurred when there is only a straight line of echoes in the endometrial cavity or a complete absence of internal uterine echoes. Patients with an ultrasonically "empty" uterus may be sent home without routine curettage (45).

ECTOPIC PREGNANCY

Investigation of ectopic pregnancy requires precise history taking and skillful scanning with attention to the ultrasonic appearance of the fetal parts and placenta. A thorough knowledge of the progressive uterine changes and stages of the developing fetus is necessary. The best sign of conception is detection of the fetal head. Present equipment allows differentiation of the fetal head from other fetal parts only if the head diameter is greater than 2 cm (Fig. 3.84). Clinical problems with ectopic pregnancy usually occur before this

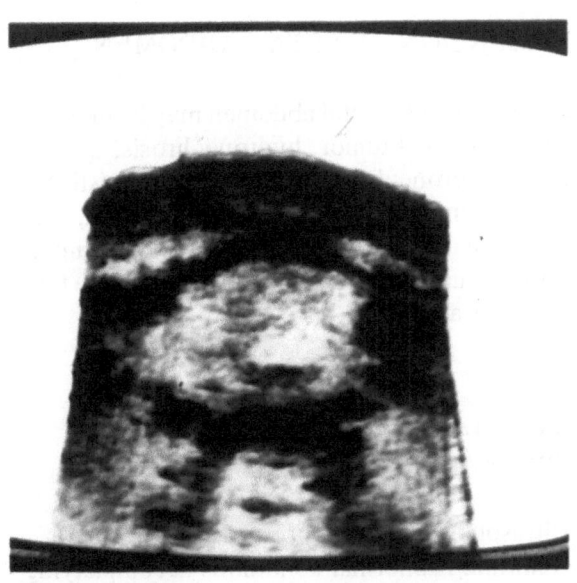

FIGURE 3.83
Supine transverse scan. Gray scale. Midline echo-free area within the uterus. The sharp distal wall should be mistaken for part of gestational sac. Retained blood clot from spontaneous abortion.

FIGURE 3.84
Supine transverse scan. Gray scale. The uterus is normal in size. An echo-free adnexal cyst was noted on serial scans. No hemoperitoneum was noted. Ectopic pregnancy at surgery.

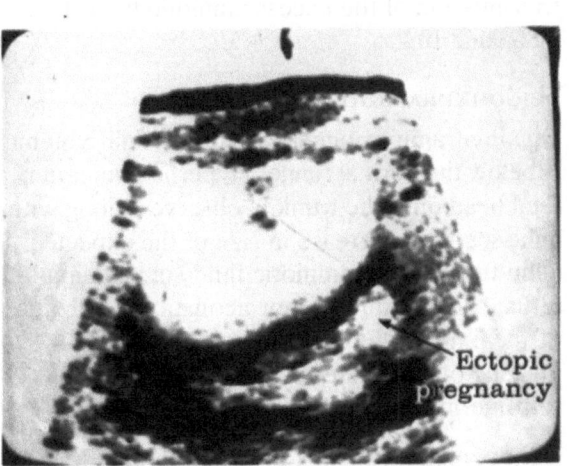

Ectopic
pregnancy

stage of fetal development is reached. Since investigation of the fetal head of less than 2 cm diameter is not possible in ectopic pregnancy, other criteria are used.

The uterus in ectopic pregnancy is enlarged to a moderate size. No definite intrauterine echo pattern of a gestational sac or fetal head is demonstrable. If there has been no history of the passage of fetal tissue products, the finding of an empty uterus with a positive pregnancy test is strongly suggestive of an ectopic pregnancy.

Various extrauterine signs are noted in the determination of ectopic gestation. The identification of a gestational sac or fetal head outside the uterus is positive proof of ectopic pregnancy; however, this finding is rarely observed. More often, a cystic, irregular mass, with or without internal echoes in the adnexal region or cul de sac is seen.

If the pregnancy sac ruptures, the resulting hemoperitoneum will produce a cystic pattern in the cul de sac which will usually change in shape and position due to gravitational forces. The chronically ruptured ectopic pregnancy appears as a complex mass. The uterus often cannot be separately imaged from the conglomerate pelvic mass.

INTRAABDOMINAL PREGNANCY

In intraabdominal pregnancy, there are irregular, widespread echoes throughout the entire abdomen, and multiple sections must be made to obtain a recognizable echo pattern. The ultrasonographer must differentiate the uterus from the fetal parts, since an enlarged uterus contains numerous echoes and in longitudinal scan may have the same ultrasonic appearance as the fetal body. Extrauterine localization of the fetal head and intraabdominal extrauterine position of the placenta are important findings; however, detection of the placenta and chorionic plate is hindered by the interfacing echo patterns from bowel loops, adhesions, inadequate amniotic fluid, and tangential placental slicing.

ABNORMAL FETUSES

HYDROCEPHALUS

Ultrasound has become a reliable method for the investigation of hydrocephalus. The biparietal diameter is greater than 10.5 cm and there is a relative disproportion between the size of the fetal trunk and the enlarged head. The distended ventricular system and associated brain atrophy allow better sonic penetration and increased through transmission is noted. Early in pregnancy, a BPD much larger than the expected size for date associated with a relatively smaller-than-normal fetal thorax raises a strong suspicion of hydrocephalus. A dead hydrocephalic fetus in utero may be surgically decompressed allowing for vaginal delivery rather than cesarian section. When the diagnosis of hydrocephalus is made, a cannula may be inserted into the fetal cranium under ultrasonic guidance. Drainage of the dilated ventricles permits serial decrease in cephalic size. Vaginal delivery may then be accomplished.

ANENCEPHALY

In normal gestation, the fetal head is usually demonstrable by 12 to 14 weeks' gestation. Anencephaly may be diagnosed after 15 weeks' gestation when scanning fails to reveal a normal fetal head despite use of multiple scanning planes. When the abnormal skull is definable, poor through transmission is noted due to the lack of sonolucent brain tissue and a relative overgrowth of the bony craniofacial structures (Fig. 3.85). The fetal outline is generally easily imaged due to the frequently associated polyhydramnios. When polyhydramnios is present the fetus and placenta are more sharply identifiable, and in many situations the placenta seems to be compressed by a massive amount of fluid.

DISTENSION OF FETAL ABDOMEN

Distension of the fetal abdomen may be due to intraabdominal tumor, hydronephrosis, or ascites. Hydronephrosis is the most interesting cause from an ultrasonographic viewpoint, since as time passes increased dilation is discernible. This is usually due to low obstruction of the fetal urinary tract.

ASSOCIATED ABNORMALITIES IN PREGNANCY

Ultrasonography is important in detecting or confirming abnormal conditions accompanying intrauterine pregnancy.

ASSESSMENT OF AMNIOTIC FLUID

POLYHYDRAMNIOS

Polyhydramnios exists when the fluid volume of the amniotic cavity exceeds 2000 ml. This condition is first clinically detectable when roughly 3000 ml of fluid is present within the uterine cavity. Ultrasonographically, a large area of sonolucency inside the uterus is noted with separation of the limbs from their usual position closely adjacent to the fetal body. The freely floating fetal parts are due to the large fluid volume in which the fetus lies. The fetal outline is sharply delineated due to the high through transmission of the excess amniotic fluid (Fig. 3.86a and b).

OLIGOHYDRAMNIOS

Oligohydramnios occurs when the fluid volume is below the normal range. Hyperflexion of the fetal head onto the trunk is observed along with an associated decrease in size of the expected echo-free zone of amniotic fluid surrounding the fetus. This produces poor acoustic visualization of the external fetal contours and impaired imaging of the posterior uterine wall and retrouterine structures.

Either polyhydramnios or oligohydramnios may reflect fetal abnormality. Anencephaly is

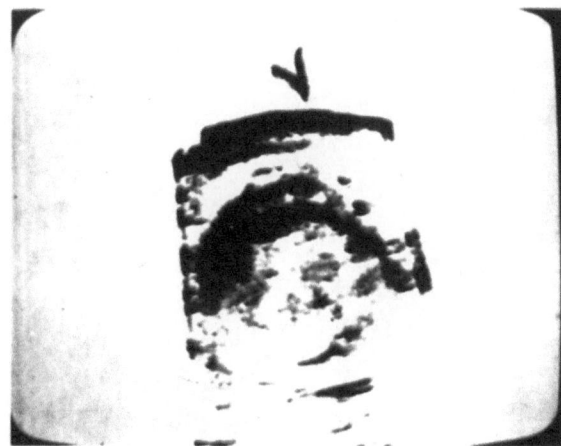

FIGURE 3-85

FIGURE 3.85
Supine transverse scan. Gray scale. Section through the fetal head shows total deformity of the usually rounded calvarial echoes. Paired echogenic oval structures represent the abnormally enlarged orbits. Through transmission is low due to the hypertrophy of the facial bones that occurs in anencephaly.

FIGURE 3.86(a)
Supine longitudinal scan. Gray scale. The uterus is markedly distended with a large echo-free area due to polyhydramnios. Note the thin rim of placental tissue from rapid uterine expansion.

FIGURE 3.86(b)
Supine longitudinal scan. Gray scale. The freely floating parts are due to the large fluid volume in which the fetus lies. The fetal outline is sharply delineated due to the excess amniotic fluid.

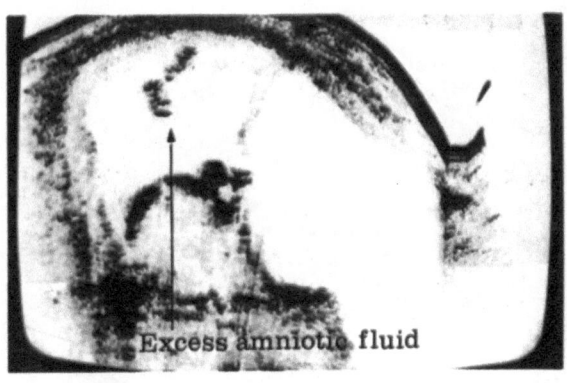
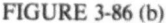

Excess amniotic fluid

FIGURE 3-86 (a)

FIGURE 3-86 (b)

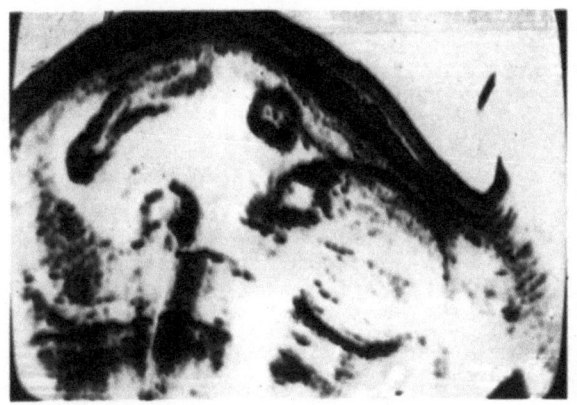

generally seen with polyhydramnios and renal agenesis occurs with oligohydramnios.

HYDATIDIFORM MOLE

Hydatidiform mole or molar pregnancy occurs when the fertilized ovum produces a rapidly growing mass of grapelike structures instead of a normal fetus. This creates a uterus larger than expected for the calculated gestation.

When a patient at 10 to 14 weeks of gestation is bleeding and has a larger uterus than that expected for the date, a mole can easily be suspected; but confirmation needs further investigation, because in positive cases the uterine cavity must be evacuated promptly. Before the advent of ultrasonography, the diagnosis was based on clinical data, an enlarged uterus beyond the normal size for the period of amenorrhea, absence of fetal parts on X ray, and increased urinary chorionic gonadotrophin. The first sign was the passage of vesicles from the vagina, possibly accompanied by abortion. By the usage of ultrasonography, the diagnosis can easily be made.

The ultrasonic appearance of a molar pregnancy shows no evidence of echoes from a fetus or placenta. Typically, a snowstorm echo pattern is noted at high gain settings and is caused by the numerous tissue interfaces occurring within the

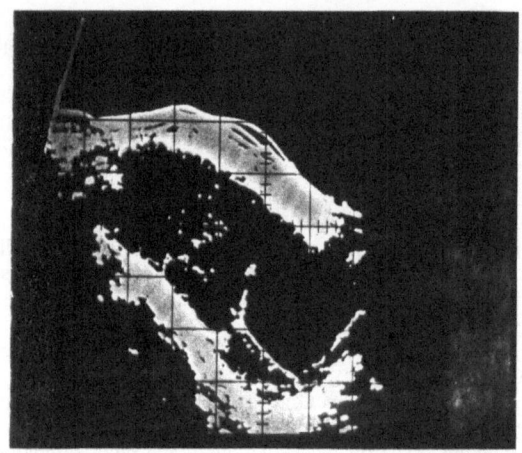

FIGURE 3-87 (a)

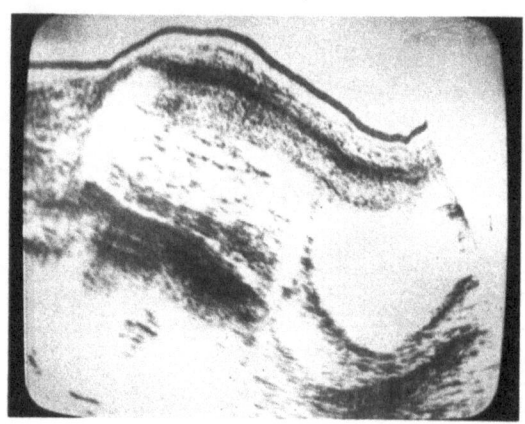

FIGURE 3-87 (d)

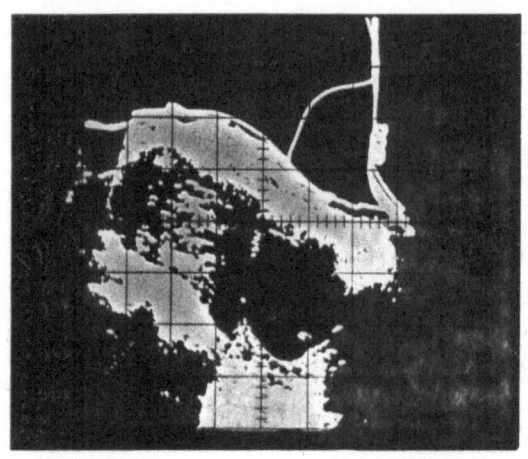

FIGURE 3-87 (b)

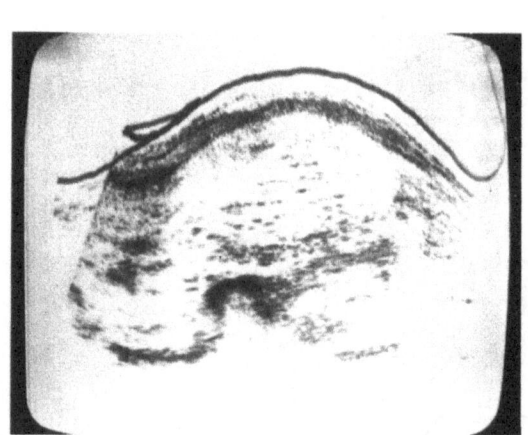

FIGURE 3-87 (e)

FIGURE 3-87 (c)

FIGURE 3-87 (f)

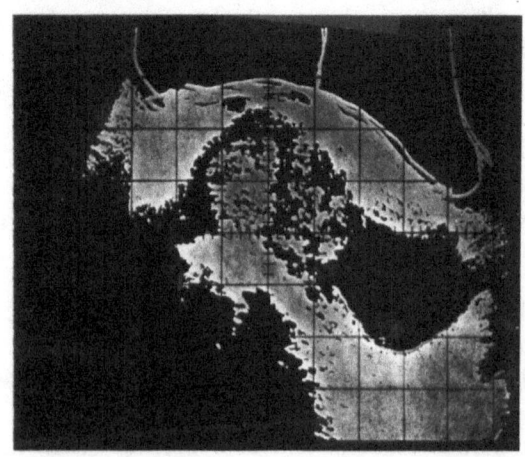

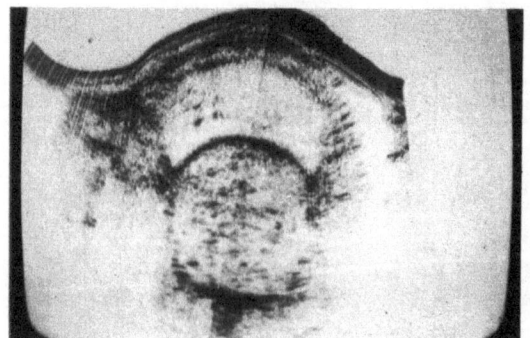

FIGURE 3.87(a)
Supine longitudinal scan. B-mode. Low-sensitivity scan shows a few scattered amorphous internal echoes within the uterus. Hydatidiform mole with low gain setting.

FIGURE 3.87(b)
Supine longitudinal scan. B-mode. Medium-sensitivity scan shows scattered amorphous internal echoes within the uterus. Hydatidiform mole with medium gain setting.

FIGURE 3.87(c)
Supine longitudinal scan. B-mode. High-sensitivity scan shows scattered amorphous internal echoes within the uterus. Hydatidiform mole with high gain setting.

FIGURE 3.87(d)
Supine longitudinal scan. Gray scale. The uterus is enlarged with an irregular echo pattern. High through transmission is noted. Snowstorm appearance of hydatidiform mole.

FIGURE 3.87(e)
Supine transverse scan. Gray scale. Same case as in Fig. 3.87d. The uterus is completely filled with echoes. Scattered anechoic spaces are noted and represent blood-filled regions. Hydatidiform mole.

FIGURE 3.87(f)
Supine transverse scan. Gray scale. The uterus is completely filled with echoes. Scattered anechoic spaces are noted and represent fluid-filled regions. Hydatidiform mole.

uterine cavity filled with the molar vesicular mass. At lower gain settings, the echo pattern from the internal echoes is noted at low sensitivity (Fig. 3.87a,b,c,d,e, and f). The theca lutein cysts frequently associated with hydatidiform mole are readily detected as multilocular or unilocular echo-free masses (Fig. 3.88a and b). These decrease in size following evacuation of the mole. Echo-free intrauterine spaces are observed and represent either large cystic areas or blood clots. Previously, when amniography was a common method of diagnosing this condition, usually puncture was made into a hematoma and the clinical picture was extremely difficult to interpret.

Early diagnosis is imperative due to this condition's potential for malignant transformation. The question of coexisting pregnancy is best answered by using gray scale (Fig. 3.89) or the real-time scanner to demonstrate fetal motion. More laboriously, an attempt may be made to define characteristic fetal structures.

At 10 to 14 weeks' gestation, difficulties may be encountered during scanning because neither the gestational sac nor the fetal head are detectable, and the only clue to a normal pregnancy may be

FIGURE 3.88(a)
Supine transverse scan. Gray scale. The enlarged uterus is filled with a snowstorm echo pattern. Bilateral cystic lesions with septations are characteristic of the luteal cysts associated with hydatidiform mole.

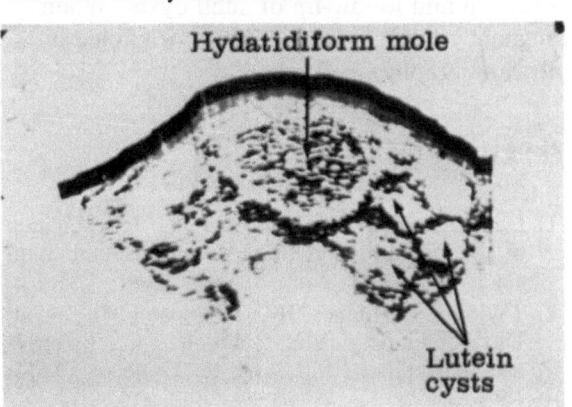

FIGURE 3.88(b)
Supine transverse scan. Gray scale. The snowstorm pattern within the uterus with moderate through transmission is sometimes noted in recurrent molar pregnancy. The increasing size of the bilateral luteal cysts indicates recurrence of this disease.

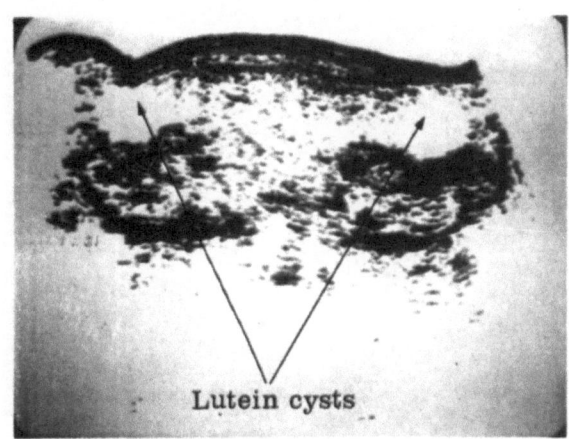

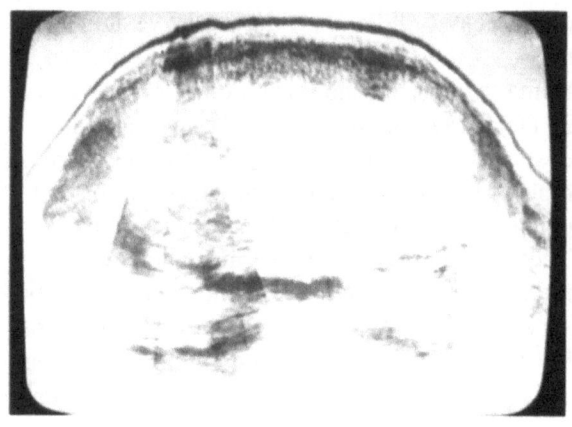

FIGURE 3.89
Supine transverse scan. Gray scale. There is a gestational sac with a 10-week-old fetus inside to the right of the enlarged uterus. The left part of the massively enlarged uterus is full of low-amplitude snowstorm echoes characteristic of hydatidiform mole coexistent with pregnancy.

FIGURE 3.90
Supine longitudinal scan. Gray scale. The uterus is globular in shape with an 8-week-old gestational sac in position. An irregularly margined echo-free sac is situated dorsal to the body of the uterus due to a pelvic abscess.

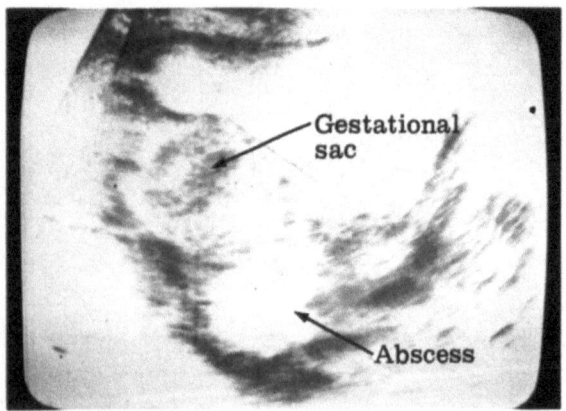

the presence of a placenta. Missed abortion with retained products of conception may simulate a mole. In missed abortion that produces molelike pictures a number of criteria are helpful, eg, the uterus will be small for date and the pregnancy test is negative. Other conditions mistaken for a hydatidiform mole include multiple pregnancy before appearance of the fetal heads, ovarian tumors, and degenerating fibroids. In such situations, clinical data and laboratory tests must be coupled with ultrasonographic findings.

A condition known as hydropic degeneration of pregnancy also exists. This is a proliferative form of fetal demise, in which fetal structure has disappeared and the placenta has already developed hydropic degeneration. This condition also may mimic hydatidiform mole, but the uterus is small for date. Only 25 percent of moles present small-for-date uteri. The pregnancy test is not reliable but chorionic gonadotrophin levels are usually not as high as in hydatidiform mole. In both conditions, the uterus should be evacuated.

MASSES IN PREGNANCY

Masses associated with pregnancy can easily be detected (Fig. 3.90). Masses such as cervical fibroids may block and interfere with normal delivery. The usage of ultrasound not only for detection of these masses but also for determination of their relationship to the pregnant uterus and growing fetus is extremely vital. For example, cysts may develop in the ovary following hormone therapy. Ultrasound may be used for detection and follow-up of such cysts. When pregnancy exists, the procedure of choice is ultrasonography.

REFERENCES

1. Donald I, MacVicar J, Brown TG: Investigation of abdominal masses by pulsed ultrasound. Lancet 1:1188, 1958
2. Taylor ES, Holmes JH, Thompson HE, et al: Ultrasound diagnostic techniques in obstetrics and gynecology. Am J Obstet Gynecol 90:655, 1964

3. Thompson HE: Ultrasonic diagnostic procedures in obstetrics and gynecology. J Clin Ultrasound 1:160, 1973

4. Donald I, Morley P, Barnett E: The diagnosis of blighted ovum by sonar. J Obstet Gynaecol Br Commonw 79:304, 1972

5. Hellman LM, Kobayashi M, Fillisti L: Human fetus prior to the twentieth week of gestation. Am J Obstet Gynecol 103:789, 1969

6. Leopold G: Diagnostic ultrasound in the detection of molar pregnancy. Radiology 98:171, 1971

7. Sabbagha RE, Barton BA, Barton FB, et al: Cephalometry. Predictive of three fetal growth patterns. In: Proceedings of the 1st World Federation of Ultrasound in Medicine and Biology. New York, Plenum, (in press

8. Flamme P: Ultrasonic fetal cephalometry. Percentile curve. Br Med J 3:384, 1972

9. Levi S: The use of ultrasonic biparietal diameter measurement of the fetus in assessing gestational age. Acta Obstet Gynecol Scand 50:179, 1971

10. Thompson H, Holmes J, Gottesfeld K, et al: Fetal development as determined by ultrasonic pulse echo technique. Am J Obstet Gynecol 92:44, 1965

11. Kossoff G, Garrett WJ, Radovanovich G: Gray-scale echography in obstetrics and gynecology. Australas Radiol 18:63, 1974

12. Robinson HP: Early detection of fetal heart movement by sonar. Ultrasonics 11:52, 1973

13. Jouppila P, Piiroinen O: Ultrasonic diagnosis of fetal life in early pregnancy. Obstet Gynecol 46:616, 1975

14. Thompson HE, Makowski EL: Estimation of birth weight and gestational age. Obstet Gynecol 37:44, 1971

15. Eule J, Bockenstedt F, Salzman E: Diagnostic ultrasound scanning. A valuable aid in radiation therapy planning. Am J Roentgenol Radium Ther Nucl Med 117:139, 1973

16. Flanigan DJ: Prediction of fetal sex by diagnostic ultrasound. In: Proceedings of the 1st World Federation of Ultrasound in Medicine and Biology. New York, Plenum, (in press)

17. Stephens B, Birnholz JC: The clinical significance of fetal movement patterns. Proceedings of the 1st World Federation of Ultrasound in Medicine and Biology. New York, Plenum, (in press)

18. Garrett W, Robinson D: Ultrasound in Clinical Obstetrics. Springfield, Ill, Thomas, 1970

19. Garrett W, Robinson D, Kossoff G: Ultrasonic echoscopy in transverse lie. J Obstet Gynacol Br Commonw 76:679, 1966

20. Donald I, MacVicar J, Brown TG: Investigation of abdominal masses by pulsed ultrasound. Lancet 1:1188, 1958

21. Donald I: Diagnostic uses of sonar in obstetrics and gynecology. J Obstet Gynaecol Br Commonw 72:907, 1965

22. MacVicar J, Donald I: Sonar in diagnosis of early pregnancy and its complications. J Obstet Gynaecol Br Commonw 70:387, 1963

23. Robinson DE, Garrett W, Kossoff G: Ultrasonic echoscopy in clinical obstetrics and gynecology. Call Report No. 40. Sydney, Commonwealth Acoustic Laboratories, 1967

24. Donald I, Abdulla U: Placentography by sonar. J Obstet Gynaecol Br Commonw 75:993, 1968

25. Gottesfeld K, Thompson H, Holmes J: Ultrasonic placentography. A new method for placental localization. Am J Obstet Gynecol 108:740, 1970

26. King D: Placental ultrasonography. J Clin Ultrasound 1:21, 1973

27. Kohorn E, Secker-Walker R, Morrsion J, et al: Placental localization. Am J Obstet Gynecol 103:868, 1969

28. Kobayashi M, Hellman L, Fillisti L, et al: Placental localization by ultrasound. Am J Obstet Gynecol 106:279, 1970

29. Kossoff G, Garrett W: Ultrasonic film echoscopy for placental localization. Aust NZ J Obstet Gynaecol 12:117, 1972

30. Sunden B: Ultrasonic placentography. Acta Obstet Gynecol Scand 48:161, 1969

31. Fisher CC, Garrett W, Kossoff G: Placental aging monitored by gray-scale echography. Am J Obstet Gynecol 124:483, 1976

32. Sanders RC, Conrad MR: Sonography in obstetrics. Radiol Clin North Am 13:435, 1975

33. Leopold G, Asher WM: Fundamentals of Abdominal and Pelvic Ultrasonography. Philadelphia, Saunders, 1975

34. Hing DL: Placental ultrasonography. J Clin Ultrasound 1:21, 1973

35. Horger EO, Kreuter AK, Underwood PB: Low implanted gestational sac producing placenta previa. Am J Obstet Gynecol 120:1119, 1974

36. Kurjak A, Olajos I, Breyer B, et al: Changes of placental site diagnosed by repeated ultrasonic examination. In: Proceedings of the 1st World Federation of Ultrasound in Medicine and Biology. New York, Plenum, (in press)

37. Winsberg F: Echographic changes with placental aging. J Clin Ultrasound 1:52, 1973

38. Rushmer RF, Baker DW, Johnson WL: Clinical applications of a transcutaneous ultrasonic flow detector. JAMA 199:326, 1967

39. Hon EH: An Introduction to Fetal Heart Rate Monitoring. New Haven, Yale Cooperative Corporation, 1971

40. Shenker L, Kane R: Doppler ultrasonic fetal heart monitoring during labor. Obstet Gynecol 39:609, 1972

41. Paul RH, Hon EH: Clinical fetal monitoring versus effect on perinatal outcome. Am J Obstet Gynecol 118:529, 1974

42. Ray M, Freeman R, Pine S: Clinical experience

with the oxytocin challenge test. Am J Obstet Gynecol 114:1, 1972

43. Gottesfeld K: The ultrasonic diagnosis of intra-uterine fetal death. Am J Obstet Gynecol 108:623, 1970

44. Ultrasound in the management of clinically diagnosed threatened abortion. Br Med J 102:424, 1975

45. Donald I: I In King DL (ed): Obstetric Ultrasonography in Diagnostic Ultrasound. St Louis, Mosby, 1974

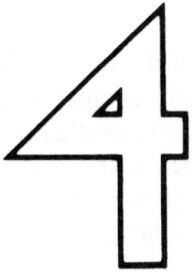

ultrasonography of gynecologically and obstetrically related medical and surgical disorders

ULTRASONOGRAPHY OF THE URINARY TRACT IN GYNECOLOGIC DISORDERS

In pelvic diseases, the urinary tract is the system most frequently secondarily involved. Both benign and malignant pelvic tumors may produce hydronephrosis of the obstructive type (Fig. 4.1a and b). Hydronephrosis may be readily diagnosed by ultrasound and has been previously discussed. Cystitis and ureterovesical reflux may cause hydronephrosis and renal scarring from pyelonephritis. Additionally, primary diseases of the kidneys often occur in patients in the older gynecologic age group. Renal tumors are frequently encountered during routine urography. Ultrasonography is particularly useful in the diagnosis and treatment of many genitourinary disorders.

RENAL CYST

The following criteria are used to diagnose a renal cyst (Fig. 4.2a and b).

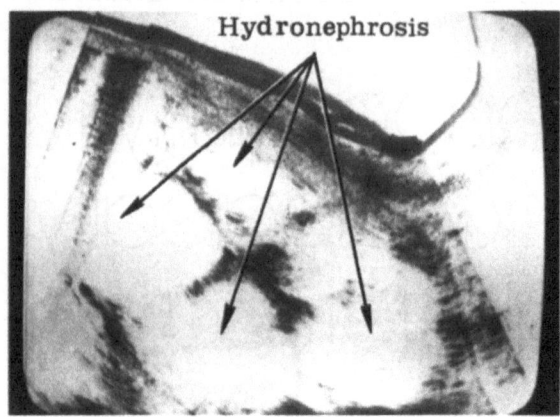

FIGURE 4-1 (a)

1. Presence of an echo-free zone within the mass due to a homogeneous medium.

2. Sharp definition of the distal wall of the mass with a smooth contour to this surface, due to the large change in acoustic impedance at the cyst wall interface and the parabolic shape reflecting more sound back to the transducer.

3. Greater energy of the sound beam due to minimal attenuation of sound traversing the homogeneous fluid-filled medium, resulting in increased through transmission and, therefore, increased echo density distal to the lesion. This

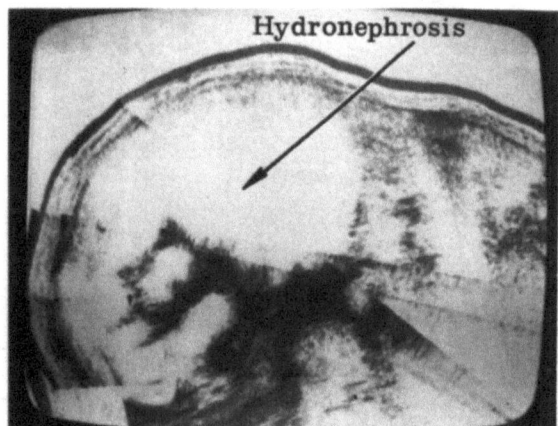

FIGURE 4-1 (b)

FIGURE 4.1(a)
Supine longitudinal scan. Gray scale. Marked hydronephrosis thins the renal parenchyma and produces sacs of fluid with septa radiating centrally.

FIGURE 4.1(b)
Supine transverse scan. Gray scale. Marked hydronephrosis thins the renal parenchyma and produces sacs of fluid with multiple septations.

FIGURE 4.2(a)
Prone longitudinal scan. Gray scale. Echo-free lower-pole renal cyst with sharp demarcation from renal substance.

FIGURE 4.2(b)
Prone longitudinal scan. Gray scale. Two anechoic areas are visualized in one slice. The outline of the kidney is severely distorted. Multiple renal cysts are common in elderly patients. The opposite kidney should be studied for cystic changes.

FIGURE 4-2 (a)

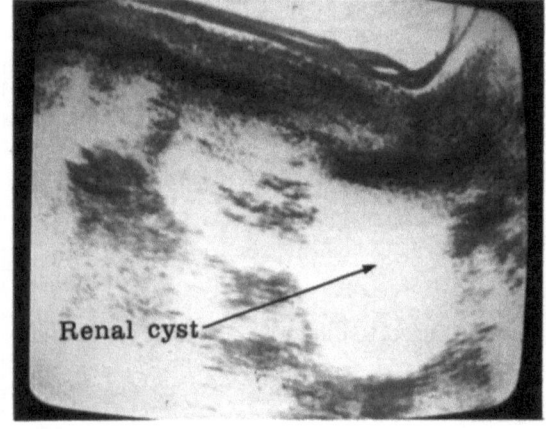

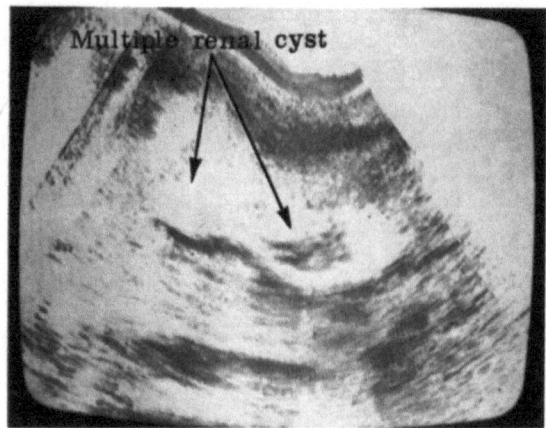

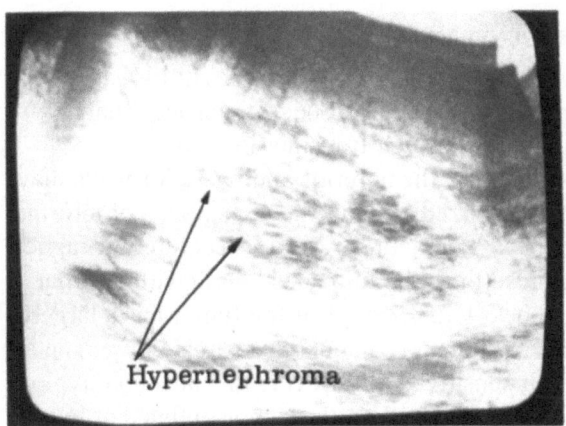

FIGURE 4-3 (a)

FIGURE 4.3(a)
Prone longitudinal scan. Gray scale. Space-occupying mass in upper pole. Solid hypernephroma with high through transmission, and area of cystic necrosis.

FIGURE 4.3(b)
Erect position. Gray scale. Same case as in Fig. 4.3a. Note space-occupying mass in upper pole. Solid hypernephroma with high through transmission, and area of cystic necrosis.

FIGURE 4.3(c)
Prone transverse scan. Gray scale. Irregular mass in upper pole of kidney. Scattered internal echoes of low amplitude are noted, and a high through transmission pattern is observed when compared with the opposite side. Degenerating hypernephroma.

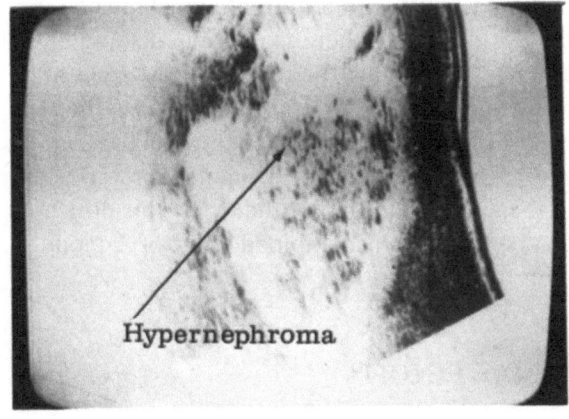

FIGURE 4-3 (b)

FIGURE 4-3 (c)

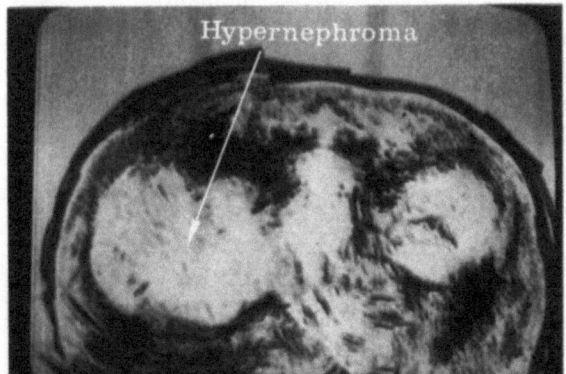

effect is more pronounced with a larger cystic mass.

Determination of the precise gain setting that fills in a cyst with artifactual echoes is a matter of experience with a specific instrument. A suspected cyst should be compared with a known cystic mass standard, such as the bladder.

SOLID TUMORS

Solid tumors occur with some frequency in older female patients (Fig. 4.3a and b). The following criteria are used to diagnose a solid neoplasm.

1. The distal wall is irregular in contour.
2. The distal wall is not sharply defined and has echoes of a lower level than those of the proximal boundary, due to small changes in acoustic impedance.
3. Poor through transmission, since a large amount of sonic energy is attenuated in passing through the tumor mass.
4. Presence of internal echoes that define the acoustic nonhomogeneity of the mass. It may be necessary to increase the sensitivity setting to demonstrate internal echoes from an acoustically heterogeneous lesion. The tumor may arise in any portion of the kidney.

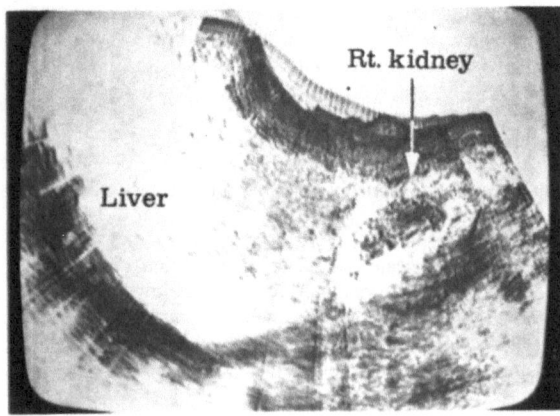

FIGURE 4.4
Supine longitudinal scan. Gray scale. The kidney lies in an extremely caudal position in the liver edge. This condition must be differentiated from a displaced kidney due to a mass lesion.

FIGURE 4.5
Erect longitudinal scan. Gray scale. Change in position of a mobile kidney is best demonstrated by scanning in the prone position and then rescanning in the erect position to document maximum renal excursion.

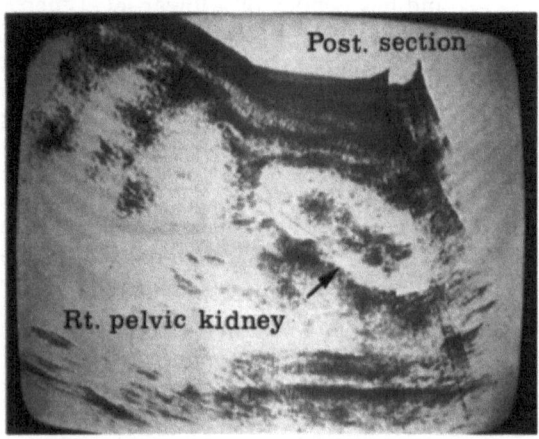

DEGENERATING SOLID TUMORS

As a tumor enlarges it outgrows its blood supply, producing fluid-filled necrotic spaces that increase through transmission. At low sensitivity, the anterior and posterior walls may be visualized without the appearance of internal echoes, simulating a cystic structure. At higher gain settings the tumor will fill in with internal echoes (Fig. 4.3c) (1). If the tumor has a largely necrotic center, an echo-free area will remain at high sensitivity. However, this anechoic region will be smaller than the tumor outlined at low sensitivity.

Thus, by varying the sensitivity of the receiver, ultrasound differentiates a fluid-filled cyst from a solid mass with a high degree of accuracy. This method is reliable for differentiating between the two lesions when there is continued sonic homogeneity within the margin of the mass at different gain settings and no change in the sharpness of the margins. Electric noise and reverberation may cause artifacts on the B-scan in the anterior portion of the cyst. This difficulty can be resolved by combined usage of A-mode with the B-scan.

RENAL ECTOPIA

Renal ectopia may be a surprising finding to the clinician who is evaluating a patient for other disorders such as hepatomegaly, splenomegaly, or abdominal or pelvic mass. The displaced kidney may be located immediately under the inferior liver edge and be clinically indistinguishable from true enlargement of the liver (Fig. 4.4). Horseshoe kidneys may simulate a variety of abdominal masses. The pelvic kidney may be normal (Fig. 4.5) or obstructed and hydronephrotic.

The surgeon must be aware that such a pelvic mass may be the patient's only functioning renal tissue. Ultrasonography will delineate the characteristic renal outline and calyceal echoes. The expected renal echo pattern in the retroperitoneum will be absent. Diseases such as hydronephrosis in the ectopic kidney may also be diagnosed by ultrasonography.

BLADDER INVOLVEMENT

The clinician is frequently concerned with bladder function or the effect of pelvic diseases upon the bladder.

The distal wall of the fluid-filled bladder is distinctly outlined by either conventional scanners or real-time units. Volume is readily assessed with a standard nomogram, and postvoiding residual urine may be measured without resorting to intravenous urography or catheterization techniques. Fluid-filled diverticulae of the bladder may be seen when they are about 2 cm in diameter. The evolution of this entity may be followed sequentially and atraumatically. Laterally placed diverticulae are best examined by sector scanning through the opposite bladder wall. Large diverticulae must not be confused with pelvic cystic lesions.

The contour of the bladder is studied for symmetry, distensibility, and tumor masses. Extravesical lesions such as uterine fibroids and ovarian cysts may distort the normal contour of the bladder wall. The expected uniform expansion of the bladder is evaluated by monitoring its shape with increasing urine or fluid volumes. Alterations in distensibility occur with infiltrating carcinoma and chronic inflammatory disease. Masses adherent to the wall of the bladder are most often malignant.

Using ultrasonic guidance, percutaneous puncture of the bladder for diagnostic or therapeutic purposes may be performed quickly and simply.

ULTRASONOGRAPHY OF THE LIVER IN GYNECOLOGIC DISORDERS

The enlarged liver in the gynecologic patient with a pelvic mass may represent metastatic enlargement (Fig. 4.6a,b,c,d, and e). Common causes of hepatomegaly are metastatic disease, hepatitis, congestive heart failure (2), and biliary obstruction (2). However, the liver may be palpable without coexistent hepatomegaly. Emphysema and asthma, with low diaphragms, or aberrant lobes, such as Riedel's lobe, would produce such a condition (Fig. 4.7). The liver may be enlarged but not palpable in cirrhosis, posterior enlargement, and marked obesity.

METASTASES

Metastases to the liver have two basic patterns (2). At low sensitivity, the presence of a round collection of echoes or a ring-shaped pattern in a sonolucent background of normal liver parenchyma is characteristic. At high sensitivity, areas of sonolucency in diffusely echogenic hepatic tissues comprise the second typical appearance. Any abnormality in echographic anatomy must be documented in both longitudinal and cross section.

A different pattern occurs when the liver is almost completely replaced by metastatic tumor (Fig. 4.6e), or by an infiltrating tumor such as a lymphoma. In massive metastases with necrosis the liver appears cystic with irregular borders. Substitution of tumor for liver parenchyma may produce an acoustically homogeneous medium that strongly attenuates sound energy. The liver appears echo free at medium and high sensitivities and the posterior wall is poorly defined.

It has been stated that the most common appearance of metastases on gray scale is that of low-amplitude echoes within the higher-amplitude echoes of the normal hepatic substance. We have found that high-amplitude echoes more often represent metastatic disease (2) or hepatoma. The majority of hepatomas occur in cirrhotic livers. Multiple irregular thick echoes represent diffuse liver disease, such as chronic inflammatory disease or metastases.

Liver metastases are a frequent complication of gynecologic malignancies. Metastatic disease

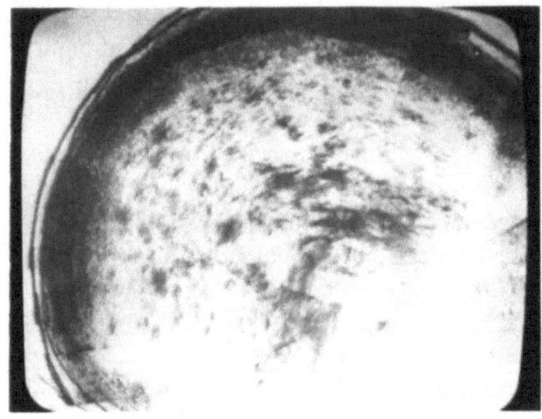

FIGURE 4-6 (a)

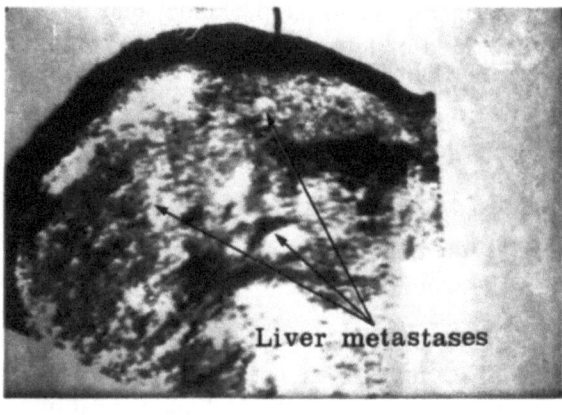

FIGURE 4-6 (d)

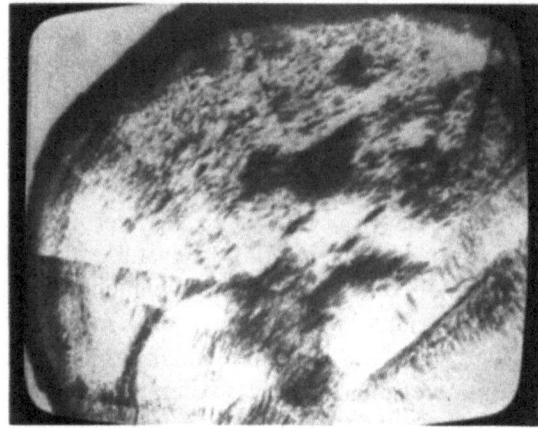

FIGURE 4-6 (b)

FIGURE 4.6(a)
Supine transverse scan. Gray scale. The liver is diffusely enlarged. Scattered echogenic foci of small to moderate size are within the liver parenchyma. Liver metastases from ovarian carcinoma.

FIGURE 4.6(b)
Supine longitudinal scan. Gray scale. Enlarged liver with multiple echogenic metastases due to ovarian carcinoma.

FIGURE 4.6(c)
Supine longitudinal scan. Gray scale. Large areas of degenerating metastatic foci are noted within the liver.

FIGURE 4.6(d)
Supine transverse scan. Gray scale. Note multiple anechoic regions within the liver parenchyma at high senstitivity. Sonolucent areas represent foci of necrotic metastatic adenocarcinoma.

FIGURE 4.6(e)
Supine transverse scan. Gray scale. Huge sonolucent zone with high through transmission. This cystic-appearing region represents a massive area of tumor replacement in the liver. Note the irregular distal wall.

FIGURE 4-6 (c)

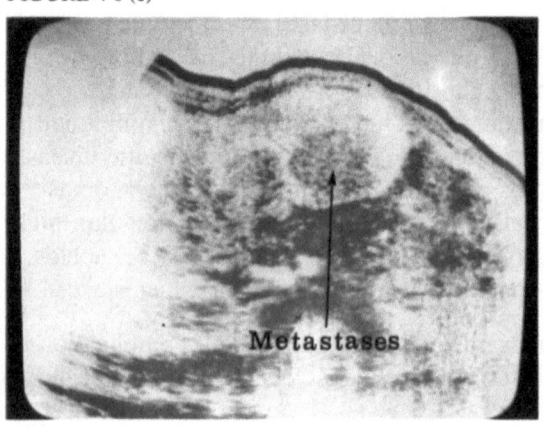

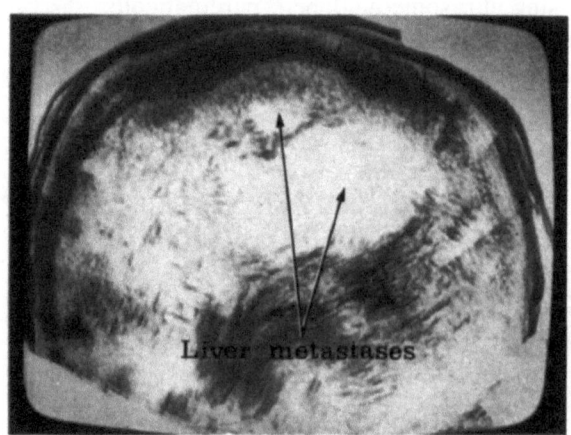

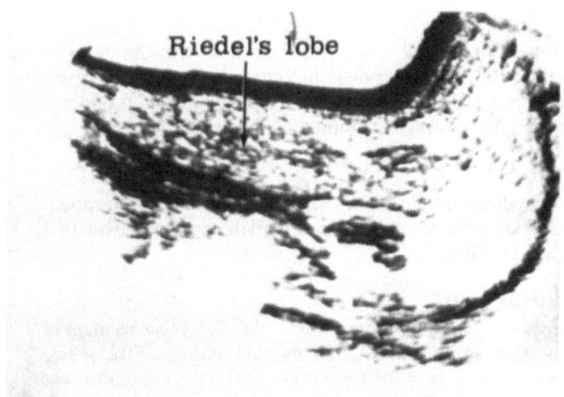

FIGURE 4.7
Supine longitudinal scan. Gray scale. Riedel's lobe is a normal variation of the right lobe of the liver. This right lobe extends into the right pelvis and may be mistaken for hepatomegaly or a mass lesion.

FIGURE 4.8
Supine longitudinal scan. Gray scale. In massive ascites without adhesions, the liver floats in the fluid and is lifted off the liver bed. Ascites with adhesions generally holds the liver adjacent to the kidney. The appearance of the thumblike kidney and the "four finger" shape of the liver produce the "mitten sign" characteristic of cirrhotic ascites.

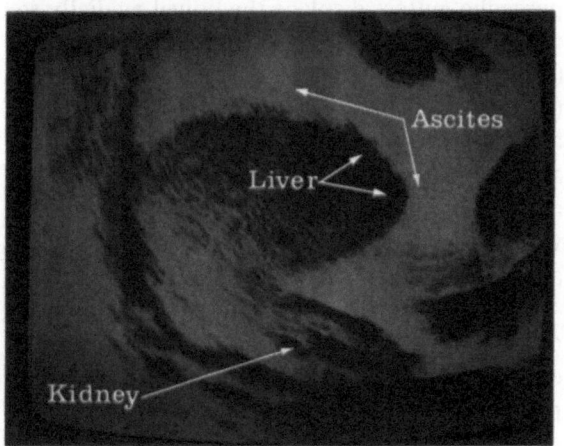

has a variety of ultrasonic appearances. The most common form is that of rounded echogenic multiple foci within the liver (Fig. 4.6a). The liver is often enlarged. Large metastatic foci may have necrotic centers which image as cystic centers to echogenic lesions (Fig. 4.6d). Another frequent form is the echo-poor focus within the echogenic liver parenchyma. Within larger metastatic zones, an echogenic center may be noted presumably related to cystic necrosis within the inner parts of the tumor (Fig. 4.6e).

ULTRASONOGRAPHY OF ASCITES IN GYNECOLOGIC DISORDERS

Ascites is a frequent complication of inflammatory processes and pelvic tumors. Intraperitoneal fluid assumes the form of either a transudate (low protein) or exudate (high protein). A common cause of transudates is portal obstruction, either intrahepatic or extrahepatic. Intrahepatic disease usually refers to cirrhosis of diverse etiology. Extrahepatic obstruction occurs with portal vein obstruction. Congestive heart failure, renal disease, and benign tumors of the ovary also cause ascites.

Exudates usually occur with inflammatory conditions of the peritoneum. The usual entities noted are infectious peritonitis and metastatic carcinoma, generally from the stomach, pancreas, and ovary. The peritoneum reacts to inflammation with a fibroblastic exudate that causes the peritoneum to adhere to other peritoneal surfaces, causing adhesions.

Ascites may be free (Fig. 4.8) or loculated (Fig. 4.9a and b). Free ascites is a transudate, except in the case of chylous ascites resulting from thoracic duct obstruction. Loculated ascites is seen with inflammatory conditions in which fluid is trapped in compartments sealed by peritoneal adhesions. This may be localized to one area or diffusely situated throughout the intraabdominal cavity,

Minimal ascites may be detected with A-mode. As little as 100 ml of free fluid may be detected with the patient in the hand-knee position with

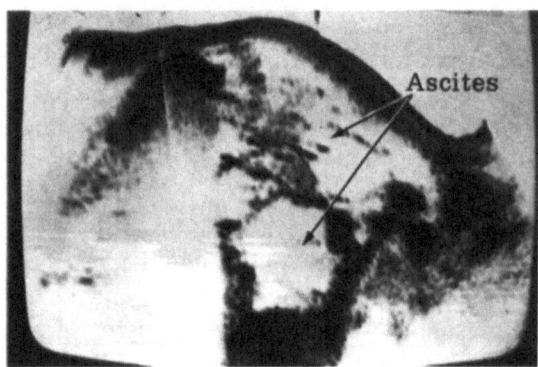

FIGURE 4-9 (a)

FIGURE 4.9(a)
Supine longitudinal scan. Gray scale. Moderate amounts of ascites collect in the pelvis in the supine position. Bowel loops projecting into the fluid are echogenic and produce a characteristic irregular outline to the ascitic fluid.

FIGURE 4.9(b)
Supine longitudinal scan. Gray scale. Note small, trapped, loculated peritoneal effusion. Ovarian carcinoma was the cause of effusion.

FIGURE 4.10
Supine longitudinal scan. Gray scale. Echo-free triangle of moderate amount of ascites. As fluid overflows the pelvic cavity it appears in the flank bordered by the abdominal wall, psoas, and displaced bowel loops.

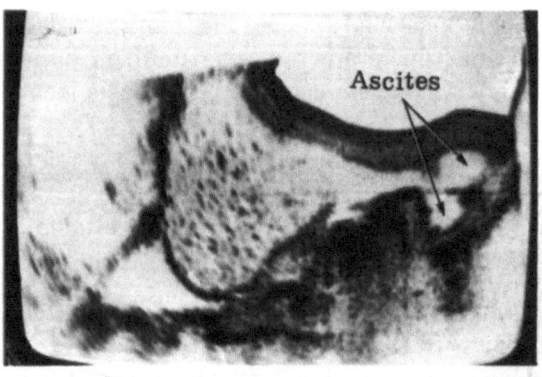

FIGURE 4-9 (b)

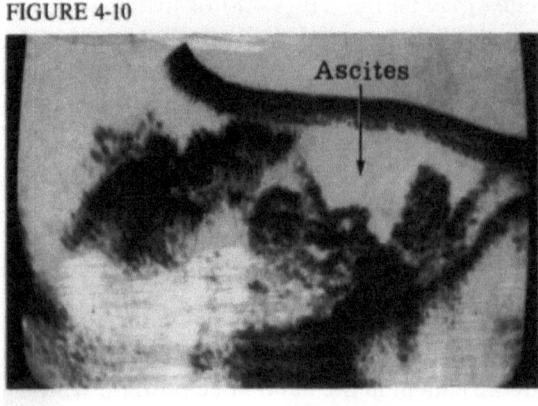

FIGURE 4-10

the transducer placed under the anterior abdominal wall (3). Usually several minutes are allowed for the fluid to gravitate ventrally before the area is scanned.

Small amounts of ascites first collect in the pelvis by gravity. This collection appears as a sonolucent mass with angular borders anterosuperiorly due to indentation from overlying bowel. Larger amounts overflow the pouch of Douglas and are directed by mesenteric reflections to specific regions (Fig. 4.10). These regions include the right paracolic gutter, the right lower quadrant at the lower end of the small bowel mesentery, and, with large amounts of fluid, the left lower quadrant along the superior border of the mesocolon (4). Ascites with tumor seedings or bacteria tends to loculate preferentially in these areas.

Large amounts of fluid that extend up the paracolic gutters displace the bowel medially so that the scan resembles an atomic explosion (Fig. 4.11) and can distort the outline of the liver (Fig. 4.12). The air-containing intestine causes artifacts in supine scanning over the anterior abdomen. However, a moderate amount of ascitic fluid provides an excellent scanning window. When flank areas are scanned, large amounts of fluid prevent proper scanning (Fig. 4.13). The lateral border of the medially displaced liver and spleen can often be clearly delineated, and elevation of the liver from the posteriorly located right kidney may be demonstrated.

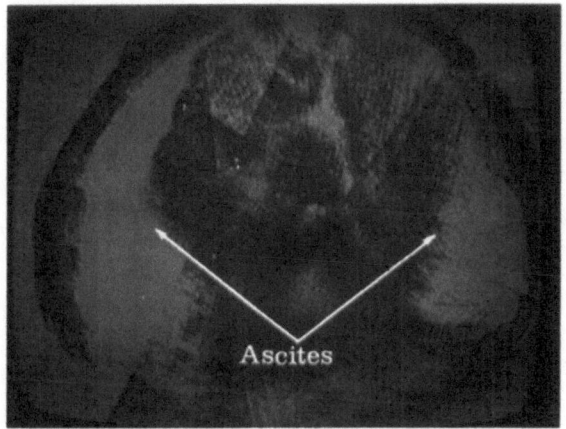

FIGURE 4-11

FIGURE 4.11
Supine transverse scan. Gray scale. Note atomic explosion configuration of massive ascites. The bowel and intraabdominal organs are displaced medially. It is difficult to obtain information of diagnostic value in such a case. Rescanning when ascites is decreased is useful.

FIGURE 4.12
Supine transverse scan. Gray scale. The liver is shrunken and floats in an echo-free zone of ascites. Note elevation of the inferior liver edge from the retroperitoneal organs. Cirrhosis with ascites.

FIGURE 4.13
Supine transverse scan. Gray scale. Massive ascites usually prevents proper scanning. Echogenic bowel loops project into the ascitic fluid. The bowel loops usually float freely in the ascitic fluid and change with position. Fixation of bowel occurs in malignant and chronic inflammatory processes.

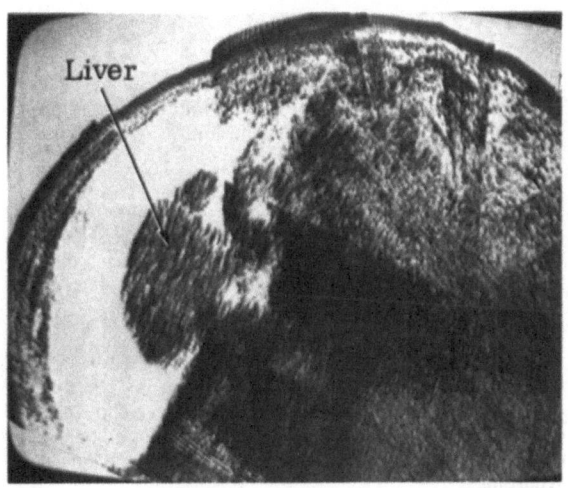

FIGURE 4-12

FIGURE 4-13

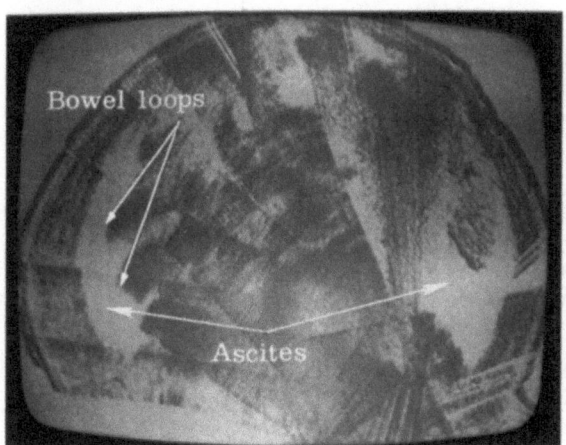

In our experience, it is sometimes possible to differentiate between benign and malignant ascites. Benign fluid usually is free intraperitoneal fluid and will change position with gravitational maneuvers. Malignant ascites tends to loculate and causes adhesions (Fig. 4.14) and will not alter its location with positioning. When ascites is in loculated cavities, the walls of the cavities will be seen as septations, which appear as linear echo patterns, in the echo-free fluid. Ascites with underlying carcinomatosis causes adhesion. As a result, fluid is trapped, loops of bowel are fixed, and there is no change in the position of the fluid by changing patient's position. Inflammatory changes in the walls or tumor deposits cause irregularity, so that the posterior wall of the region scanned will not be smoothly outlined. Appropriate clinical data and ultrasonographic findings almost yield enough information to differentiate benign from malignant ascites.

Free fluid ascending the paracolic gutters may be tapped over the lower quadrants without perforating the medially displaced bowel. Loculated ascites implies that adhesions are preventing normal separation of bowel from the peritoneal surface. Ultrasonic detection of loculated ascites is very important when paracentesis is planned, because the risk of bowel perforation is then increased. Indeed, since the transducer may be easily placed over

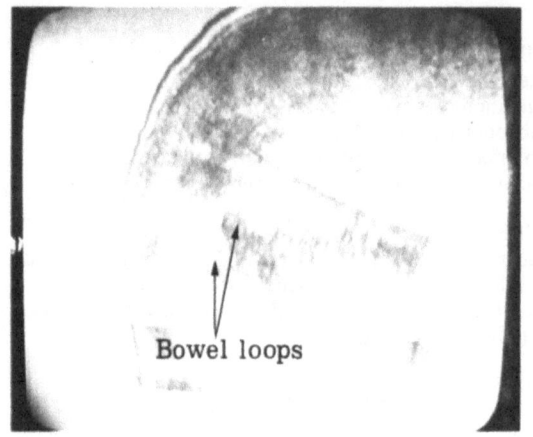

FIGURE 4-14

the pocket of trapped ascites, ultrasonically guided paracentesis is the method of choice when loculated fluid is present (Fig. 4.15a).

Excessive ascites prevents proper scanning of the abdomen. The examination should be repeated after the fluid is aspirated, either blindly or through ultrasonically guided paracentesis.

The etiologies of ascites are diverse, but when ascites and pleural effusion coexist this is most likely due to fibroma with an ovarian origin.

Ovarian fibroma accounts for about 5 percent of all ovarian tumors. About 90 percent are

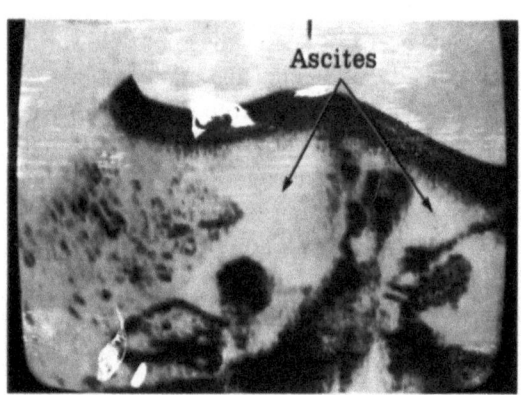

FIGURE 4-15 (a)

FIGURE 4.14
Supine transverse scan. Gray scale. Note the bowel loop fixed in peritoneal fluid due to adhesion.

FIGURE 4.15(a)
Supine longitudinal scan. Gray scale. Large amounts of ascites collect in the pelvis in the supine position. This echo-free fluid has the same echo pattern as does the urine-filled bladder. Bowel loops projecting into the fluid are echogenic and produce a characteristic irregular outline to the ascitic fluid.

FIGURE 4.15(b)
Prone posterior longitudinal scan. Gray scale. Echo-free area above the renal and liver outline is due to a large benign pleural effusion secondary to an ovarian tumor. Meigs's syndrome.

FIGURE 4.15(c)
Erect posterior longitudinal scan. Gray scale. Echo-free area above the renal outline is due to a large benign pleural effusion secondary to an ovarian tumor. Meigs's syndrome.

FIGURE 4-15 (b)

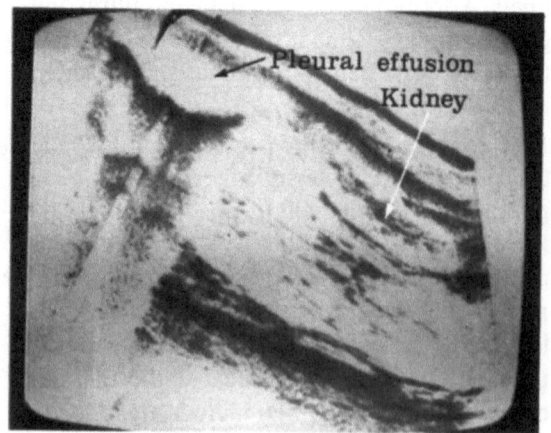

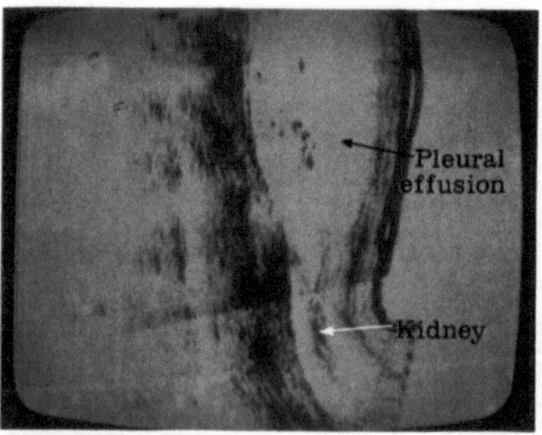

unilateral, and they occur usually after menopause. In 25 percent of cases the tumor is complicated by ascites and hydrothorax (Meigs's syndrome) (Fig. 4.15b and c). The effusions regress after removal of the tumor. The cause of the hydrothorax and ascites is not clear.

ULTRASONOGRAPHY OF THE RETROPERITONEAL AREA IN GYNECOLOGIC DISORDERS

The retroperitoneum must often be studied carefully for any pathology or, mostly, for the staging of pelvic tumors. It is difficult to evaluate the retroperitoneal area by ordinary radiographic methods, since space-occupying lesions must be well advanced in this region before they can be detected. In addition, despite the standard roentgenographic work-up, which includes intravenous urography, barium enema, lymphangiography, retroperitoneal air insufflation, and angiography, the nature of the lesion may remain unclear. This is especially true of avascular masses and surgery may be required for definitive diagnosis. However, sonolaparotomy, as a noninvasive, safe, and simple technique for detecting, evaluating, and differentiating retroperitoneal lesions, has been rewarding.

Ultrasonographically, the retroperitoneal space is divided into upper and lower sections at the plane of the umbilicus or iliac crest (5). The ultrasonographer should identify as many structures as possible in the supine, prone, or lateral projections. The bony pelvis prevents visualization of the lower compartment in posterior projections. Details of the sonoanatomy of each retroperitoneal organ are described separately.

In the upper abdomen enlarged lymph nodes are usually seen as rounded masses in close proximity to the abdominal aorta (Fig. 4.16a,b,c, and d). Lymph node masses may be detected in any part of the abdomen; lymphadenopathy generally appears sonolucent. These masses

may retain an echo-free pattern even at high gain settings (Fig. 4.17a,b, and c) because the diseased lymph nodes are acoustically homogeneous.

During the scan, every attempt is made to image the spine in order to establish a boundary distal to the lesion. A lymph node mass adjacent to the wall of the aorta makes it difficult to verify the position of this vessel within the tumor mass (Fig. 4.16b). The echo silhouette sign of lymphadenopathy adjacent to the aorta, actually obliterating the anterior aortic wall, has been noted with B-scan, gray scale, and real-time scanner. Indeed, such a cluster of periaortic lymph nodes may mimic an aortic aneurysm. Generally, these nodal aggregates have an irregular, lobulated outline as compared to an abdominal aortic aneurysm. Scanning other areas of the abdomen or retroperitoneum may demonstrate other sonolucent lesions distinct from the abdominal aorta. The presence of other foci of lymphadenopathy rules against the possibility of an aortic aneurysm. We have noted lymphadenopathy appearing as discrete masses, sonolucent layers covering the aorta, and multiple tumors that may elevate the aorta and inferior vena cava anteriorly (Fig. 4.18).

Retroperitoneal tumors may be demonstrated either by prone or supine sonolaparotomy. These masses may displace the kidneys and intraabdominal organs by spread into the mesentery. Tumors with internal degeneration may be observed to have multiple internal echoes with high through transmission.

Retroperitoneal fluid collections may be noted by an echo-free zone. It may be difficult to differentiate between hemorrhage, abscess (Fig. 4.19), and sterile fluid (5). However, if the patient is symptomatic, collating ultrasonographic information can yield excellent results. For example, in a patient with diabetes and fever, who is nonresponsive to antibiotics, and who has evidence of a space-occupying lesion in the retroperitoneum, the usual diagnosis would be an abscess rather than a tumor or hematoma.

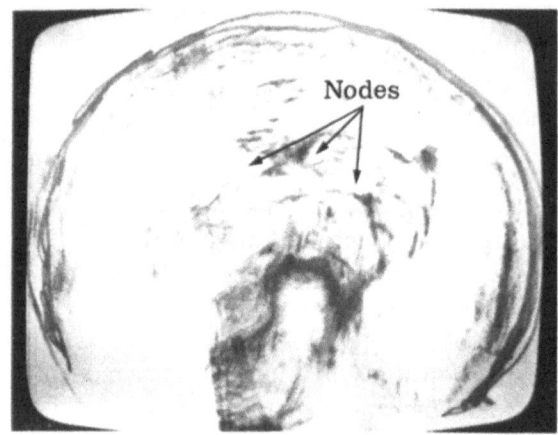

FIGURE 4-16 (a)

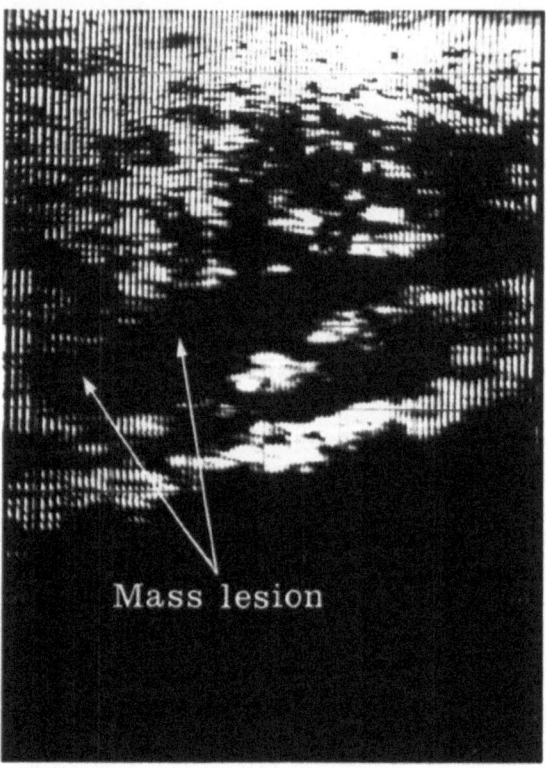

FIGURE 4-16 (d)

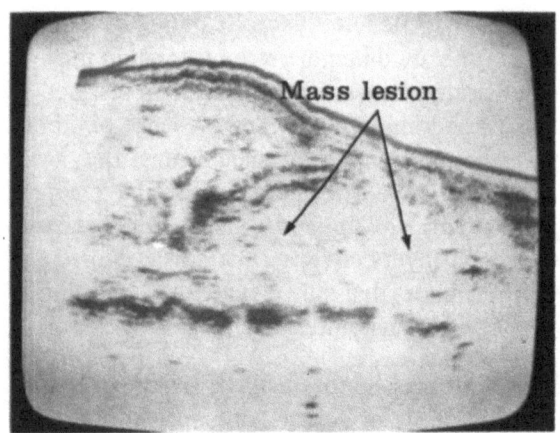

FIGURE 4-16 (b)

FIGURE 4-16 (c)

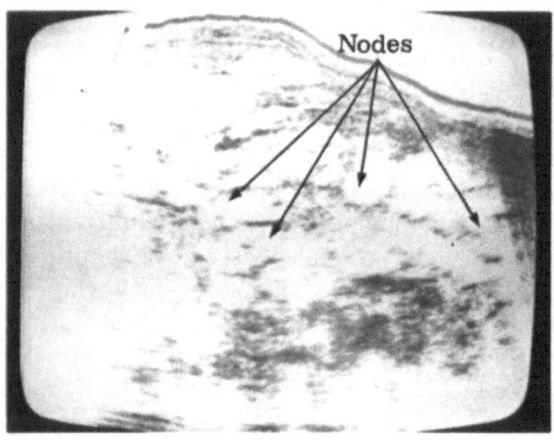

FIGURE 4.16(a)
Supine transverse scan. Gray scale. The liver and spleen are enlarged. The spleen is echo poor. Multiple matted lymph nodes are noted in the retroperitoneum and mesenteric lymph node chains due to Waldenström's macroglobulinemia.

FIGURE 4.16(b)
Supine longitudinal scan. Gray scale. The superior mesenteric artery is markedly displaced anteriorly by a mass of echo-poor lymph nodes. The celiac axis is also noted cephalicaly.

FIGURE 4.16(c)
Supine longitudinal scan. Gray scale. The aortic silhouette is poorly defined due to the large adjacent lymph nodes in this advanced case of Waldenström's macroglobulinemia. The real-time scanner is used to locate the aorta in this situation.

FIGURE 4.16(d)
Supine longitudinal scan. Real-time scanner. The aorta is displaced dorsally by echo-free matted lymph nodes. Note the concave shape of the normally straight anterior aortic wall.

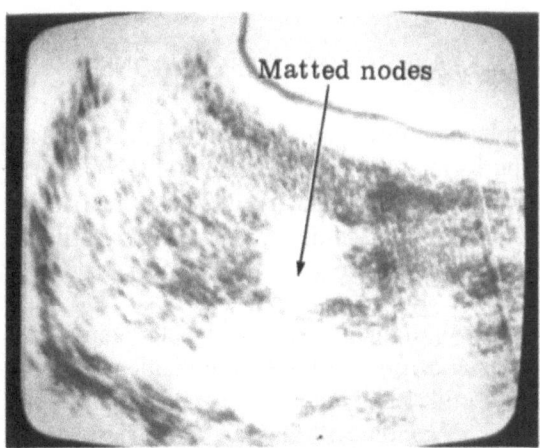

FIGURE 4-17 (a)

FIGURE 4.17(a)
Supine longitudinal scan. Gray scale. Discrete clusters of anechoic and echogenic masses above the normal aortic outline are noted. Hodgkin's disease.

FIGURE 4.17(b)
Supine longitudinal scan. Gray scale. Discrete clusters of anechoic and echogenic masses obscure the normal aortic outline. Hodgkin's disease.

FIGURE 4.17(c)
Supine transverse scan. Gray scale. Periaortic lymphadenopathy presenting as multiple anechoic masses. Left paraaortic lymph nodes displace the left kidney laterally.

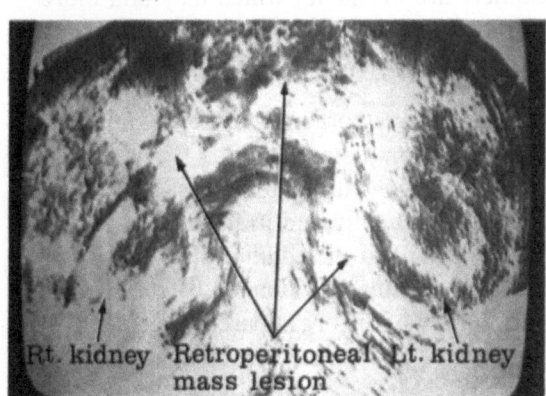

FIGURE 4-17 (b)

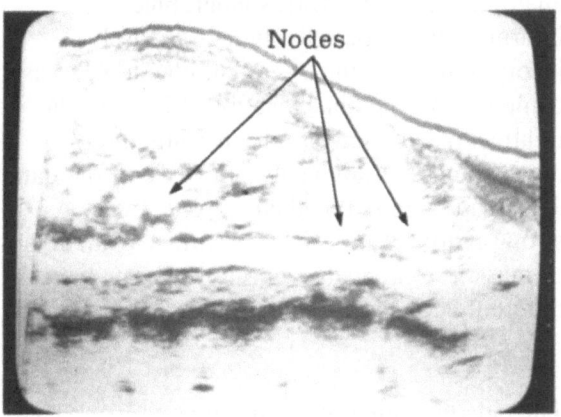

FIGURE 4.18
Supine longitudinal scan. Gray scale. The inferior vena cava is well demarcated from the mass of lymph nodes immediately adjacent to the vessel.

FIGURE 4.19
Prone longitudinal scan. Echo-free retroperitoneal hematoma displaces the lower pole of the kidney anteriorly. Leaking aortic aneurysm.

FIGURE 4-17 (c)

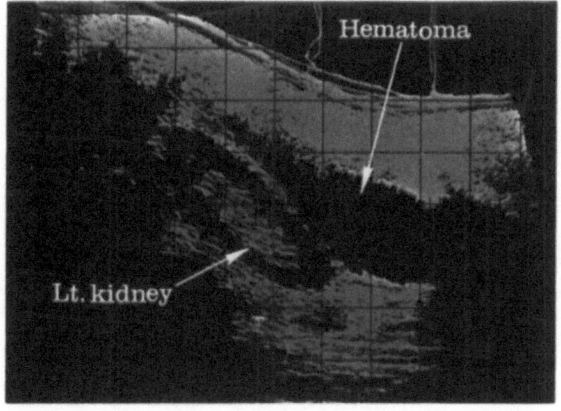

ULTRASONOGRAPHY IN PLANNING RADIATION THERAPY IN GYNECOLOGIC DISORDERS

Radiation therapy planning is an essential aspect of the treatment of certain pelvic malignancies. In gynecologic malignancy, B-scan or gray scale ultrasonography is practical and accurate for demonstrating cross-sectional anatomy and displaying the morphology of organs altered by pathologic processes. Deep-seated tumors can be localized and tissue characteristics determined. Consequently, a plan for radiation therapy can be based on recording the patient's anatomic contours. Ultrasonographic information can be reliably and precisely incorporated into the treatment plan to decrease complications and increase the efficacy of the treatment. Ultrasonography permits three-dimensional therapy analysis by use of the data displayed from perpendicular sonograms. A strong echo will appear at the surface of an organ or mass lesion because different tissues have different acoustic characteristics.

The patient's anatomic contour can be obtained in any desired plane simply and accurately. At a very low gain setting, a single sweep of the transducer over the area of interest will give a contour tracing (6, 7). Ultrasonographic marking is more accurate than mechanical jigs, lead solder, plastic templates, or plaster. The transducer can be swept over a given region repeatedly. If the area of pathology is complex, multiple sections can be made for additional information.

Lung lesions, at present, cannot be evaluated by ultrasonography because sound does not transmit through pulmonary tissue that contains air. However, the thickness of the chest wall can be displayed, so that treatment can be planned for carcinoma of the breast. This measurement is important because it is used to calculate beam energy and for tangential planning, so that underlying lung tissue receives minimum irradiation (6).

LOCALIZATION OF DEEP LESIONS

Sonolaparotomy with different gain settings can be performed at the same time that the patient's anatomic contour is scanned. Thus, the location and size of a space-occupying lesion relative to regional anatomy can be recorded.

Ultrasonographic study to delineate deep-seated lesions and retroperitoneal lymphadenopathy is very useful. Enlarged lymph nodes in this area appear as sonolucent masses, with sharp margins anterior or anterolateral to the spine. This information may be obtained in both longitudinal and transverse scans.

Ultrasonography is also valuable for staging carcinoma of the cervix, since it detects enlarged lymph nodes in the pelvis and abdomen. Similarly, ultrasonography is important in assessing the extent of Hodgkin's disease and other lymphomas. Ascites, both free and loculated, can also be diagnosed.

Pelvic malignancy, especially in the uterus and cervix, can be outlined and tumor size and contour used to plan treatment. If intracavitary applicators are to be used, their position can be monitored by ultrasound. The echo from a radium-loaded tandem is quite strong. To calculate dosage, the positon of the applicator with respect to the bladder as well as the uterine width must be known.

Ultrasonography detects bladder tumors and determines the degree to which the bladder wall is involved. Special transurethral and transrectal scanners are available, which may add more information for staging malignancies of the bladder and prostate.

Upper abdominal organs are also outlined and necrotic tumors demonstrated (1). The enlarged spleen in malignant disorders can be mapped three dimensionally and irradiated accordingly. The development of radiation fibrosis within irradiated organs is evidenced by the increased echogenicity of the organ parenchyma (8). The kidneys can be localized and their size and

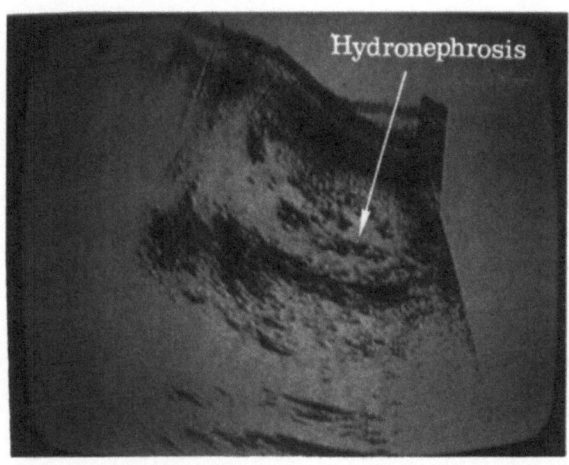

FIGURE 4.20
Prone longitudinal scan. Gray scale. Minimal hydronephrosis. Note multiple echo-free sacs. This is physiologic hydronephrosis of pregnancy.

position determined so that they can be shielded appropriately during treatment (9).

The portal of treatment can be outlined over the abdomen, retroperitoneum, or pelvis. Breaking the contact between transducer and skin surface produces a mark on the scan. Thus, the periphery of a specific region can be marked on the scan and the skin painted with indelible ink. In every step of marking, the transducer should be elevated slightly from the skin surface; the margin is obtained by visual display. A Polaroid is taken as a baseline and compared with Polaroids of future examinations. In this manner portal margins can be decreased as needed.

ULTRASONOGRAPHY OF RENAL DISORDERS IN OBSTETRICS

RENAL DISEASE IN PREGNANCY

The physiologic hydronephrosis of pregnancy occurs early in gestation and lasts through the puerperium. This produces moderate dilatation of the calyces, pelves, and ureters which is more pronounced on the right side (Fig. 4.20). We note that this dilatation usually clears in normal patients within 3 months of delivery. During pregnancy, radiologic investigation of the genitourinary tract must of necessity be limited. Ultrasound is a superb noninvasive means of assessing the physiologic and pathologic changes of the kidneys in gravid females. The size, shape, and position of the kidneys are easily determined. Ptosis may be simply evaluated with positional changes. The ratio of the renal parenchyma to the calyceal complex and the extent of parenchymal damage may be assessed in the diagnosis of chronic renal disease.

The kidney has an ovoid configuration in the transverse plane and is elliptic in the longitudinal axis. In the normal kidney, the renal parenchyma appears echo free (colorless or light gray), and calyceal echoes extend to the ventral and medial borders of the kidney. The image of the kidney with the real-time scanner is similar to that with the conventional B-scan.

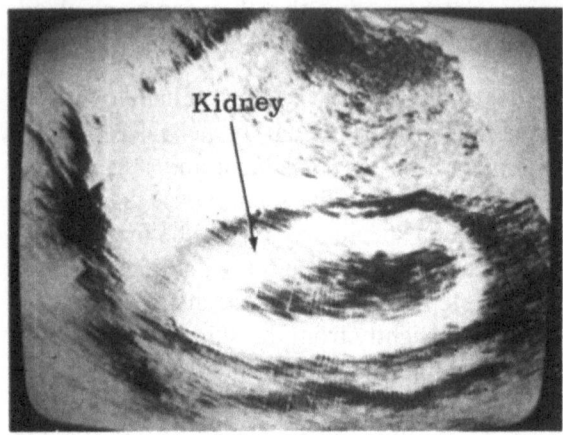

]FIGURE 4-21 (a)

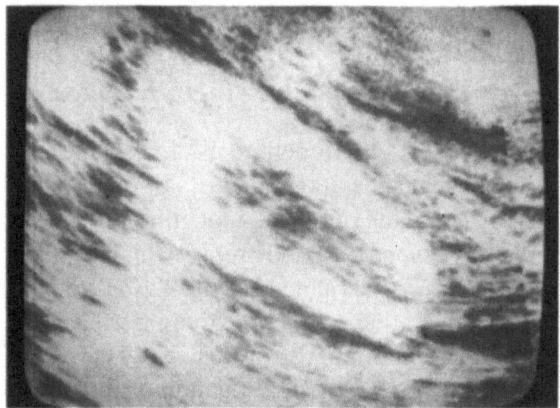

FIGURE 4-21 (b)

FIGURE 4-22

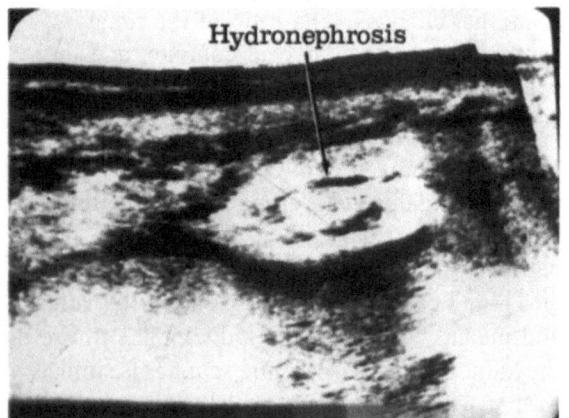

FIGURE 4.21(a)
Supine longitudinal scan. Gray scale. The edematous kidney is better delineated. The through transmission is higher than normal.

FIGURE 4.21(b)
Prone longitudinal scan. Gray scale. Patient with acute nephritis. Note renal parenchyma produces higher through transmission.

FIGURE 4.22
Prone longitudinal scan. Gray scale. Splitting of the renal sinus echoes forming an ovoid echo pattern. Obstructive hydronephrosis.

Acute nephritis is an uncommon complication of pregnancy. Often the kidney cannot be satisfactorily imaged with routine intravenous pyelography. Nephrotomography is often needed to outline the kidney satisfactorily and substantially increases the radiation exposure. We note by ultrasound that the kidney is swollen and increased in its anteroposterior diameter. The through transmission pattern is higher than normal due to the edematous renal parenchyma (Fig. 4.21a and b). The chronic renal diseases include chronic glomerulonephritis, chronic interstitial nephritis, chronic pyelonephritis, collagen diseases, and renal tuberculosis. Chronic renal disease may appreciably increase the risk of toxemia of pregnancy. Ultrasonography shows that chronic renal disease generally produces a smaller kidney than normal. The kidney may be affected diffusely or focally. Chronic pyelonephritis and systemic lupus erythematosus tend to produce areas of focal scarring pathologically, although smooth and contracted renal outlines may be noted ultrasonographically. However, at present, in our experience, it is not possible to demonstrate focal scarring or to differentiate medical disorders of renal parenchyma ultrasonically. The diagnosis of chronic renal disease is best made by renal biopsy. Upon deep inspiration, the kidneys are outlined on the skin with indelible ink or by scratch marks made with a scalpel or needle tip. Biopsy may be performed under ultrasonic guidance, since the kidney appears in the line of sight of the sonic beam from the transducer and the depth to the renal parenchyma may be read off the oscilloscope directly. The ultrasonically guided renal biopsy uses a needle which will fit through the center of the puncture transducer. Follow-up examination after 24 hours may be added to evaluate the possibility of local hematoma formation. Basically, renal biopsy with a puncture transducer needs extensive experience and patient cooperation.

OBSTRUCTIVE UROPATHY

Routine evaluation of obstructive uropathy includes a plain X-ray film of the abdomen and intravenous urography. Nephrotomography, retrograde pyelography, arteriography, and renal isotope studies are frequently added for further information. The poor function of the obstructed kidney generally necessitates delayed films, multiple injections of contrast medium, significant radiation exposure, and patient discomfort associated with long waiting periods on a hard table. In addition, osmolality of the contrast medium may increase intrapelvic pressure sufficiently to produce pyelosinus reflux or even peripelvic extravasation of urine and contrast medium into the retroperitoneum (10). The routine study of the kidney in pregnancy is limited due to exposure. Ultrasonography may yield extensive information; however, for urinary stasis or determination of the site of obstruction the contrast study is necessary.

Urinary stasis may have obstructive (Fig. 4.22) and nonobstructive mechanisms. Impedance to urine flow commonly occurs with tumors and calculi of the kidneys, ureters, and bladder. Other ureteral problems include anomalies of insertion, stricture, stenosis, and pregnancy. Abnormal ureteral compression is associated with retrocaval ureter, lymphadenopathy, abscess, hematoma, or aberrant vessel. Nonobstructive stasis follows neurogenic dysfunction of the bladder, chronic inflammatory conditions, atony of the ureters with high urinary output, and vesicoureteral reflux (11).

The size of the obstructed kidney may appear increased, normal, or decreased. Interstitial edema of acute obstruction tends to enlarge the renal parenchyma. Back pressure atrophy of the cortex associated with chronic obstruction produces a small kidney in most cases (11). Thus, renal size may only be interpreted diagnostically with reference to sequential studies over a known period of time.

Pathophysiologic changes in the pelvicalyceal system reflect the degree and duration of increased pressure and damage from superimposed infection. Dilatation of the calyces, infundibula, and pelves usually progresses proportionately. However, the extrarenal pelvis acts as a hydraulic buffer, sparing infundibula and calyces as it dilates to dissipate the increased pressure.

The earliest pathologic changes of chronic increased pressure occur in the calyceal system. Blunting of the acute forniceal angle is followed by flattening and eventual clubbing of the calyx. Subtle calyceal alterations often escape ultrasonic detection (12) due to the resolution of the 2.25-MHz transducer routinely used in renal scanning. The renal sinus is the invagination of the renal hilus and contains the renal pelvis, major caylces, and main renal vessels. The principle ultrasonic observation in early obstruction is dilatation of the renal sinus produced by intrarenal enlargement of the renal pelvis and adjacent major calyces.

The first ultrasonographic finding in hydronephrosis is "splitting" of the renal pelvicalyceal echoes (13). This corresponds to distension of the calyces and infundibula, so that distinct echoes are reflected by each inner wall surrounding the anechoic collected urine. As dilatation proceeds, degeneration of renal tissue distorts the calyces into pockets of urine retained within compressed atrophic bands of renal tissue. This produces the picture of thick septa dividing a large cystic collection, with a shell of remaining sonolucent cortex discernable at medium sensitivity (14). Further destruction of the cortex by back pressure atrophy and infection may result in a lobulated renal periphery, simulating a multilocular cyst (15). Eventually, only a fluid-filled sac of variable size can be visualized (13). Differentiation between hydronephrosis and pyonephrosis may be suggested by observing irregularity of tissue septa dividing cystic collections within the kidney (14). However, in our experience, differentiation of these two conditions by ultrasonography is extremely difficult, and again appropriate clinical data and laboratory findings are more informative.

Polycystic renal disease is a disorder transmitted by an autosomal dominant gene and is frequently found in many members of an affected family. Since the clinical manifestations of this disease usually appear in the early forties, it is usually not a common problem in pregnancy.

Polycystic disease is generally diagnosed by observing bilaterally enlarged renal outlines with a markedly lobulated outer contour, as contrasted to the smoother surface produced by hydronephrosis. In addition, septa in the polycystic kidney have a random distribution, as opposed to the central radiation noted in the obstructed and dilated calyceal system (Fig. 4.23a and b) (15). It is difficult to distinguish a hydronephrotic sac from a massive renal cyst severely compressing the remaining renal parenchyma.

Ultrasound is an excellent screening procedure for the diagnosis and follow-up of polycystic disease. Early cystic changes will enlarge the kidney, but will not distort the calyces sufficiently to be detected on routine intravenous urograms. Gray scale may identify cystic lesions before calyceal changes appear. Other affected organs may also be studied. Thus, ultrasonography is ideal for evaluating asymptomatic family members.

Anuria may accompany acute renal failure or calculous disease with obstructive uropathy. Both have approximately the same overall low incidence in pregnancy. Renal failure is often due to septic abortion or toxemia. The resultant nonfunctioning kidney cannot be diagnosed by routine radiography. Ultrasonography quickly distinguishes between the swollen kidney of acute renal failure and the dilated pelvicalyceal system of the obstructed kidney.

The high calcium content of the usual radioopaque calculus markedly reflects sound waves. The echo from the stone will appear to be stronger than the surrounding calyceal echoes, if it acts as a specular reflector. An irregular or amorphous calculus will act as a diffuse reflector and will be difficult to image. The lack of through transmission may cause a sonic shadow (Fig. 4.24) (16). A secondary observation may be splitting of the renal sinus echoes due to concurrent hydronephrosis. In the presence of a dilated renal collecting system, renal calculi of lower reflecting qualities may be demonstrated as low-amplitude echogenic masses lying against the dependent wall of the dilated collecting system.

The advent of renal transplantation techniques now allows previously infertile females with chronic renal disease to bear children. As surgical and immunosuppressive techniques improve, some women with renal transplants will become pregnant. The usual site of transplantation is in the pelvis. Because of this location, during delivery, the transplant may be compressed and injured by the fetal head. Ultrasonography may now replace the previous combined usage of renal urography and pelvimetry in showing the fetal head in relation to the transplanted kidney.

If contraceptive devices are not employed, the transplanted patient may become pregnant soon after surgery. Ultrasonography is excellent for monitoring the possible complications of renal transplants.

Serial measurements of the size of renal transplants are useful for detecting acute or intermediate rejection and shrinkage secondary to progressive fibrosis of the transplanted kidney. Magnification on X-ray film (approximately 20 percent) should be corrected before the film is compared with the undistorted scan. The transplanted kidney is located in the iliac fossa

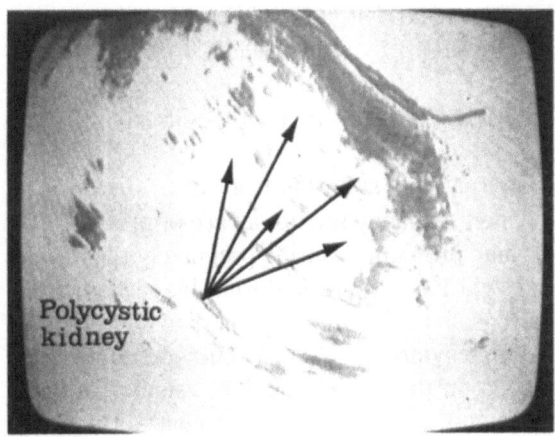

I FIGURE 4-23 (a)

FIGURE 4.23(a)
Prone longitudinal scan. Gray scale. Enlarged and distorted renal outline. Multiple anechoic regions are noted in a diffuse arrangement. Septations between anechoic cysts are random in distribution. Opposite kidney with similar appearance. Polycystic disease.

FIGURE 4.23(b)
Prone transverse scan. Gray scale. The enlarged renal outline has sonolucent regions with random septations.

FIGURE 4.24
Prone longitudinal scan. Gray scale. A very dark echo complex within the gray renal collecting system echoes represents a calcified renal calculus. The distal wall of the kidney is not imaged. Sonic shadowing may be produced by highly reflecting renal stones. Head is toward the right.

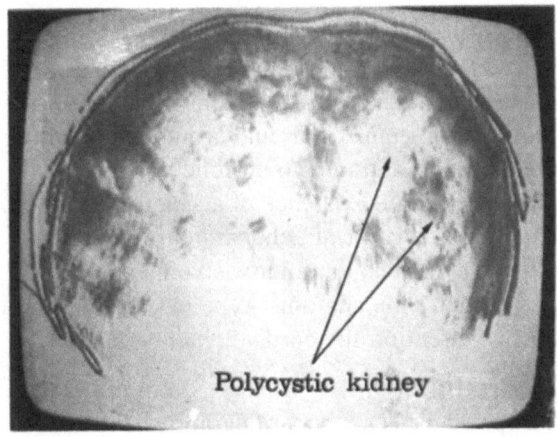

FIGURE 4-23 (b)

FIGURE 4-24

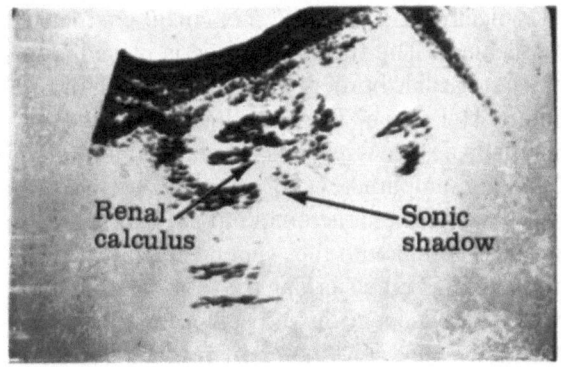

obliquely. The A-mode or B-mode may be used. More accurate measurements are possible when the A-mode echoes are superimposed on a calibrated scale. Newly devised electronic calipers may also be employed.

Longitudinal and transverse scans are made with respect to the lie of the transplanted kidney; length, width, and volume can be calculated. When the kidney becomes edematous, the sonolucency and through transmission are increased compared with the previous sonogram; size and volume are also increased.

Asymptomatic infections often appear since the immune mechanisms of these patients are altered by steroids, cytotoxic drugs, or radiation therapy. The infections are commonly perirenal abscesses at the site of renal transplantation. Scanning may demonstrate collections of serum, lymph, blood, or pus as sonolucent areas that may fill in with echoes at high sensitivity, depending on the contents of the fluid (17, 18). Morphologic changes in renal transplants are of diagnostic value. A sudden increase in renal size implies acute rejection. Absence of expected hypertrophy of the transplant after several months suggests chronic rejection and fibrosis. Dilatation of the calyceal system indicates ureteral obstruction (2). Renal agenesis may also be detected ultrasonically (Fig. 4.25). Pelvic lipomatosis can easily be investigated and serial studies may be used to follow its course (Fig. 4.26).

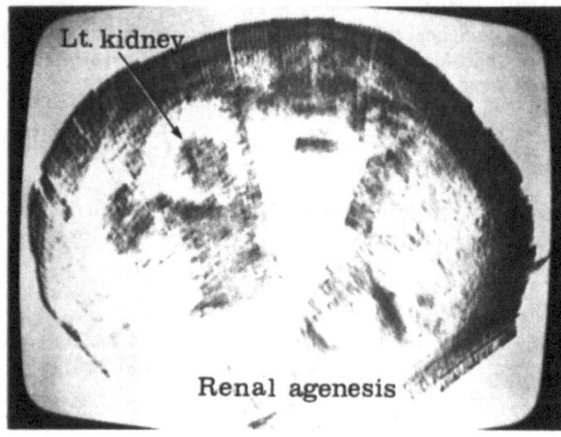

FIGURE 4.25
Prone transverse scan. Gray scale. The ovoid outline of the left kidney is clearly imaged. The right renal outline is not visible and the low-level echoes of the hepatic parenchyma fill the region normally reserved for the right kidney. Congenital absence of the right kidney.

FIGURE 4.26
Prone longitudinal scan. Gray scale. The echo pattern of the renal collecting system is heterogeneous due to accumulation of fatty substance in the renal tissue. This echo pattern is usually seen in pelvic lipomatosis.

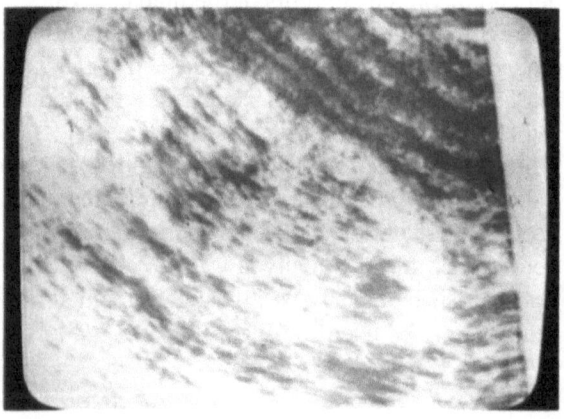

ULTRASONOGRAPHY OF CARDIAC DISORDERS IN OBSTETRICS

CARDIAC DISEASE IN PREGNANCY

Many patients suffering from heart disease during pregnancy are not aware of preexisting cardiac problems. During pregnancy the heart rate, cardiac output, and total blood flow are increased, so that marginal cardiac function may become symptomatic due to the greater stress placed on the cardiovascular system. Cardiac signs and symptoms which appear during pregnancy, such as hyperventilation, pedal edema, and various murmurs and unusual heart sounds, may be associated with normal gestation. The obstetrician is thus faced with a patient who may have significant cardiac disability.

The established criteria for evaluating heart disease in pregnancy include the presence of a diastolic murmur, clear-cut cardiomegaly on the chest X ray, a grade 3/6 systolic murmur or greater, and the existence of a severe arrythmia. The recent advent of echocardiography has given the clinician a noninvasive means of categorizing the anatomic type of cardiac lesion and its effect on the cardiac chambers and valves.

The principles of echocardiography have been well discussed in the literature (19). The unit is operated in A-mode and M-mode or gray scale, with the specially designed cardiac transducer placed over the precordium. A coupling agent consisting of a thick gel is generally applied to the chest wall. The transducer for the adult heart is typically a 2.25-MHz, 7.5-cm or 10-cm focused transducer. The transducer face is placed along the left cardiac border between the fourth or fifth intercostal space. The transducer is angled medially as the A-scope is constantly monitored. The high-amplitude echo pattern of the aortic valve with its characteristic to-and-fro structure is easily found with the A-mode display. This is then verified by observing the M-mode tracing which may appear on an oscilloscope face, television tube, or strip-chart recorder. After locating this echo pattern the transducer is angled inferolaterally to identify the "jerky" motion of the anterior mitral valve leaflet. Tracings are then recorded in these positions and intermediate angulations are performed to completely outline the entire cardiac apparatus in a one-dimensional read-out.

The cardiac valves and chambers may also be observed with specially designed real-time scanners. These consist of an array of transducers which produce a two-dimensional, real-time image. Sonofluoroscopy of the heart is proving to be a useful adjunct in cardiac diagnosis. This extra dimension gives the ultrasonographer much more data which serve to produce a three-dimensional representation with greater ease than is possible with the unidimensional mental tracing. Indeed, ventricular contractility abnormalities, valvular deformities, and chamber enlargements may be readily studied.

RHEUMATIC HEART DISEASE

Although there has been a continuing decrease in the incidence of rheumatic fever and its associated short-term and long-term cardiac disorders, rheumatic heart disease is still the most common cause of organic heart disease in pregnant females. Mitral stenosis by itself or with associated valvular abnormalities is the most frequently encountered sequel of previous rheumatic disease. This abnormality may be clinically confused with other disorders such as atrial septal defect, primary pulmonary hypertension, and left atrial myxoma. These conditions may be separated by their distinctive appearances on the echocardiogram.

The normal echocardiogram shows an ice-pick slice of the heart. The aortic root appears as a series of parallel lines with a to-and-fro motion. Within the aortic root in its lower portion, the echoes of the opened and closed aortic leaflets are noted. Distal to the aortic root is the left atrial cavity, which may be measured from the calibrated tracing. The motion of the interventricular septum is readily outlined and its synchrony with the posterior left ventricular wall is seen. The characteristic M-shaped diastolic motion of the mitral valve leaflet and the systolic apposition of the anterior and posterior mitral valves are readily documented.

The pathologic changes of mitral stenosis exacerbated by pregnancy are easily observed on the echocardiogram. The increased cardiac output along with the shortened diastolic filling time serve to increase the left atrial pressure and chamber size. Not only are the chamber dimensions visible, but the presence or absence of clot is detectable. The right ventricular overload results in an increase in the chamber size of the right ventricle. Most important is the shape of the mitral valve echo pattern. The scarring produced by the rheumatic endocarditis produces shortening of the chordae tendineae, fusion of the fissures, and retraction of the valve leaflets. These latter present as a reversal of the opposite motion of the posterior mitral valve leaflet, so that it now follows the path of the anterior mitral valve leaflet. Also, the normal diastolic flutter of the mitral valve with fluctuation of pressure changes between the left atrium and left ventricle is severely limited, producing flattening of the M-shaped valve outline. The presence of calcification of the valves due to longstanding fibrosis is also demonstrable by the echogenic nature of the calcific valve. The degree of stenosis of the mitral valve orifice is not well quantified by ultrasound. However, the presence of a normal echocardiogram rules out the presence of mitral stenosis.

Ultrasound is helpful in detecting aortic stenosis of either the congenital bicuspid or rheumatic type. As with mitral stenosis, rheumatic aortic stenosis is due to commissural fusion. This presents as poor opening motion of the aortic valve leaflets with incomplete excursion to the walls of the aortic root. The left ventricular outflow obstruction produces left ventricular hypertrophy and left ventricular chamber enlargement, which appear as a widened left ventricular cavity with a thickened left ventricular wall dimension.

Insufficiency of the mitral and aortic valves scarred by rheumatic endocarditis is due to shortening of the valve cusps and chordae

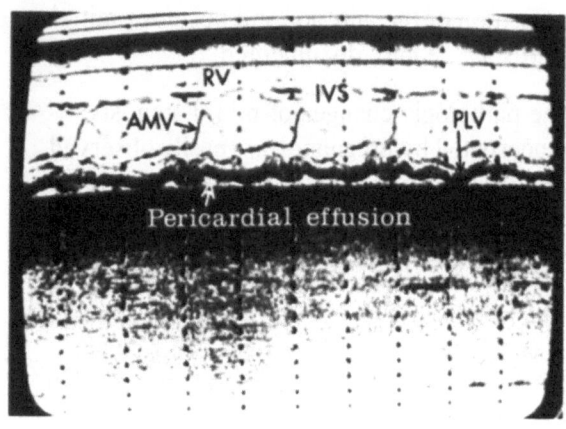

FIGURE 4.27
M-mode. Echocardiogram shows echo-free zone behind the strong epicardial echo complex. Pericardial effusion.

tendineae. Mitral regurgitation is more common in males than in females, in contrast to mitral stenosis which is most common in females. However, the apical systolic murmur associated with pregnancy may be difficult to distinguish from the murmur of mitral insufficiency. Echocardiography in mitral insufficiency shows dilatation of the left heart, especially of the left atrium.

Most cases of aortic insufficiency are due to rheumatic inflammatory disease. Aortic insufficiency is also seen in ankylosing spondylitis, lues, and old bacterial endocarditis. Regurgitation produces dilatation of the left ventricular chamber associated with left ventricular hypertrophy. Echocardiography documents this as a distinctive fluttering of the anterior mitral valve leaflet, due to the eddy produced in the left ventricle by the stream of regurgitant blood.

A significant contribution to cardiac diagnosis is the ability of echocardiography to detect pericardial effusions in quantities between 100 and 150 ml of free or loculated pericardial fluid. It is radiologically difficult to differentiate small to moderate-sized effusions from other causes of cardiomegaly. Ultrasound shows the fluid as an echo-free space between the posterior left ventricular wall and the pericardium (Fig. 4.27). Pericardial effusion may be due to rheumatic carditis, trauma, hypothyroidism, malignant disorders, tuberculosis, ischemic heart disease, and metabolic disorders. Pericardial effusion or cardiac tamponade may be treated by percutaneous insertion of a special aspiration needle under ultrasonic visual guidance. The distance of the beating epicardium to the needle tip may be continually monitored to prevent cardiac laceration.

Ultrasound is specific in differentiating between left atrial myxoma and mitral stenosis, a clinically difficult procedure. The echocardiogram shows flattening of the M-shaped valve with a series of echoes projecting distally from the valve in diastole. This finding is pathognomonic of a left atrial tumor. Prolapse of the mitral valve is a common condition due to myxomatous degeneration of the mitral valve apparatus. Clinical variations range from asymptomatic patients to patients with severe arrythmias. This entity is more common in females and the average age of onset is 37 years. The prolapse appears on echo-cardiograms as a distal swing of the valve in systole. This may involve the anterior mitral valve, posterior mitral valve, or both in various combinations.

Another lesion that is specifically diagnosed by ultrasound is asymmetric septal hypertrophy, which is a generalized category that includes idiopathic hypertrophic subaortic stenosis. The pathologic change is that of marked and asymmetric thickening of the interventricular septum, which narrows the left ventricular outflow cavity and simultaneously produces abnormal mitral valve motion. The characteristic echocardiographic picture is that of a thickened interventricular septum larger than the left ventricular wall thickness by a certain degree, accompanied by a paradoxic systolic anterior motion of the mitral valve so that it almost touches the interventricular septum.

CONGENITAL HEART DISEASE

Due to the effective treatment of streptococcal infections by antibiotics, the incidence of rheumatic heart disease is decreasing. The obstetrician is thus faced with a greater percentage of patients with congenital cardiac abnormalities. The most common cardiac lesion in the clinical practice of obstetrics is the atrial septal defect. The physiologic right heart overload caused by the lesion produces a large right ventricular cavity with a left ventricular chamber correspondingly decreased in size. A paradoxic motion of the interventricular septum is often demonstrable.

Other common types of congenital heart disease include ventricular septal defect, patent ductus arteriosus, congenital aortic stenosis, and Ebstein's anomaly. In each of these suspected disorders, echocardiography may either confirm the clinical diagnosis or discover another cardiac disorder simulating the physician's impression.

VASCULAR DISEASE IN PREGNANCY

The diagnosis of vascular disorders in pregnancy is somewhat different than in the nongravid patient, due to the need to avoid the ionizing radiation inherent in X-ray and radioisotopic procedures. Use of gray-scale and real-time scanning together with Doppler ultrasound may add significant contributions to the study of disease entities with vessel pathology.

ARTERIAL DISEASES

The gravid term uterus lies upon the abdominal aorta when the patient is in the supine position. A series of aortograms performed for the diagnosis of placenta previa before the advent of diagnostic ultrasound showed anterior compression by the uterus on the wall of the aorta. Reduced blood flow to the peripheral vessels was noted. None of the patients were symptomatic for arterial vascular disease. However, it is logical to anticipate that younger patients with collagen disease or other forms of arterial insufficiency may have their symptoms aggravated by gestational pressure. The aorta may be imaged during gestation either with the real-time scanner or with gray scale instruments. The degree of compression of the aortic lumen in the anteroposterior diameter may be measured.

Aneurysms of the abdominal aorta may be identified easily. Although the cystic medial necrosis responsible for dissecting aneurysm most often produces a dissection in the thoracic aorta, this may extend into the abdominal aorta. Widening of the anterior aortic root is demonstrable with echocardiography in the usual positions. Dissection of blood may be noted at higher gain settings. The aneurysm of the descending thoracic aorta may be studied if the aneurysmal dilatation comes into contact with the posterior pleura–chest wall interface. This may then be demonstrated with M-mode, gray scale, or real-time scanning. The complications of rupture into the pleural space or into the pericardial sac may be easily documented with conventional ultrasonic techniques.

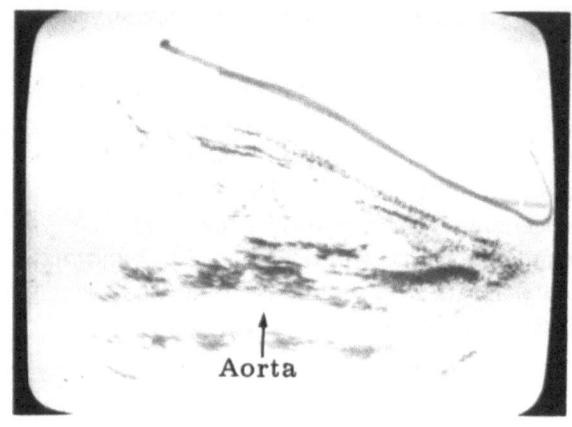

FIGURE 4.28(a)
Supine longitudinal scan. Gray scale. The aorta appears as a linear echo-free structure that tapers smoothly. It usually may be imaged from the xiphoid process down to the level of the umbilicus. Generally, the distal wall is more sharply outlined than is the proximal wall.

FIGURE 4.28(b)
Supine longitudinal scan. Real-time scanner. The aorta may be studied easily with the real-time scanner. The characteristic systolic contraction wave may be observed. This verifies the aorta and distinguishes it from other echo-free regional structures.

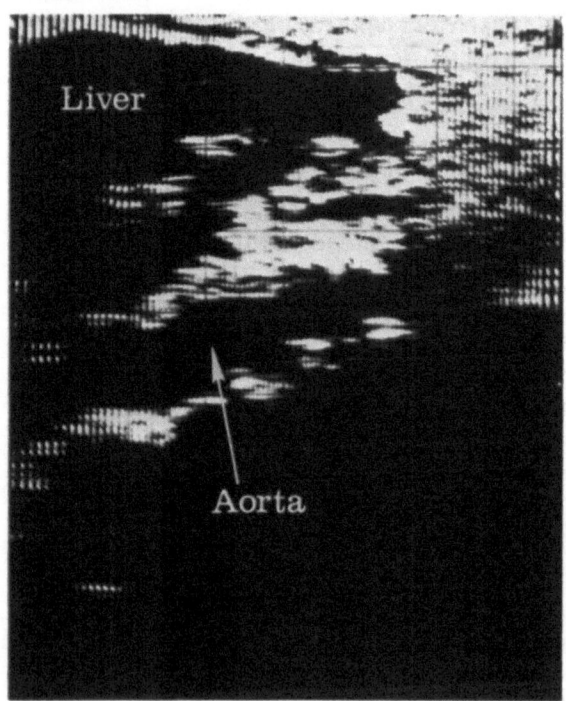

Ultrasonography of the abdominal aorta is performed in the transverse and longitudinal planes. Combined use of the real-time scanner with gray scale is particularly appropriate in pulsating structures. Ultrasonography is not only an excellent diagnostic modality, but is also the least invasive for the detection and follow-up of aortic aneurysms. Indeed, this was one of the first uses of ultrasound in the upper abdomen. Improved diagnostic techniques have revealed a greater incidence of asymptomatic abdominal aortic aneurysms in the elderly than was previously recognized (20, 21).

Abdominal aortic ultrasonography assumes increased importance since this may be the only method available for examining the geriatric patient or the pregnant patient with suspected dissecting aneurysm.

Blood is a good transonic medium. Consequently, the aorta can be detected easily by abdominal sonolaparotomy. The aorta is located anterior to the spine, generally slightly to the left (Fig. 4.28a and b). Its walls reflect strong echoes, with an anechoic region representing the blood-containing lumen. The diameter of the normal aorta is approximately 3 cm and tapers off as the aorta descends. On gray scale, blood does not have the same homogeneity as does clear fluid.

There is no magnification, and the size of the aorta may accurately be determined. Simple measurement may be accomplished by calculating the anterior-to-posterior diameter in the longitudinal or transverse planes. Traditionally, the aorta has been studied with contrast angiography by the translumbar approach or through percutaneous, retrograde, femoral artery catheterization. However, serious consequences may result from these methods. A known incidence of thrombosis and embolization is associated with arterial catheterization, especially after a plaque, in patients with severe atherosclerosis. Since systemic hypertension is frequently associated with atherosclerosis, hematomas may form at the puncture site.

ANEURYSM

Arteriography can only show the lumen of an aneurysm; the clotted portion obviously cannot be seen. The true size of an aneurysm is assessed by measuring the width of the lumen on the angiogram and adding to it the distance from the lumen to the outer calcified wall. If calcification cannot be seen radiologically, the true dimensions of the aneurysm cannot be accurately estimated. In fact, if there is no wall calcification and the laminated thrombus completely fills the aneurysmal sac, the contrast-opacified lumen of the aortic aneurysm may be mistaken for a normal distal aorta and the diagnosis completely missed (22, 23). The outer diameter is an important preoperative parameter for the surgeon. Elective operation is considered when this measurement exceeds 7 cm (21, 23, 24).

Abdominal aortic aneurysms may assume a variety of forms (Fig. 4.29a,b,c,d, and e). Dilatation may be localized and the aneurysm saccularly shaped. It usually has a sharp anterior wall, and may easily be confused with a cystic lesion. However, the outer wall of a cyst is generally not as sharply defined as is that of an aneurysm. Fusiform aneurysms typically originate below the level of the renal arteries in the region of the inferior border of the liver, but they may involve the entire abdominal aorta. Fusiform aneurysms may extend into the iliac arteries and may involve long segments of the aorta, beginning in the thoracic aorta and extending into the abdominal aorta. This thoracoabdominal aneurysm appears on the abdominal scan as dilated lumen that tapers in size as it descends into the lower abdomen.

Various layers of the aneurysm can be detected by adjusting the sensitivity of the ultrasonic unit. At low sensitivity, only the outer walls of the aneurysm are seen. Higher sensitivity will show echoes from the clot or thrombus. The true lumen, filled with blood, remains echo free.

Dissecting aneurysm occurs less often in the abdominal than in the thoracic aorta. Intimal necrosis permits blood to course in the media of the vessel (Fig. 4.30). External rupture may occur or the channel may reenter the aortic lumen. The intima is pushed into the blood-filled true lumen by the intramural hemorrhage, which appears as a septation in the echo-free aorta, generally best seen on the longitudinal scan. At higher sensitivities, the thrombus in the false channel may fill in with echoes. Thrombus is best demonstrated with gray scale equipment.

PARAAORTIC LYMPHADENOPATHY

Paraaortic lymphadenopathy occurs in benign and malignant states. Large preaortic masses are seen in lymphoma and retroperitoneal lymph node metastases. These conglomerates of nodal tissue silhouette the normal outer wall of the aorta, sonographically creating a false outer wall. Lymphadenopathy is difficult to differentiate from aortic aneurysm. Usually, the anterior border of the aneurysm is more sharply delineated than is the lobulated anterior border of lymph node masses. To confirm paraaortic lymph nodes, other areas of lymphadenopathy must be sought.

A confusing artifact frequently occurs when the plane of the scanning beam passes through the fibrocartilaginous intervertebral discs of thin patients. Although the body of the vertebra blocks sonic transmission, the disc structure appears echo free at low sensitivities and may be echogenic at higher gain settings. The neural arch elements may be partly visualized, forming an outline of the spinal canal. In transverse scanning, the anechoic disc may be mistaken for a cystic or vascular structure. This problem can be resolved by sensitivity studies and M-mode or real-time scanners.

VENOUS DISORDERS

Venous thrombosis and embolic phenomena are among the most common serious vascular disorders in pregnancy. The combined use of gray scale and real-time scanning may be of particular value in these situations.

A less serious but more common problem is the venous insufficiency syndrome in pregnancy due to uterine compression of the inferior vena cava.

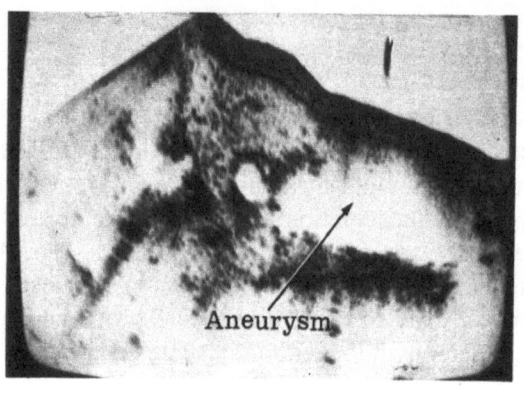

FIGURE 4-29 (a)

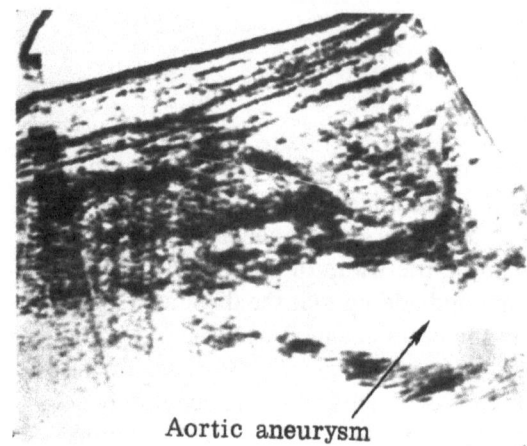

Aortic aneurysm

FIGURE 4-29 (d)

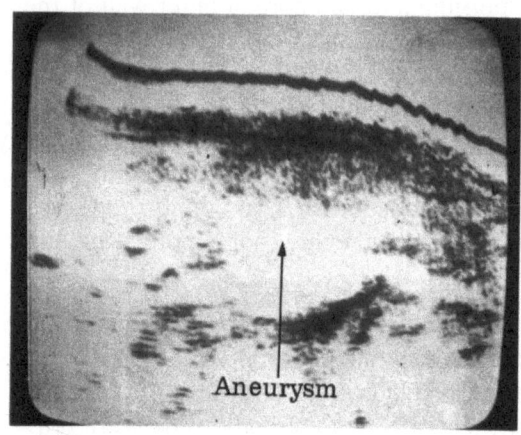

FIGURE 4-29 (b)

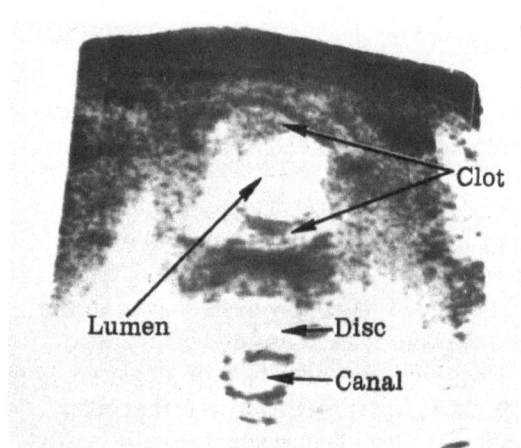

FIGURE 4-29 (e)

FIGURE 4-29 (c)

FIGURE 4-30

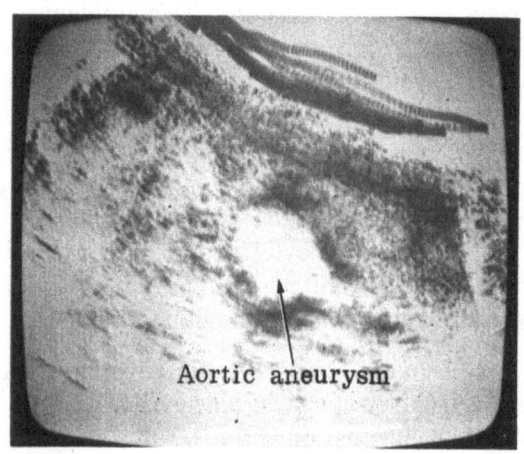

Aortic aneurysm

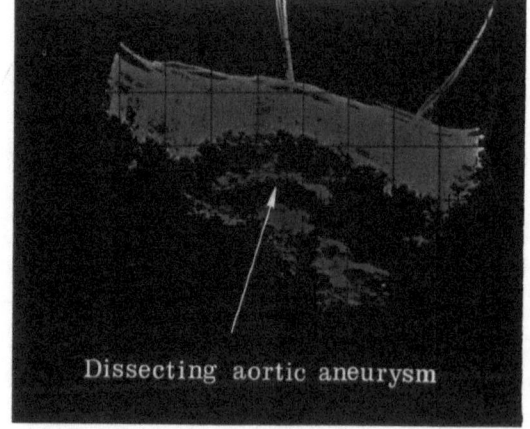

Dissecting aortic aneurysm

FIGURE 4.29(a)
Supine longitudinal scan. Gray scale. The abdominal aortic aneurysm appears as a dilatation of the lumen of the aorta and tapers to the normal aortic caliber. Note posterior sharp border.

FIGURE 4.29(b)
Supine longitudinal scan. Gray scale. Aneurysm of aorta may be confused with other cystic structures. The entrance of the aorta into the dilatation and its exit from the aneurysmal sac are important in definitively diagnosing a saccular abdominal aortic aneurysm.

FIGURE 4.29(c)
Supine longitudinal scan. Gray scale. Aneurysm of the aorta may be confused with other cystic structures. The entrance of the aorta into the dilatation and its exit from the aneurysmal sac are important in definitively diagnosing a saccular abdominal aortic aneurysm.

FIGURE 4.29(d)
Supine longitudinal scan. Gray scale. The thoracoabdominal aortic aneurysm appears as a dilatation of the lumen of the aorta at the level of the diaphragm and tapers to the normal aortic caliber. Head is toward the right.

FIGURE 4.29(e)
Supine transverse scan. Gray scale. Three anechoic regions are noted. An aortic aneurysm is seen anteriorly with an inner layer of thrombus producing an echo-free lumen. Distal to the aneurysm is the echo-poor intervertebral disc. Distally are noted parts of the arch forming the spinal canal.

FIGURE 4.30
Supine longitudinal scan. B-mode. Dissection of the wall of the aneurysm displaces the intimal wall centrally as blood runs in the media of the vessel. This appears as a linear echo band paralleling the lumen of the aorta. Motion of the intimal wall may be observed with M-mode or the real-time scanner.

Although this may be documented by observing total anteroposterior compression of the walls of the vena cava, this problem is generally not one of clinical difficulty. It is, however, of great importance to the ultrasonographer who may examine a patient for an extended period of time in the supine position (Fig. 4.31a,b, and c). After the study is completed, the patient must be returned gradually to the sitting position. After the removal of uterine pressure allows restoration of circulating blood volume, the patient may assume an erect posture and ambulate with an attendant nearby.

Imaging of the inferior vena cava and simultaneous measurement of its diameter are valuable in conditions that cause this vessel to distend. The cause of the turgescent vessel, such as right heart failure, can be determined by evaluating the dilated inferior vena cava. Hepatomegaly due to right heart failure can also be diagnosed by scanning the inferior vena cava. The normal vessel collapses during the expiratory phase of respiration, but does not do so in the patient with heart failure. This phenomenon is best studied with the real-time scanner. Inferior vena cava imaging can also be used to detect a thrombus or tumor in this structure.

The image of the inferior vena cava in longitudinal section is usually very difficult to visualize when the scan is performed with conventional equipment, but is easily demonstrated by the real-time scanner and gray scale. In a normal subject, during inspiration the vena cava reaches a maximum diameter after several seconds. Study performed with the real-time scanner in the paramedian approach shows the vessel's complex motion, which corresponds to the respiratory cycle. The liver and aorta transmit systolic pressure to the inferior vena cava, so that the anterior wall of the vein has even more intense motion than does the anterior wall of the aorta (25). During inspiration, it is well filled and prominent; during expiration it is collapsed and not easily visualized.

Shifting method
Where uncertainty exists in verification of the inferior vena cava, the aorta can easily be found with the real-time scanner. The applicator of the machine is then shifted toward the right side to locate the inferior vena cava. This maneuver can also be done from the location of the inferior vena cava toward the aorta when this artery is difficult to identify.

Evaluation of the inferior vena cava
In right-sided cardiac conditions, the respiratory motion of the vena cava diminishes and, in severe cases, completely disappears; the vein, however, will be seen clearly, measuring at least 2 cm in anteroposterior diameter. Increased diameter of the inferior vena cava usually signifies right-sided heart failure.

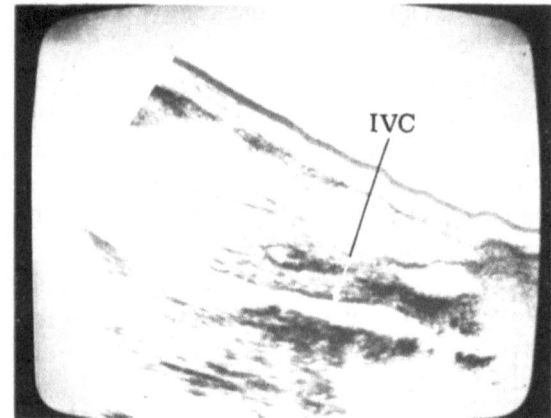

FIGURE 4-31 (a)

FIGURE 4.31(a)
Supine longitudinal scan. Gray scale. Fast scanning speed over the inferior vena cava (IVC) may demonstrate the changes in the outline of this vessel due to inherent motion.

FIGURE 4.31(b)
Supine longitudinal scan. Gray scale. The ovoid portal vein may be distinguished from an enlarged common bile duct by noting its confluence from the splenic vein and the superior mesenteric vein. This may be observed with gray scale or the real-time scanner. Note typical location of the portal vein anterior to the inferior vena cava.

FIGURE 4.31(c)
Supine longitudinal scan. Gray scale. The echo-free lumen of the inferior vena cava extends into the right atrium. The vena cava may be completely surrounded by the substance of the liver as a normal variant. The kinking of the midportion of the inferior vena cava is due to the pressure of the musculotendinous diaphragm on deep inspiration. This kink may disappear on expiration.

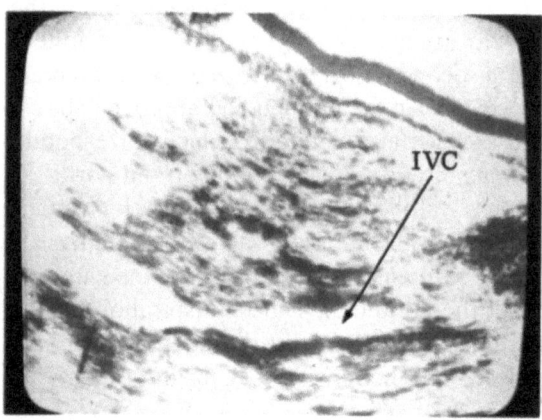

FIGURE 4-31 (b)

Tumor or thrombus within the inferior vena cava may be demonstrated with gray scale or real-time scanners. Internal echoes and the absence of normal pulsatile motion indicate invasion by tumor or areas of clotted blood (26). The inferior vena cava may be displaced anteriorly by retroperitoneal tumors, lymphadenopathy, and adrenal masses. The vena cava or the aorta may be displaced posteriorly by pancreatic lesions. Extrinsic obstruction by masses in or near the pancreas may cause the superior mesenteric vein to distend. The venous system distends in pericardial effusion or right heart failure. Study of the venous system may suggest a cardiac or hepatic etiology for hepatomegaly.

THROMBOEMBOLIC DISEASE

Treatment of thromboembolic disease with anticoagulants is common and the expected complications are few. However, when a gravid female suffers from thromboembolic disorders or other hypercoagulable states and is treated with standard doses of anticoagulant drugs, certain problems generally occur at the time of delivery.

The trauma of birth may precipitate fetal intracranial hemorrhage with resulting neurologic sequelae or even death. Optimally, the fetus should have normal coagulation mechanisms during delivery while the mother should remain in a hypocoagulable state.

FIGURE 4-31 (c)

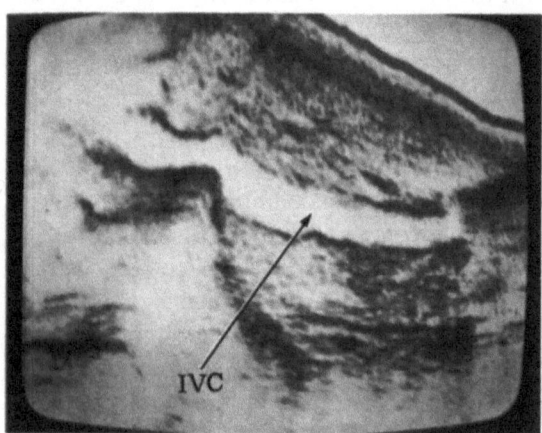

Experimental intrauterine fetal injection of vitamin K (phytomenadione) demonstrated the feasibility of this approach (27). Vitamin K was administered to the mother intravenously or intraamniotically, producing a subclinical rise in the prothrombin-proconvertin level. Vitamin K was then injected into the fetus under ultrasonic guidance (27). (The motion of the fetus may be observed with A-mode or rapid B-scanning with a variable persistence oscilloscope. The best imaging occurs with the multielement real-time scanner.) Injections with a fine needle were made into the fetal thigh shortly before delivery. The injection is performed while the fetal thigh is continually monitored with the real-time scanner; the needle enters the plane of the sound beam and fetal limb and produces a high-amplitude echo which is then monitored. Any alteration in fetal position is instantly noted and adjustments are made in needle insertion as needed. Postdelivery coagulation values were within normal limits in the fetuses previously injected in utero.

ULTRASONOGRAPHY OF GASTROENTERIC DISORDERS IN OBSTETRICS

GASTROENTERIC DISEASES

The common symptoms of nausea, vomiting, and epigastric pain or burning are frequently nonspecific for gastrointestinal (GI) disorders and may even be a normal part of gestation, as in the clinical entity of morning sickness. The large variety of serious disorders that may mimic the simple nausea and vomiting of pregnancy are basically divided into two types: those related to gestation and those unrelated to pregnancy.

Aside from the normal variations of morning sickness, other GI disorders secondary to pregnancy may stem from hydatidiform mole, multiple gestation, and hydramnios. These may be readily diagnosed by ultrasound. Other causes of GI disorders as hyperemesis gravidarum, preeclampsia, and the onset of labor are supported by the lack of positive ultrasonic evidence of definitive pathologic conditions.

Gastrointestinal complaints in the pregnant female may stem from such disorders as cholecystitis, biliary obstruction, appendicitis and appendiceal abscess, peritonitis, hepatic abscess, perinephric abscess, and subdiaphragmatic abscess. Also, ruptured or twisted ovarian tumors may cause nausea and vomiting. Diagnosis of the above entities may be either specifically confirmed or substantiated with ultrasonographic scanning. Disease processes such as ulcers, metabolic disorders, and gastroenteritis and colitis are not diagnosable with ultrasound.

Disorders of the bowel occurring during pregnancy, such as peptic ulcer disease, regional enteritis, and ulcerative colitis, are best diagnosed by radiographic barium examinations. Ultrasonography is useful to document and locate exacerbations or complications of intestinal diseases.

Regional enteritis may involve all parts of the alimentary tract. It mainly affects the small bowel and the most frequent complication that is demonstrable by ultrasound is the tendency for mass formation with the production of fistulas and the adherent masses of matted small bowel loops. These masses appear as poorly localized areas which are usually transonically complex due to the presence of edematous bowel wall and its fluid-filled contents.

The development of amyloidosis and chronic renal failure may show small contracted kidneys with conventional renal ultrasonography. Regional enteritis is not exacerbated by pregnancy.

Ulcerative colitis is primarily an intrinsic colonic lesion and only the secondary complications are diagnosable with ultrasound. Colonic cancer with metastases, fatty liver infiltration and hepatitis, renal disease, and ocular complications may be verified with ultrasonography. Colitis may be exacerbated by pregnancy.

In a similar manner to the nausea and vomiting of pregnancy, constipation may be an associated aspect of gestation. However, there may be serious underlying causes for constipation which may demand further investigation. Internal lesions of the colon, either of the intrinsic or the submucosal type, are able to produce complete obstruction of the lumen of the large bowel. Similarly, inflammatory disorders of the chronic or acute type may produce spasm of the colon or extracolonic abscesses which will obstruct either from extrinsic pressure or reflex atony. Neuromuscular problems and systemic diseases such as scleroderma may be encountered. Anorectal lesions are painful and may cause reflex constipation. Such problems as thrombosed hemorrhoid and anal fissure are common causes of fecal disorders.

Ultrasonography of the constipated colon is difficult since there may be great variety in the size, shape, and localization of the fecal products. If the area of fecal tumor is small and in the cul de sac, its bizarre echo pattern may be mistaken for a dermoid. Fluid contents backing up behind an impacted colon may simulate a cyst. In severe cases of fecal impaction, the air-containing stool may completely block sonic transmission, producing a characteristic picture.

Intestinal obstruction may occur during pregnancy. The obstructed small or large bowel enlarges as the intraluminal contents accumulate. The ultrasonic appearance depends upon the presence of fluid or air within the dilated bowel loops. Bowel that is fluid filled will appear as an echo-free region separated by multiple septations corresponding to the walls of the bowel. Bowel filled with air (eg, from gas swallowing) will produce a sonic shadow. Certain areas of the colon may produce diagnostic difficulty in abdominal ultrasonography. The fluid-filled cecum and sigmoid, especially in inflammatory conditions of the colon or adjacent to the colon, will produce hypotonic segments of bowel which appear as cystic lesions. The real-time scanner may be used to document peristaltic activity. If uncertainty exists, a water enema will show changes in size in bowel loops simulating cystic lesions.

Appendicitis in pregnancy is unique in that the appendix is usually located in the right upper quadrant. Inflammation limited to the appendix

may produce a localized reflex ileus resulting in fluid accumulation in regional bowel loops. This may appear as a cystic mass with septations. Perforation of the appendix may result in localized abscess formation (Fig. 4.32) which appears as an echo-free area surrounding the appendix. Generally, the walls are somewhat irregular due to inflammatory edema and necrotic debris. Through transmission is high.

ULTRASONOGRAPHY OF HEPATIC DISORDERS IN OBSTETRICS

HEPATIC DISORDERS IN PREGNANCY

Hepatic disorders are common in pregnancy. Since the normal liver is positioned almost entirely beneath the ribs, ultrasonic scanning is technically difficult due to sonic attenuation and reverberation artifacts caused by the rib cage.

At low sensitivity, the liver appears as an echo-free organ with a concave distal border overlying the gallbladder, inferior vena cava, aorta, and pancreas. At higher gain settings, the liver fills with echoes. These weak echoes, shaped like dots or short lines, are reflections from larger biliary radicles and hepatic vessels. Using the gray scale, the liver is more echogenic than is the kidney or spleen and less echogenic than is the pancreas.

The increased resolution noted with scan converters shows the normal liver to be homogeneously filled with gray echoes, throughout which are scattered multiple, linear, echo-free areas with dark gray walls projecting toward the hilum.

The most common liver disease in pregnancy is viral hepatitis. The course of hepatitis is similar in the pregnant and nonpregnant states. We have noted that the liver may be enlarged; however, no consistent parenchymal echo pattern has been noted in our series.

Chronic toxic and infectious hepatitis results in cirrhosis, which is an irreversible alteration of the normal lobular architecture, with widespread fibrosis replacing atrophic liver parenchyma.

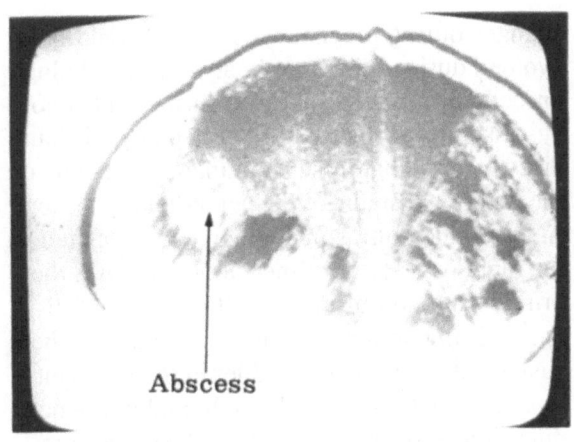

Abscess

FIGURE 4.32
Supine transverse scan. Gray scale. Appendicular abscess.
Note echo-free round area with irregular border and high
through transmission. Patient had history of appendicitis
which developed appendiceal abscess.

Areas of regenerating liver tissue are interspersed diffusely. The size of the liver varies; however, there is usually an increased echo pattern in the liver substance, which may be demonstrated on B-scan and gray scale studies. The distinctive echo pattern in cirrhotic patients is due to the wide spectrum of changes caused by fatty metamorphosis, connective tissue proliferation, regenerating nodules, and necrosis in various combinations. The cirrhotic liver may be accompanied by detectable ascites and has a contracted homogeneous appearance.

Cholestatic jaundice of pregnancy associated with pruritis is due to cholestasis with dilatation of the canaliculi which may contain bile plugs. There is no evidence of distal obstruction and it is thought that the stasis is hormone induced. Ultrasonography is nonspecific and shows an increased echo pattern to the hepatic substance. A similar echo pattern is seen in the acute fatty liver of pregnancy which is associated with fatty changes in the hepatic cells.

Abscess formation accompanying pregnancy may be pyogenic and may appear as single or multiple irregular echo-free areas within the hepatic parenchyma. An amebic abscess is usually located in the posterior portion of the right lobe of the liver. It appears as a complex mass with irregular walls and a high degree of through transmission. Liver abscesses regress more rapidly by ultrasound than by isotopic scanning. Perihepatic abscesses are noted as irregular anechoic regions in the subphrenic and subhepatic spaces. A subphrenic abscess should not be confused with subpulmonic effusion.

CYSTS

Hepatic cysts may be congenital and may be incidentally discovered in females of child-bearing age. These are usually small and associated with polycystic changes in other organs, such as the kidney. If the cysts are larger than 1.5 cm in diameter, they will be detected as echo-free areas on gray scale systems.

Hydatid cysts are usually large when detected; the simple echinococcal cyst appears echo free.

Often septa, necrotic debris, and internal cysts produce the picture of an echogenic mass.

Locating pathology in the liver by sonotomograms is relatively easy. However, it may be quite difficult to determine the nature of the lesion. Diagnostic criteria aid in differentiating benign from malignant processes and cystic from solid lesions.

Surgery may produce fetal wastage in the attempted diagnosis of focal liver lesions. A less traumatic technique uses the percutaneous puncture transducer which enables the clinician to perforate lesions with great accuracy and to aspirate their contents. This transducer has a special central bore through which puncture needles of various sizes can be passed. A fine-gauge needle produces minimal trauma to tissues.

When an echogenic zone, at low sensitivity, or a sonolucent region, at high sensitivity, is delineated, percutaneous cyst puncture may be performed with minimal patient preparation. Coagulopathy should be ruled out by history and laboratory determinations. The skin is sterilized and draped. The scanning transducer is then replaced with a sterile puncture transducer. The sound beam is directed into the zone of interest, and the depth of the lesion from the skin surface is readily measured from the echo pattern on the calibrated A-mode oscilloscope screen. After local anesthesia, the needle is advanced into the lesion to a predetermined depth. The contents of the suspected metastases are then aspirated and submitted for cytologic examination.

Ultrasonography provides a sensitive and atraumatic method for localizing and diagnosing suspected metastatic foci. The percutaneous puncture technique permits simple histologic confirmation of suspected lesions.

ULTRASONOGRAPHY OF GALLBLADDER AND BILIARY TRACT DISORDERS IN OBSTETRICS

Gallbladder and biliary tract diseases are much more common in females than in males. Hence, this organ system may be a site of pathologic changes during pregnancy. X rays should be avoided during this time. In any case, radiologic procedures are seldom useful during acute chole-cystitis, biliary obstruction, or hepatogenic jaundice since radiographic examination depends on the functional status of the hepatobiliary system. Indeed, since ultrasonic imaging is unrelated to the functional status of the gallbladder, it is the primary method of investigation for the radiographically nonfunctioning gallbladder or the suspected diseased gallbladder in the pregnant woman. Anatomically, the right and left hepatic ducts join at the porta hepatis to form the common hepatic duct, which becomes the common bile duct after giving off the cystic duct to the gallbladder. The common bile duct passes anterior to the inferior vena cava and through the superior aspect of the pancreatic head to enter the duodenum at the papilla of Vater.

The gallbladder is a distensible sac lying in a fossa on the inferior surface of the right hepatic lobe. The neck of the gallbladder and the cystic duct are near the porta hepatis, while the fundus projects inferolaterally beyond the liver edge. The fundus may contact the anterior abdominal wall.

The fluid-filled gallbladder appears echo free at low and medium sensitivities. The resolution of gray scale systems permits easier localization of the gallbladder, and fluid-filled compartments greater than 1.5 cm in width can be imaged. The gallbladder is demonstrated along the inferior surface of the liver as an oval or round echo-free structure and is roughly elliptic in its longitudinal axis (Fig. 4.33).

In the filled gallbladder the posterior wall is sharply demarcated and can be delineated in one scan sweep. As it extends caudally, the gallbladder becomes more lateral and superficial. The nonfilled gallbladder is ill defined and difficult to locate.

The patient is instructed to fast overnight to distend the gallbladder optimally. Demonstration of contractility distinguishes the duodenal bulb from the gallbladder. This is best done by A-mode or the real-time scanner (Figs. 4.34 and 4.35). The gallbladder must always be

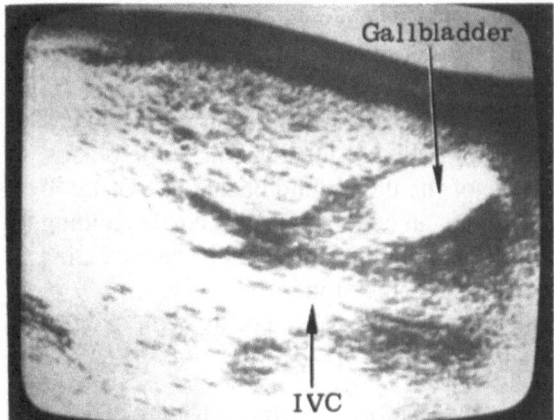

FIGURE 4-33

imaged in both planes to obtain its characteristic shape to prevent misdiagnosing this echo-free area as a cyst of the pancreas (Fig. 4.36) or a metastatic focus in the liver. The biliary tree is best appreciated with gray scale or real-time scanners. The ductal system must be dilated to 1.0 cm to be imaged clearly.

Primary acute cholecystitis is not associated with gallstones. An enlarged echo-free gallbladder is seen without internal echoes. There is no response to a fatty meal. Stones are present in chronic cholecystitis and vary from gravel-size to several centimeters in dimension. In the supine position, gallstones lie against the posterior wall and appear as echoes within the gallbladder. On B-scan, single or multiple echoes, close to the posterior wall, are noted.

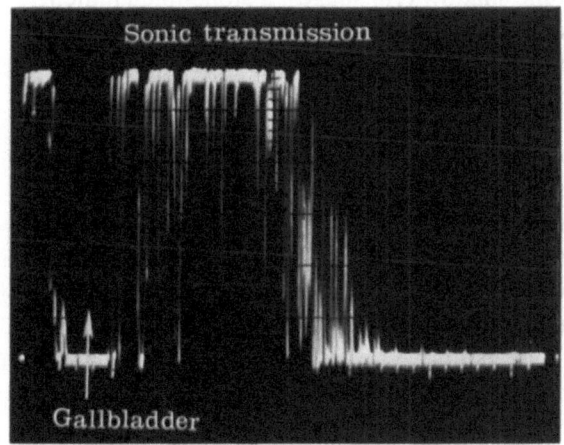

FIGURE 4-34

FIGURE 4.33
Supine longitudinal scan. Gray scale. The gallbladder usually lies in an oblique position. The neck of the gallbladder is often situated over the inferior vena cava.

FIGURE 4.34
A-mode at high sensitivity. High through transmission demonstrated as multiple echoes distal to the posterior wall of the anechoic gallbladder. No change in size will be noted when the transducer is over the gallbladder. A duodenal bulb filled with fluid will change in size with normal contractions.

FIGURE 4.35
Supine longitudinal scan. Gray scale. Dilated gallbladder over kidney. Sharply outlined anterior and posterior walls. No response to fatty meal. Acute cholecystitis.

FIGURE 4.36
Supine oblique scan. Gray scale. The gallbladder was not imaged in the routine scanning planes. Partial outline of the gallbladder appears when the oblique scanning plane is used to locate this structure.

FIGURE 4-35

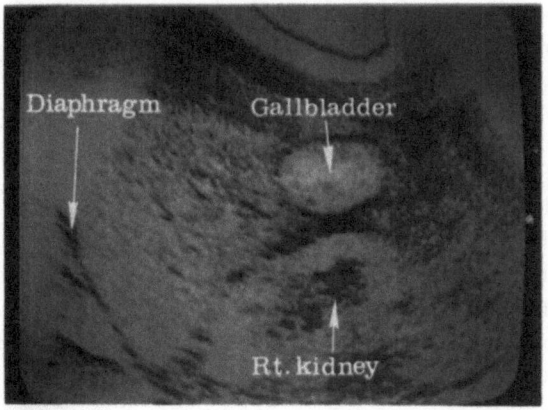

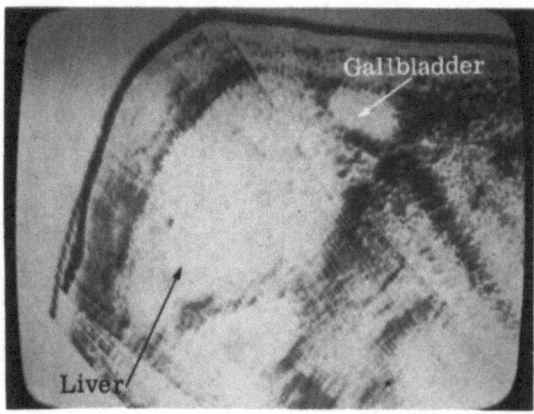

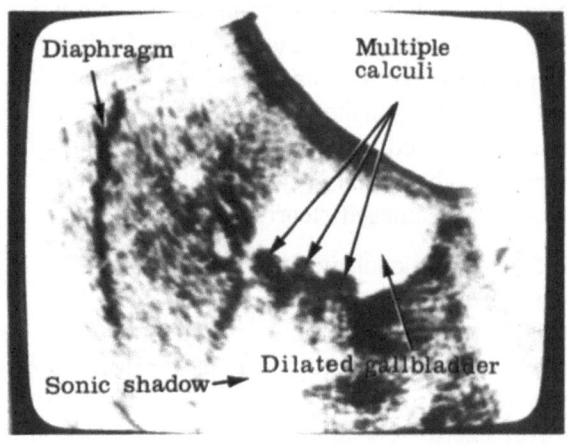

FIGURE 4.37
Supine transverse scan. Gray scale. The gallbladder is echo free. On the distal wall, high-amplitude echoes of a gallstone are noted. A sonic shadow occurs distal to the stone.

FIGURE 4.38
Supine transverse scan. Gray scale. The normal pancreas is generally situated beneath the inferior surface of the liver. The echogenic "cobblestone" appearance of the pancreatic substance is noted above the aorta and superior mesenteric artery. The pancreas is more echogenic than is the liver.

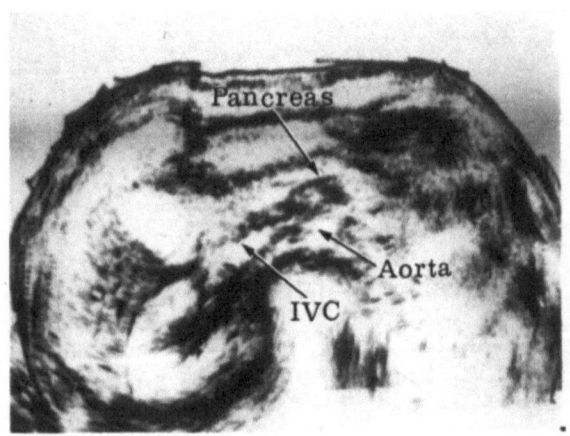

With gray scale imaging, stones as small as 0.4 cm in diameter may be visualized as dark-gray masses of echoes adjacent to the distal wall (Fig. 4.37). With careful linear scanning, a sonic shadow may be produced as the stone blocks passage of the ultrasound beam (16). Distal to the stone is an echo-free space corresponding to the dimension of the calculus in the scanning plane. Behind the stone, the posterior gallbladder wall is either poorly seen or not visualized at all.

If the gallbladder is completely filled with stones, there is insufficient fluid to produce an echo-free interface in which to detect intraluminal echoes. The presence of high-amplitude echoes in the region of the gallbladder and the appearance of a sonic shadow (16) suggest a stone-filled lumen. In chronic cholecystitis, the gallbladder may be shrunken secondary to fibrosis and may contain too little fluid to be detected.

In both chronic obstruction and acute inflammation the gallbladder is dilated and there is no response to fatty meal stimulus. Although the clinical setting is usually diagnostic, the pancreas should be investigated to rule out tumor mass or acute pancreatitis with reflex cholecystitis.

Obstruction of the distal common bile duct is usually caused by impacted gallstones, carcinoma of the head of the pancreas, strictures of the common bile duct, lymphadenopathy, and secondary tumor deposits in the porta hepatis. Carcinoma of the common bile duct is rare. Gradual obstruction causes proximal dilatation of the gallbladder and the common bile duct. The intrahepatic bile duct appears as a tubular echo-free structure on longitudinal section, connecting with the dilated, branching, echo-free major biliary radicles located cephalad (28).

The dilated common bile duct must be differentiated from the portal vein. We identify the portal vein by observing its formation from the splenic and superior mesenteric venous tributaries. The splenic vein posterior to the pancreas is first demonstrated and then followed to the right upper quadrant to its confluence with

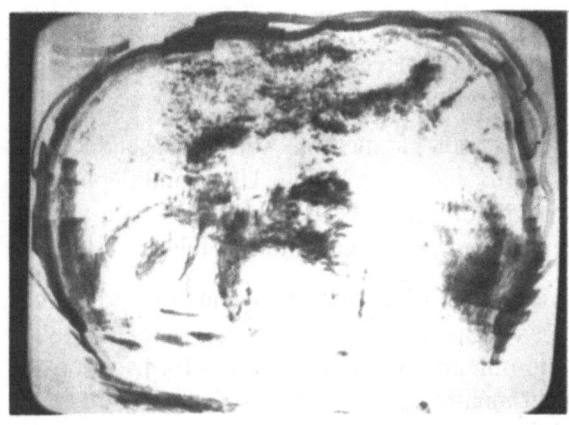

FIGURE 4.39(a)
Supine transverse scan. Gray scale. The acutely inflamed pancreas appears as a sonolucent band above the aorta and inferior vena cava. The edema of acute inflammation produces high through transmission and the margins of the gland are distinctly outlined. The distal wall is well seen.

FIGURE 4.39(b)
Supine longitudinal scan. Gray scale. Enlarged transonic pancreas due to pancreatitis.

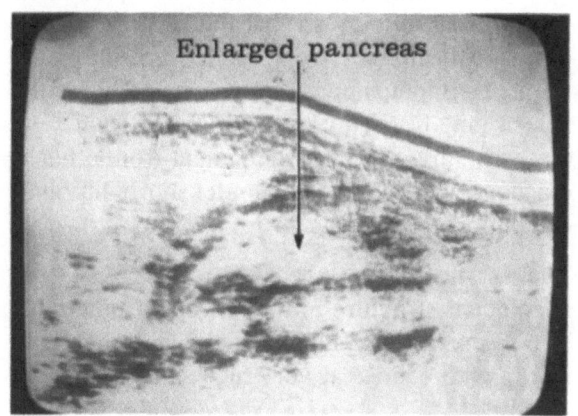

the portal vein. Although this may be done with gray scale, we and others (29) utilize the real-time scanner for speed and accuracy.

ULTRASONOGRAPHY OF PANCREATIC DISORDERS IN OBSTETRICS

Pancreatitis may complicate pregnancy. Either the acute or chronic form may occur in the gravid patient. Pseudocyst formation may result secondary to this disease process. Ultrasonography is now being accepted as the best method for imaging inflammatory processes of the pancreas. Serial examinations may be performed without risk to the patient or discomfort, and are useful in documenting the size of the pancreas in acute pancreatitis. Determination of changes in pancreatic volume is helpful in following the course of chronic pancreatitis.

The pancreas has numerous blood vessels, ducts, and a lobular architecture. The many interfaces in this organ produce internal echoes at medium sensitivity. Ultrasonographically, it is usually ill defined due to the normal irregularity of the gland and the absence of a well-defined pancreatic capsule. The normal pancreas is more echogenic than is the liver, spleen or kidney. It has a "pebbly" gray echo pattern on gray scale systems (Fig. 4.38). The location and shape of the pancreas vary considerably. It is positioned rather anteriorly and may assume a sigmoid, L-shaped, V-shaped, or horseshoe configuration.

PANCREATITIS

Ultrasonography is extremely helpful in the acute stage of pancreatitis when the gland is edematous and usually well visualized (30). The margin of the inflamed pancreas is smooth and the gland becomes highly transonic (Fig. 4.39a and b).

We have noted that turgescence of the superior mesenteric vein frequently accompanies pancreatic enlargement. Other studies show that inflammation of the pancreas is accompanied by increased fluid content, which permits better sound transmission and sharp definition of boundaries (31). Solid organs surrounding the pancreas are filled in with echoes and the pancreas stands out in contrast. The enlarged head of the pancreas may be mistaken for a pseudocyst; however, it does not have the same degree of through transmission nor the sharp posterior wall of a cyst.

Some authors (32,33) feel that ultrasonography is frequently inconclusive in chronic pancreatitis. However, large pancreatic stones may occasionally be demonstrated in the parenchyma of the gland, appearing as strong echoes within the organ indicative of chronic calculous pancreatitis. We have demonstrated the sonic shadow sign (16) in several patients with this disorder. In chronic pancreatitis the entire gland may appear as an echogenic mass; however, delineation of the gland deteriorates as fibrosis and contraction progress.

PSEUDOCYST

Pseudocyst formation in acute pancreatitis may be demonstrated by echography as early as 2 weeks after onset (31), although pseudocysts usually appear 8 weeks after acute inflammation. Some investigators (30,31) described the application of sonotomography in diagnosing pseudocyst of the pancreas. Their studies revealed that the pseudocyst presents as a rounded sonolucent or transonic area, with a strong posterior wall echo. Our series shows that these cysts may be located in any part of the pancreas and may contain septa, pus, or necrotic debris. After drainage, the cyst becomes irregular and fills in with echoes at higher sensitivity settings.

It is stated that pseudocysts may be multiple or lobulated (31,34). We use A-mode in conjunction with B-scan to prove total transonicity of the pseudocyst to differentiate it from solid tumors. The natural course of pseudocystic development can be followed by sonotomography. Spontaneous rupture of a pseudocyst into the duo-denum has been documented by ultrasonography (35). The pseudocyst may resemble ascites in the region of the flank.

Other radiologic methods evaluate pseudocysts by a process of exclusion. Ultrasonography not only directly detects the pseudocyst, but also permits temporal evaluation of this disorder.

Since ultrasound is atraumatic and may safely be repeated as often as necessary, we feel that sonotomography of the pancreas for pseudocyst determination is the method of choice. In addition, complications such as infection or rupture may be documented.

ULTRASONOGRAPHY OF SPLENIC DISORDERS IN OBSTETRICS

Ultrasound is useful in outlining the size, shape, and position of the spleen when splenectomy is considered as a treatment for various hematologic disorders. This is the case in the coagulation disease of idiopathic thrombocytopenic purpura when steroid therapy has failed. We have noted that the spleen may be massively enlarged and yet not project under the left costal margin. Splenomegaly may be difficult to evaluate in obese patients. Ultrasonography may be used in these conditions to estimate the volume of the spleen or to verify that the left upper quadrant mass is indeed splenic in origin. The displacement of the intraabdominal organs by the gravid uterus may displace the spleen in unexpected directions, and ultrasonography may be used to outline the position of the spleen and its regional anatomy so that the surgeon may optimize the operative approach. In addition, the ultrasonographic appearance of the pathologic spleen may be highly diagnostic of certain diseases, and may save the patient from other diagnostic procedures of greater morbidity and discomfort.

The normal spleen appears as a concave sonolucent structure in the left upper quadrant. The splenic pulp is homogeneous and the organ fills in with echoes at very high sensitivity settings. It is much more sonolucent than is the liver and slightly more sonolucent than is the renal parenchyma.

While scanning the pregnant female, certain anomalies may be encountered. Congenital variations of the spleen include asplenia, splenic separations, accessory spleens, and polysplenia with multiple small spleens. Rather large spleens have been incidentally noted as a normal variation in both adults and children.

True cysts of the spleen are rare and may be due to parasites (Echinococcus) or teratoma. False cysts are more common and usually occur in the young adult. These may produce splenomegaly in the pregnant woman. They may be serous or hemorrhagic and are believed to represent organizing hematomas (36,37). The cyst has a sharp posterior border and high through transmission. If the cyst is hemorrhagic or septate, internal echoes may be demonstrated. An attempt is made to visualize the remaining compressed splenic tissue. At higher sensitivity settings, the echogenic spleen will contrast with the echo-free cyst.

Hyperplastic splenomegaly occurs in hemolytic anemias, which are a common problem for the obstetrician. The size and internal echo pattern depend on the chronicity of the disorder and the extent of fibrosis or calcification of the parenchyma. For example, in early sickle cell disease the gland is generally large and anechoic but later contracts and becomes echogenic.

Primary malignant tumors of the spleen are of the lymphoma family. The spleen may contain discrete foci of tumor, with or without necrosis. In advanced disease complete replacement of the organ may occur. Multiple foci of tumor may appear echogenic. The diffusely infiltrated spleen is homogeneous and generally anechoic unless areas of necrosis exist. Most of these spleens highly attenuate the ultrasound beam so that the posterior border is poorly demonstrated. Differentiation of this echo-free tumor from a cyst depends upon the through transmission pattern (1).

In leukemia cellular infiltration is diffuse. Small spleens are generally noted in acute leukemia, while larger spleens occur in chronic leukemia. Infarction and fibrosis are more common in chronic myelogenous leukemia than in chronic lymphatic leukemia. These spleens tend to have anechoic or low-level echo–producing parenchyma. However, we have observed echogenic spleens in chronic myelogenous leukemia (Fig. 4.40).

Trauma may produce splenic injury in pregnant women. The enlarged spleen is more easily traumatized. The lacerated spleen will usually maintain its size and shape as blood spills intraperitoneally. If the capsule is intact, a splenic hematoma will result, enlarging and distorting the splenic outline. Following trauma, ultrasonography is performed, so that use of X rays will be avoided. Inspection is made for intraperitoneal blood. The spleen is examined for breaks in the continuity of the cortical outline, or areas of hemorrhage that appear separated from the normal tissue by a band of echoes corresponding to the blood-spleen interface. At higher sensitivity, the compressed spleen will fill in with echoes, while the subcapsular blood remains echo free (30).

INFLAMMATORY PROCESS

The spleen may enlarge in the presence of extrasplenic inflammatory disease, such as pelvic inflammatory disease or puerperal sepsis, or may be the site of septic infarcts resulting in abscess formation. Splenic abscesses may appear as irregular sonolucent foci as the spleen becomes sonopaque at higher gain settings. Tuberculosis, brucellosis, sarcoid, and other chronic infections tend to produce echogenic spleens (8).

INFILTRATIVE DISORDERS

In benign infiltrative disorders that cause deposition of metabolic products within the cells, such as Gaucher's disease, the enlarged

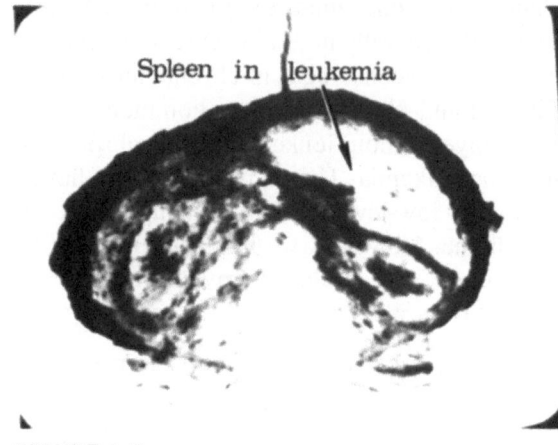

FIGURE 4-40

FIGURE 4.40
Supine transverse scan. Gray scale. The spleen is enlarged, echo poor, and transonic. The spleen crosses the midline of the body. Chronic leukemia.

FIGURE 4.41
Supine longitudinal scan. Gray scale. Echo-free zone above the right hemidiaphragm. Note the high through transmission associated with the pleural fluid. One liter of pleural effusion was evacuated.

FIGURE 4.42
Supine longitudinal scan. Gray scale. The left hemidiaphragm is well imaged. The gas-containing organs in the left upper quadrant are displaced by the enlarged spleen of chronic leukemia.

spleen has an echo pattern consistent with the degree of internal necrosis and fibrosis. Our case material showed moderately echogenic parenchyma in patients with such disorders.

VOLUME DETERMINATION

In general, medical disease of the spleen diffusely enlarges the organ (36), while space-occupying lesions distort the splenic outline and compress normal parenchyma.

The spleen may be enormously enlarged and yet not project below the left costal margin (38). Splenic volume can be determined by analyzing the scans with a pencil-following device linked to a computer system (38). Massive splenomegaly occurs in chronic leukemia, portal hypertension, Gaucher's disease, Hodgkin's disease, myelofibrosis, lymphosarcoma, and some chronic hemolytic anemias. Accurate determination of splenic volume is useful in the diagnosis and management of hematologic disorders.

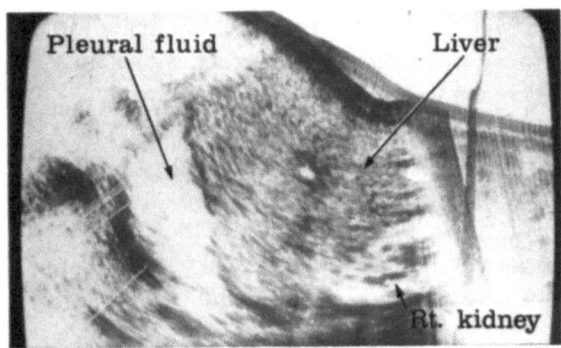

FIGURE 4-41

ULTRASONOGRAPHY OF DIAPHRAGMATIC DISORDERS IN OBSTETRICS

The diaphragm separates the lungs from the abdomen and is affected in diseases of both regions. Both diaphragmatic motion and contour may be demonstrated by ultrasound. Fluid

FIGURE 4-42

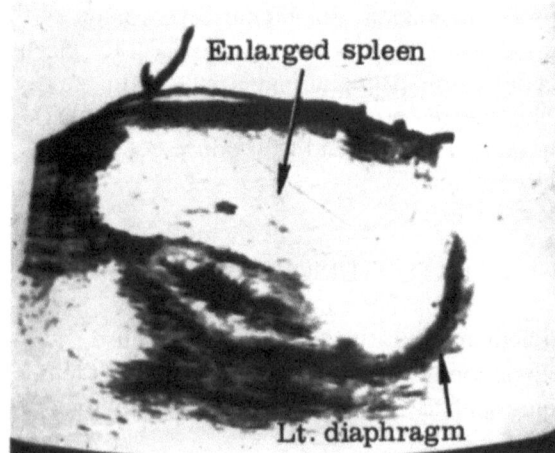

collections above and below this muscular septum are easily identified.

The presence of the liver allows sound to reach the midsagittal plane of the right hemidiaphragm from the posterior aspect almost to the anterior attachment. The sonogram shows a smooth, mobile arc of dense echoes at the periphery of the liver. Normally, the left hemidiaphragm cannot be imaged from the anterior aspect, and the portion that may be visualized by posterior scanning appears as a short, concave, echo-dense structure. Basically, in pregnant females, in the early stage, the diaphragm can be properly evaluated. In later pregnancy, its motion has been restricted due to the gravid uterus, and pathologic conditions are more difficult to evaluate.

Supradiaphragmatic fluid appears as an echo-free area above the liver echoes of the diaphragm. This zone ceases at the pleural interface where another linear arc of echoes is noted (Fig. 4.41). The echo-free area, or free pleural fluid, will decrease in size as the patient is moved from the erect to the recumbent position. Loculated fluid or abscess will not change in shape as the patient's position is altered.

A space-occupying mass in the left upper quadrant makes the left hemidiaphragm easy to image. Indeed, if the left hemidiaphragm is visualized without special effort, a sound-transmitting mass in contact with the left hemidiaphragm must be suspected (Fig. 4.42). This has also been seen when sonic windows were created by marked hepatomegaly, ascites, and left subphrenic abscesses (39).

ULTRASONOGRAPHY OF THYROID DISORDERS IN OBSTETRICS

THYROID DISEASES

Disorders of the thyroid are more common in women than in men. Consequently, thyroid disease is not uncommon in pregnancy. It is well known that the stroma of the thyroid is altered by the hormonal and metabolic changes in pregnancy. During gestation the thyroid gland has large follicles and actively secretes thyroid hormone.

The occurrence of tumors of the thyroid in the pregnant female presents particular problems, since the usual diagnostic modality of radioactive thyroid uptake is associated with the risk of radiation exposure both to the mother and the developing fetus. The fetal thyroid concentrates iodine much more than does the maternal thyroid, and cases of congenital hypothyroidism have been documented following exposure to radioactive iodine (40).

The fetus is more sensitive to radiation effects since irradiation has a more marked effect on rapidly dividing tissue. It is well established that a higher percentage of offspring of mothers exposed to X rays die from leukemia or cancer before the age of 10 years (41). In addition to malignancy, microcephaly has been noted with increased incidence in children irradiated in utero. Retardation in growth and development during adolescence has also been noted.

The superficial position of the thyroid gland in the neck allows inspection and palpation by the clinician and permits soft tissue X-ray examination and isotopic imaging by the radiologist. Since thyroid accumulation of radioactive iodine is histologically specific and thyroid tissue may be ectopic, radionuclide imaging is the best screening procedure for the detection of thyroid pathology. (The application of radioisotopes to the localization of the solitary cold thyroid nodule has greatly aided the physician. However, a poorly functioning area on the scan may represent primary or secondary carcinoma, benign adenoma, cyst, thyroiditis, hyperplasia, or hemorrhage.)

Thyroid tumors may be studied with high resolution ultrasound. Gray scale systems and real-time scanners permit differentiation between benign cysts and solid thyroid tumors. Ultrasound is safe, atraumatic, and may be performed serially, providing important data on the progression of the disease or its response to treatment.

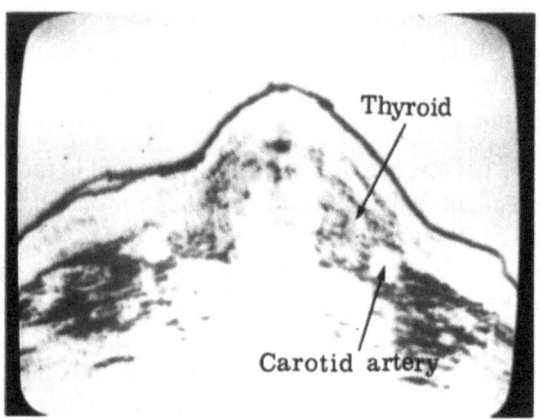

FIGURE 4-43 (a)

FIGURE 4.43(a)
Supine transverse scan. Gray scale. The normal thyroid appears as moderately echogenic tissue bounded by the trachea, carotid sheath, and anterior strap muscles.

FIGURE 4.43(b)
Supine longitudinal scan. Gray scale. The normal carotid artery appears as an echo-free structure. It should be identified to determine the normal position of the thyroid gland.

FIGURE 4.44
Supine transverse scan. Gray scale. Adenoma of the thyroid usually presents as a tumor with a core of high-amplitude echoes surrounded by a periphery of low-amplitude echoes.

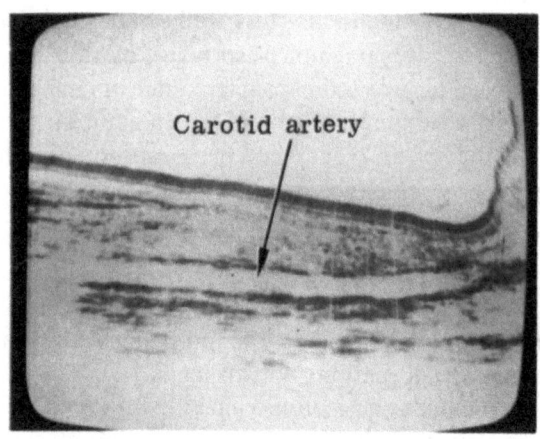

FIGURE 4-43 (b)

The small size and subsurface location of the gland permit the ultrasonographer to use a 5-MHz transducer of limited range but high resolution for the examination. Better contour scanning may be achieved by separating the transducer from the neck surface with a plastic bag filled with water or oil. The patient is studied with the neck hyperextended. The anterior neck is scanned by moving the transducer across the neck transversely in 1-cm intervals from the hyoid bone to the thoracic inlet. Our system of identification uses the thyroid cartilage as a reference point with all sections above it indicated as plus (+) and all sections below indicated as minus (−). A longitudinal scan is performed to complete the examination along the greatest length of the lobe or area of pathology. This results in a three-dimensional representation of the organ.

NORMAL ANATOMY

The thyroid gland occupies the compartment bounded by the trachea, carotid sheath, and neck muscles. The trachea lies posteriorly to the body of the thyroid and is medial to the lateral and posterior extensions of the individual lobes. The air-filled trachea blocks the transmission of sound waves, creating a sonic shadow distally. The common carotid artery and distended jugular vein (due to the gravitational venous filling of the hyperextended neck) appear as

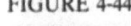

FIGURE 4-44

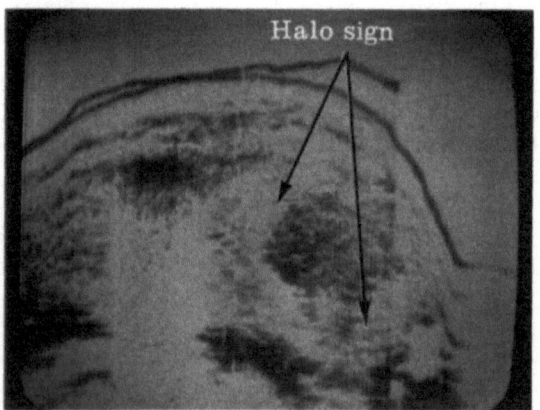

bilaterally symmetric, discrete echo-free structures posterolaterally (Fig. 4.43a and b). Anteriorly is the superficial and lateral cervical musculature. At a given gain setting the thyroid parenchyma fills in with a characteristic "pebbly" echo pattern of predominantly low-amplitude gray tones within the above anatomic boundaries.

THYROID CYSTS

At standard gain settings the cyst of the thyroid is echo free with high through transmission, resulting in many echoes distal to the posterior wall of the cyst. The cyst remains echo free at high gain and the size of the lesion is unchanged. Cysts are generally rounded lesions with smooth walls.

A recently designed percutaneous puncture transducer (2) now enables the clinician to perforate cysts as the transducer is centered over the echo-free zone and aspirate their contents. This transducer has a central lumen allowing passage of a fine-gauge needle which produces minimal trauma to the tissues. In our experience in the past 3 years, there have been no complications of thyroid cyst puncture (40). Most benign cysts contain serous fluid. Only a small percentage of malignant lesions have enough cystic or hemorrhagic degeneration to be confused with a cyst at ultrasonic investigation (41). Before cyst puncture, we generally check the location of the carotid artery and jugular vein with the real-time scanner.

THYROID ADENOMA

Adenoma of the thyroid usually presents as a tumor with a core of high-amplitude echoes surrounded by a periphery of low-amplitude echoes (Fig. 4.44). Although the majority of benign simple adenomas will demonstrate this typical appearance, other ultrasonic pictures may also occur. We call this echo-poor rim of the thyroid

adenoma the "halo" sign. At the present time, this sign should be cautiously interpreted, pending further evaluation. Adenomas larger than 4 cm in diameter have a tendency to degenerate. Cystic necrosis produces echo-free, fluid-filled spaces within the adenoma of varying size and location. The echo pattern of the thyroid adenoma and the halo sign is best imaged with gray scale. The appearance of cystic degeneration is more easily shown with the real-time scanner. The higher fluid content of the degenerating adenoma produces a high through transmission pattern. The tumor tends to displace the carotid artery in various directions. The halo sign most likely represents the capsule of the thyroid adenoma (42).

THYROID CARCINOMA

The infiltrating and homogeneous nature of thyroid malignancies produces the ultrasonic appearance of a lesion that is echo poor. There is generally an irregular distribution to the echo pattern and some echogenic areas may be randomly noted. The outer capsule is frequently irregular and we have not observed the halo sign in any thyroid carcinomas to date.

THYROID VOLUME

Knowledge of the total volume of the thyroid gland is important due to the increasing emphasis on medical therapy of thyroid disorders. Three-dimensional reconstruction of the thyroid lobes during scanning may be further refined by computer analysis. Special computer-linked pencil-following devices are available to give a digital read-out of the glandular volume. Improved estimation of thyroid mass allows better ^{131}I dose calculation for the hyperthyroid patient being considered for radiation therapy. Similarly, the course of suppressive drug treatment may be followed more precisely.

The noninvasive nature of thyroid echography makes it an ideal modality for the study of cold nodules detected by isotopic imaging.

REFERENCES

1. Hassani N, Bard R, von Micsky LI: Through transmission patterns in solid tumors. In: Proceedings of the 20th Annual Meeting of the American Institute of Ultrasound in Medicine. New York, Plenum Press, 1975.

2. Hassani N, Bard R: Ultrasonography of the Abdomen. New York, Springer-Verlag, 1976

3. Goldberg BB, Goodman GA, Clearfield HR: Evaluation of ascites by ultrasound. Radiology 96:15, 1970

4. Meyers MA: Distribution of intra-abdominal malignant seeding. Dependency on dynamics of flow of ascitic fluid. AM J Roentgenol 119:198, 1973

5. Leopold GR: A review of retroperitoneal ultrasonography. J Clin Ultrasound 1:82, 1973

6. Brascho DJ: Diagnostic ultrasound in radiation treatment planning. J Clin Ultrasound 1:320, 1973

7. Brown RE, Sartin M, Bogardus CR: Patient contours in radiation therapy planning. Presented at the 17th Annual Meeting of the American Institute of Ultrasound in Medicine, November 16–20, 1972

8. Taylor KJW: Gray scale ultrasonography in the differential diagnosis of chronic splenomegaly. In: Proceedings of the 20th Annual Meeting of the American Institute of Ultrasound in Medicine. New York, Plenum Press, 1975

9. Porrath S, Avallone LT: Radiation planning using ultrasound. In: Proceedings of the 20th Annual Meeting of the American Institute of Ultrasound in Medicine. New York, Plenum Press, 1975

10. Rabinowitz JG, Keller RJ, Wolf BS: Benign peripelvic extravasation associated with renal colic. Radiology 86:220, 1966

11. Hodson JC, Craven DJ: The radiology of obstructive atrophy of the kidney. Clin Radiol 17:305, 1966

12. Goldberg BB, Ostrum BJ, Isard HJ: Nephrosonography. Ultrasound differentiation of renal masses. Radiology 90:1113, 1968

13. Sanders RC, Bearman S: B-scan ultrasound in the diagnosis of hydronephrosis. Radiology 108:375, 1973

14. Mountford RA, Ross FGM, Burwood RJ: The use of ultrasound in the diagnosis of renal disease. Br J Radiol 44:733, 1971

15. Damascelli B, Lattuada A, Musumeci R: Two-dimensional ultrasonic investigations of the urinary tract. Br J Radiol 41:837, 1968

16. Hassani N: Sonic shadow sign. J Natl Med Assoc 67:307, 1975

17. Ben-ora A: Ultrasound diagnosis of lymphoceles following renal transplantation. In: Proceedings of the 20th Annual Meeting of the American Institute of Ultrasound in Medicine. New York, Plenum Press, 1975

18. Leopold GR, Asher WM: Diagnosis of extraorgan retroperitoneal space lesions by B-scan ultrasonography. Radiology 104:133, 1972

19. Feigenbaum H, Chang S: Echocardiography. Philadelphia, Lea and Febiger, 1972

20. Halpert B, Willms RK: Aneurysms of the aorta. Arch Pathol 74:163, 1962

21. Steinberg I, Stein HL: Visualization of abdominal aortic aneurysms. Am J Roentgenol 95:684, 1965

22. Rogoff MS, Lipchick OE: Aneurysms of the abdominal aorta. In Abrams LH (ed): Angiography. Boston, Little, Brown, 1971, pp 759–772

23. Segal LB: Ultrasound diagnosis of an abdominal aortic aneurysm. Am J Cardiol 17:101, 1966

24. Goldberg BB: Ultrasound aortography. JAMA 119:353, 1966

25. Weill F, Maurat P: The sign of the vena cava. Echotomographic illustration of right cardiac insufficiency. J Clin Ultrasound 2:27, 1974

26. Greene D, Steinback HL: Ultrasonic diagnosis of hypernephroma extending into the inferior vena cava. Radiology 115:676, 1975

27. Jensen FI, Jacobsen B, Larsen JF, et al: Intrafetal Injection of Vitamin K. In: Proceedings of the 20th Annual Meeting of the American Institute of Ultrasound in Medicine. New York, Plenum Press, 1975

28. Taylor KJW, Carpenter DA: The anatomy and pathology of the porta hepatis demonstrated by gray scale ultrasound. J Clin Ultrasound 3:117, 1975

29. Weill F, Elsenschar A, Aucent D, et al: Ultrasonic study of venous patterns in the right hypochondrium. An anatomical approach to differential diagnosis of obstructive jaundice. J Clin Ultrasound 3:23, 1975

30. Holm HH: Ultrasonic scanning in the diagnosis of space-occupying lesions of the upper abdomen. Br J Radiol 44:24, 1971

31. Leopold GR: Pancreatic echography. A new dimension in the diagnosis of pseudocyst. Radiology 104:365, 1972

32. Kahn PC: Pancreatic echography. In Eaton SB, Ferrucci JT (eds): Radiology of the Pancreas and Duodenum. Philadelphia, Saunders, 1973

33. Leopold GR: Echographic study of the pancreas. JAMA 232:287, 1975

34. Filly RA, Freimanis AK: Echographic diagnosis of pancreatic lesions. Radiology 96:575, 1972

35. Leopold GR: Echographic and radiological documentation of spontaneous rupture of a pancreatic pseudocyst into the duodenum. Radiology 102:699, 1972

36. Lande A, Bard R: Arteriographic diagnosis of pedunculated splenic cysts. Angiology 25:617, 1974

37. Rosch J: Roentgenology of the Spleen and Pancreas. Springfield, Ill, Thomas, 1967

38. Rasmussen SN: Spleen volume determination by ultrasonic scanning. Scand J Haematol 10:298, 1973

39. Haber K, Asher WM, Freimanis AK: Echographic evaluation of diaphragmatic motion in intra-abdominal diseases. Radiology 114:141, 1975

40. Murray IPC: The current status of radioactive iodine. Practitioner 199:696, 1967

41. Stewart A. Webb J, Hewitt D: A survey of childhood malignancies. Br Med J 1:1495, 1974

42. Hassani N, Bard R: Gray scale and real time ultrasonic evaluation of thyroid neoplasm. In: Proceedings of the 1st Meeting of the World Federation of Ultrasound in Medicine. New York, Plenum Press, 1976

index